Alcoholic Hepatitis

Editor

PAUL Y. KWO

CLINICS IN LIVER DISEASE

www.liver.theclinics.com

Consulting Editor
NORMAN GITLIN

August 2021 • Volume 25 • Number 3

ELSEVIER

1600 John F. Kennedy Boulevard • Suite 1800 • Philadelphia, Pennsylvania, 19103-2899

http://www.theclinics.com

CLINICS IN LIVER DISEASE Volume 25, Number 3
August 2021 ISSN 1089-3261, ISBN-13: 978-0-323-89700-6

Editor: Kerry Holland
Developmental Editor: Ann Gielou M. Posedio

Clinics in Liver Disease (ISSN 1089-3261) is published quarterly by Elsevier Inc., 360 Park Avenue South, New York, NY 10010-1710. Months of issue are February, May, August, and November. Business and Editorial Offices: 1600 John F. Kennedy Blvd., Ste. 1800, Philadelphia, PA 19103-2899. Customer Service Office: 3251 Riverport Lane, Maryland Heights, MO 63043. Periodicals postage paid at New York, NY and additional mailing offices. Subscription prices are $319.00 per year (U.S. individuals), $100.00 per year (U.S. student/resident), $752.00 per year (U.S. institutions), $409.00 per year (international individuals), $200.00 per year (international student/resident), $790.00 per year (international instituitions), $371.00 per year (Canadian individuals), $100.00 per year (Canadian student/resident), and $790.00 per year (Canadian institutions). Foreign air speed delivery is included in all *Clinics* subscription prices. All prices are subject to change without notice. **POSTMASTER:** Send address changes to *Clinics in Liver Disease*, Elsevier Health Sciences Division, Subscription Customer Service, 3251 Riverport Lane, Maryland Heights, MO 63043. **Customer Service: Telephone: 1-800-654-2452 (U.S. and Canada); 314-447-8871 (outside U.S. and Canada). Fax: 314-447-8029. E-mail: journalscustomer service-usa@elsevier.com (for print support); journalsonlinesupport-usa@elsevier.com (for online support).**

Reprints. For copies of 100 or more of articles in this publication, please contact the Commercial Reprints Department, Elsevier Inc., 360 Park Avenue South, New York, NY 10010-1710. Tel.: 212-633-3874; Fax: 212-633-3820; E-mail: reprints@elsevier.com.

Clinics in Liver Disease is covered in *MEDLINE/PubMed (Index Medicus)*, Science Citation Index Expanded, Journal Citation Reports/Science Edition, and Current Contents/Clinical Medicine.

Contributors

CONSULTING EDITOR

NORMAN GITLIN, MD, FRCP (LONDON), FRCPE (EDINBURGH), FAASLD, FACP, FACG

Head of Hepatology, Southern California Liver Centers, San Clemente, California, USA

EDITOR

PAUL Y. KWO, MD

Professor of Medicine, Stanford University School of Medicine, Redwood City, California, USA

AUTHORS

AIJAZ AHMED, MD

Division of Gastroenterology and Hepatology, Stanford University School of Medicine, Stanford, California, USA

JOSEPH AHN, MD, MS, MBA

Professor of Medicine, Division of Gastroenterology and Hepatology, Department of Medicine, Oregon Health and Science University, Portland, Oregon, USA

JUAN PABLO ARAB, MD

Department of Gastroenterology and Hepatology, Escuela de Medicina, Departamento de Biología Celular y Molecular, Centro de Envejecimiento y Regeneración (CARE), Facultad de Ciencias Biológicas, Pontificia Universidad Católica de Chile, Santiago, Chile

MARCO ARRESE, MD

Department of Gastroenterology and Hepatology, Escuela de Medicina, Departamento de Biología Celular y Molecular, Centro de Envejecimiento y Regeneración (CARE), Facultad de Ciencias Biológicas, Pontificia Universidad Católica de Chile, Santiago, Chile

STEPHEN R. ATKINSON, MD, PhD

Senior Clinical Fellow, Department of Metabolism, Digestion and Reproduction, Imperial College London, London, United Kingdom

RAMÓN BATALLER, MD, PhD

Chief of Hepatology, Professor of Medicine, Division of Gastroenterology, Hepatology and Nutrition, Department of Medicine, University of Pittsburgh Medical Center (UPMC), Pittsburgh, Pennsylvania, USA

SUNDUS BHATTI, MD

Section of Gastroenterology and Hepatology, Division of Abdominal Transplantation, Baylor College of Medicine, Houston, Texas, USA

ANDREW M. CAMERON, MD, PhD

Division of Liver Transplant Surgery, Department of Surgery, Johns Hopkins School of Medicine, Baltimore, Maryland, USA

GEETANJALI CHANDER, MD, MPH
Division of General Internal Medicine, Johns Hopkins School of Medicine, Baltimore, Maryland, USA

KRISTINA CHANDLER, BS
Division of Gastroenterology and Hepatology, Department of Medicine, Indiana University School of Medicine, Indianapolis, Indiana, USA

PO-HUNG CHEN, MD
Division of Gastroenterology and Hepatology, Johns Hopkins School of Medicine, Baltimore, Maryland, USA

GEORGE CHOLANKERIL, MD, MS
Assistant Professor of Medicine and Surgery, Section of Gastroenterology and Hepatology, Division of Abdominal Transplantation, Baylor College of Medicine, Houston, Texas, USA

ANA CLEMENTE-SÁNCHEZ, MD
Division of Gastroenterology, Hepatology and Nutrition, Department of Medicine, University of Pittsburgh Medical Center (UPMC), Pittsburgh, Pennsylvania, USA; CIBERehd, Instituto de Salud Carlos III, Madrid, Spain

SALLY CONDON, MD
GI Fellow, Division of Gastroenterology, Hepatology and Nutrition, University of Louisville School of Medicine, Louisville, Kentucky, USA

TAMI DAUGHERTY, MD
Associate Professor, Department of Medicine, Stanford University, Palo Alto, California, USA

APARNA GOEL, MD
Assistant Professor, Department of Medicine, Stanford University, Palo Alto, California, USA

AHMET GURAKAR, MD
Medical Director, Liver Transplant, Division of Gastroenterology and Hepatology, Johns Hopkins School of Medicine, Baltimore, Maryland, USA

SEN HAN, MD
Division of Gastroenterology and Hepatology, Department of Medicine, Indiana University School of Medicine, Indianapolis, Indiana, USA; Key Laboratory of Carcinogenesis and Translational Research, Peking University Cancer Hospital, Beijing, China

GENE Y. IM, MD
Division of Liver Diseases, Icahn School of Medicine at Mount Sinai, Recanati/Miller Transplantation Institute, New York, New York, USA

DONGHEE KIM, MD, PhD
Division of Gastroenterology and Hepatology, Stanford University School of Medicine, Stanford, California, USA

SUTHAT LIANGPUNSAKUL, MD, MPH
Professor of Medicine, Division of Gastroenterology and Hepatology, Department of Medicine, Indiana University School of Medicine, Department of Biochemistry and Molecular Biology, Indiana University School of Medicine, Roudebush Veterans Administration Medical Center, Indianapolis, Indiana, USA

JING MA, MD, PhD
Division of Gastroenterology and Hepatology, Department of Medicine, Indiana University School of Medicine, Indianapolis, Indiana, USA

HARIPRIYA MADDUR, MD
Assistant Professor of Medicine, Department of Gastroenterology and Hepatology, Northwestern University Feinberg School of Medicine, Chicago, Illinois, USA

LUIS S. MARSANO, MD
Professor of Medicine, Division of Gastroenterology, Hepatology and Nutrition, University of Louisville School of Medicine, Department of Medicine, University of Louisville, Louisville, Kentucky, USA

CRAIG J. MCCLAIN, MD
Professor of Medicine, Associate Vice President for Health Affairs/Research, Division of Gastroenterology, Hepatology and Nutrition, University of Louisville School of Medicine, UofL Alcohol Research Center, Department of Medicine, Hepatobiology and Toxicology Center, University of Louisville, Robely Rex Veterans Affairs Medical Center, Louisville, Kentucky, USA

ARNAB MITRA, MD, MS
Assistant Professor of Medicine, Division of Gastroenterology and Hepatology, Department of Medicine, Oregon Health and Science University, Portland, Oregon, USA

MARSHA Y. MORGAN, MD
Professor, UCI Institute for Liver and Digestive Health, Division of Medicine, Royal Free Campus, University College London, London, United Kingdom

LAUREN MYERS, MMSc, PA-C
Instructor of Medicine, Division of Gastroenterology and Hepatology, Department of Medicine, Oregon Health and Science University, Portland, Oregon, USA

ALINE OLIVEIRA-MELLO, PhD
Division of Gastroenterology, Hepatology and Nutrition, Department of Medicine, University of Pittsburgh Medical Center (UPMC), Pittsburgh, Pennsylvania, USA

NIKOLAOS PYRSOPOULOS, MD, PhD, MBA, FACP, AGAF, FAASLD, FRCP (Edin)
Professor of Medicine, Chief of Gastroenterology and Hepatology, Division of Gastroenterology and Hepatology, Rutgers New Jersey Medical School, Medical Director of Liver Transplantation for University Hospital Newark, New Jersey, USA

CRISTIAN D. RIOS, MD
GI Fellow, Division of Gastroenterology, Hepatology and Nutrition, University of Louisville School of Medicine, Louisville, Kentucky, USA

STEPHANIE M. RUTLEDGE, MD
Division of Gastroenterology, Icahn School of Medicine at Mount Sinai, New York, New York, USA

MOKSH SHARMA, BSc
Medical Student, UCI Institute for Liver and Digestive Health, Department of Medicine, Royal Free Campus, University College London, London, United Kingdom

ASHWANI K. SINGAL, MD, MS, FACG, FAASLD
Professor of Medicine, University of South Dakota Sanford School of Medicine, Transplant Hepatologist, Avera McKennan University Hospital Transplant Institute, Sioux Falls, South Dakota, USA

MA AI THANDA HAN, MD, FACP
Assistant Professor, Division of Gastroenterology and Hepatology, Rutgers New Jersey Medical School, Newark, New Jersey, USA

PENG-SHENG TING, MD
Division of Gastroenterology and Hepatology, Johns Hopkins School of Medicine, Baltimore, Maryland, USA

JASON WHEATLEY, MSW
Department of Social Work, Johns Hopkins Hospital, Baltimore, Maryland, USA

ZHIHONG YANG, PhD
Division of Gastroenterology and Hepatology, Department of Medicine, Indiana University School of Medicine, Indianapolis, Indiana, USA

TING ZHANG, PhD
Division of Gastroenterology and Hepatology, Department of Medicine, Indiana University School of Medicine, Indianapolis, Indiana, USA

Contents

> Alcohol-associated liver disease (ALD) is a consequence of excessive alcohol use. It comprises a spectrum of histopathologic changes ranging from simple steatosis, steatohepatitis, and cirrhosis to hepatocellular carcinoma. The public health impact of ALD is growing because of an increase in the prevalence and incidence of ALD in parallel with liver transplant and mortalities. There are multiple factors involved in the pathogenesis and progression of ALD. Reducing alcohol consumption is the cornerstone of ALD management. The efforts to reduce excessive alcohol use at the individual and population levels are urgently needed to prevent adverse outcomes from ALD.

> Alcoholic hepatitis (AH) is a clinical syndrome of jaundice, abdominal pain, and anorexia due to prolonged heavy alcohol intake, and is associated with alterations in gene expression, cytokines, immune response, and the gut microbiome. Currently, we have limited biomarkers to diagnose and prognosticate in AH, but there are many novel noninvasive biomarkers under development. We evaluate the currently used algorithms to risk-stratify in AH (such as the Maddrey modified discriminant function), and discuss novel biomarkers in development, such as breath biomarkers, microRNAs, cytokeratin-18 fragments, and the AshTest. We also review the characteristics of an ideal biomarker in AH.

> Constitutional, environmental, and genetic risk factors influence the development of alcohol-related cirrhosis. The amount of alcohol consumed and whether excessive drinking continues after the identification of pre-cirrhotic liver damage are key risk factors. Female sex, ethnicity, obesity, coffee consumption, cigarette smoking, and exposure to other causes of liver injury also influence the risk of disease development. More recently several genetic loci have been robustly associated with the risk for developing significant alcohol-related liver disease. It remains unclear whether additional risk factors are involved in the development of the clinical syndrome of alcoholic hepatitis, but the genetic evidence is suggestive.

The natural history of moderate alcoholic hepatitis (AH) is not well known. It is a frequent disease with a probable underestimated incidence compared with its severe form. Among the different prognostic scores predicting short-term mortality in AH, MELD seems to be the most accurate. The mortality of moderate AH is 3% to 7% in the short to medium term and 13% to 20% at 1 year, mainly because of liver-related complications, including severe infections. Long-term abstinence is the main goal of the treatment. There is still need for the development of new therapies for AH, including the less severe forms.

Malnutrition is common in alcohol-associated hepatitis (AH); almost all patients with severe AH have some component of malnutrition. The classic phenotype of malnutrition in AH is sarcopenia, but this has become more difficult to discern clinically as patients have become more obese. Patients with AH are often drinking 10 to 15 standard drinks per day. This substantial alcohol consumption becomes a major source of calories, but these are considered "empty" calories that contain little nutritional value. Malnutrition is associated with liver complications, such as hepatic encephalopathy, and worse liver outcomes. Nutrition support can improve nutrition status and reduce complications.

Alcohol-associated hepatitis (AH) is a unique clinical syndrome in patients with excessive and prolonged alcohol consumption, and negatively impacts the patient outcomes. Among patients with asymptomatic alcohol-associated liver disease with elevated liver enzymes and/or steatosis, liver biopsy is required to diagnose AH. Noninvasive assessment should be performed in these patients to determine risk of advanced fibrosis. In symptomatic patients with jaundice, liver biopsy is required when the clinical diagnosis is uncertain. Liver biopsy is not recommended to determine prognosis of patients with AH. Noninvasive biomarkers are emerging for diagnosis of and determining prognosis of patients with AH.

Acute alcoholic hepatitis is a clinical entity with significant consequences. Those with severe disease can have high short-term mortality, and considerations for liver transplant candidacy may be raised. Estimating prognosis and mortality is of the utmost importance, as it can guide decision making for corticosteroid therapy and help patients gain an understanding of their illness. Maddrey's discriminant function and MELD score are 2 commonly used static models validated to help estimate severity and prognosis in acute alcoholic hepatitis. This article reviews the 2 models and others used in this difficult setting to assess these patients and guide decision making.

Alcohol-associated hepatitis is associated with poor outcomes, especially when severe. Despite extensive study with a plethora of potential therapeutic agents, treatment options remain limited, with the current standard of therapy being corticosteroids. Granulocyte colony-stimulating factor is an alternate agent that seems promising, although further study in a more heterogenous patient population is needed before implementation. Adjuncts to therapy that are often overlooked are alcohol abstinence and adequate optimization of nutrition to improve outcomes. In select patients, early liver transplantation may be an option or enrollment in clinical trials.

The incidence of alcoholic hepatitis is increasing while the mortality rate remains high. The single current available therapy for severe alcoholic hepatitis is administration of corticosteroids for patients with severe alcoholic hepatitis, which has demonstrated limited benefits, providing a short-term mortality benefit with a marginal response rate. There is a need for developing safe and effective therapies. This article reviews novel therapies targeting various mechanisms in the pathogenesis of alcoholic hepatitis, such as the gut-liver axis, inflammatory cascade, oxidative stress, and hepatic regeneration. Current ongoing clinical trials for alcoholic hepatitis also are described.

Liver transplantation (LT) for alcohol-related or alcoholic hepatitis (AH) remains a controversial treatment option. However, recent studies have shown promising outcomes for LT in a subgroup of patients with AH. Considering these emerging data, LT as definitive therapy for severe AH refractory to medical management is gaining recognition. However, concerns of alcohol recidivism pose a significant barrier to perform LT for this indication. Predictive models can be utilized to develop a selection criterion to identify suitable candidates for LT. Hence, carefully selected patients with severe AH and low risk of alcohol relapse can be considered for LT.

Severe acute alcohol-associated hepatitis that is nonresponsive to medical therapy has an extremely high mortality. Liver transplantation is a feasible treatment option and available at certain transplant centers globally. Selection criteria for liver transplantation are not, uniform but there are important key criteria shared across protocols. Of equal importance to the management of liver disease is the treatment of alcohol use disorder. A thorough assessment of candidates involves input from an addiction specialist and psychiatrist. With careful selection practices, graft and patient survival among transplant recipients with severe alcohol-associated hepatitis is similar to other etiologies of chronic liver disease.

Severe alcoholic hepatitis portends a high risk of mortality without liver transplantation. Transplant outcomes in patients with severe alcoholic hepatitis exhibit a strong inverse association with post-transplant alcohol relapse. The ingredients most central to ameliorating alcohol relapse risk may include destigmatized post-transplant alcohol monitoring, a nonpunitive clinician–patient partnership, and multimodal therapies to maintain abstinence and mitigate high-risk drinking. We here review the core principles of post-liver transplant management specific to alcohol use disorder.

CLINICS IN LIVER DISEASE

Preface

Alcoholic Hepatitis and its Many Facets

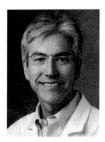

Paul Y. Kwo, MD
Editor

The field of Hepatology has seen enormous advances in the past decade. We now have therapies to effectively treat hepatitis C as well as effective therapies to suppress the hepatitis B virus. Indeed, hepatitis C, which used to be the most common indication for transplantation, has now been supplanted by alcohol-associated liver disease as the most common indication for liver transplantation. In addition, alcohol-associated liver disease accounts for 6% of all deaths worldwide, and 50% of all cases of cirrhosis have alcohol as a contributing factor.

In this issue of *Clinics in Liver Disease*, the epidemiology of alcoholic hepatitis is addressed by Dr Liangpunsakul, including the growing per-capita alcohol consumption worldwide and its relationship to increased rates of alcoholic liver disease. Practitioners routinely encounter those with alcohol use disorder, and early recognition of hepatic injury can be difficult to discern. Dr Im explores in detail our current biomarkers to detect alcoholic hepatitis and comments on future biomarkers that may provide greater sensitivity in detecting alcoholic hepatitis prior to the onset of severe complications. Dr Marsha Morgan details the genetic and environmental susceptibilities to alcoholic hepatitis that have been identified as well as emerging data on how best to identify individuals at risk for severe alcoholic hepatitis. Dr Bataller reviews the clinical diagnosis and identification of those with moderate alcoholic hepatitis who are still at risk for poor outcomes.

Nutrition in liver disease has become increasingly important, and Dr McClain and colleagues present in detail how to identify patients who are at risk for malnutrition, as well as interventions to address sarcopenia. With the growing number of diagnostic modalities to identify fibrosis, such as elastography and serum markers, the role of liver biopsy in hepatology has changed. Nonetheless, liver biopsy can still be an invaluable tool to help inform diagnosis and management options for those who may have alcoholic hepatitis, and Dr Singal addresses when a liver biopsy may be appropriate.

Clin Liver Dis 25 (2021) xiii–xiv
https://doi.org/10.1016/j.cld.2021.04.003
1089-3261/21/© 2021 Published by Elsevier Inc.

Defining prognosis is also important, and Dr Ahn and his colleagues review the available prognostic models and how they help clinicians assess those who require prioritization for therapy for alcoholic hepatitis. Historically, the treatment of alcoholic hepatitis has consisted of a finite course of corticosteroids for those with severe alcoholic hepatitis. Dr Maddur reviews our current approach to the treatment of alcoholic hepatitis and reviews adjuvant therapies currently available to clinicians who care for those with acute alcoholic hepatitis. There is an increasingly diverse group of novel therapies being evaluated to treat alcoholic hepatitis as well. Dr Pyrsopoulos reviews the emerging data with novel agents for alcoholic hepatitis, including preliminary outcomes from multiple trials.

One of the most significant changes in the past 10 years has been the approach to treatment of refractory alcoholic hepatitis with orthotopic liver transplant. Historically, a 6-month sobriety has been required prior to consideration for transplant. Dr Ahmed details the emerging trends in liver transplantation for alcoholic hepatitis that have occurred over the past decade. Dr Goel addresses the emerging data on how patients who have failed current medical therapies with acute alcoholic hepatitis may be selected for potential transplant candidacy via an exception pathway approach. Finally, Dr Gurakar details a multidisciplinary approach to ensure that alcohol use disorder is addressed after liver transplantation for acute alcoholic hepatitis.

This issue of *Clinics in Liver Disease* will be a useful resource to clinicians who care for those with alcohol-associated liver disease, allowing clinicians to not only identify patients at risk for alcoholic hepatitis but also intervene early, provide appropriate therapy for those with severe alcoholic hepatitis, and refer appropriate patients for transplantation if required.

Paul Y. Kwo, MD
Stanford University School of Medicine
430 Broadway, Pavilion C, 3rd Floor
Redwood City, CA 94063, USA

E-mail address:
pkwo@stanford.edu

Epidemiology of Alcohol-Associated Liver Disease

Sen Han, MD[a,b], Zhihong Yang, PhD[a], Ting Zhang, PhD[a], Jing Ma, MD, PhD[a], Kristina Chandler, BS[a], Suthat Liangpunsakul, MD, MPH[a,c,d,*]

KEYWORDS

- Liver diseases • Alcoholic • Epidemiology • Public health

KEY POINTS

- The public health impact of alcohol-associated liver disease (ALD) is growing, partly because of the increase in the incidence of alcoholic hepatitis and alcoholic liver cirrhosis.
- There is a direct relationship between the risk for ALD and the amount of alcohol consumed. However, other factors, such as obesity and underlying genetic variants, may also influence the progression of ALD.
- The mortality and liver transplant rates for persons with ALD have increased substantially, with a grim projection for the disease burden over the next 2 decades.
- The efforts to reduce excessive alcohol use at the individual and population levels are urgently required to prevent adverse outcomes from ALD.

INTRODUCTION

Alcohol drinking has been popular in many cultures, and fermented beverages were brewed as early as the seventh millennium BC.[1] According to the recent global status report on alcohol and health by the World Health Organization (WHO), approximately

Conflict of interest: None of the authors have any conflicts of interest relevant to this work.
Author contributions: S.H., Z.Y., and T.Z., literature review; S.H., Z.Y., J.M., and K.C., drafting the article; S.H. and S.L., a critical review of the article; and S.L., finalizing the article. All authors have read and approved the article for submission.
Sources of funding: Z.Y. is supported by NIH K01AA26385, Indiana University School of Medicine Research Support Fund Grant (IU RSFG), and the Ralph W. and Grace M. Showalter Research Trust, Indiana University School of Medicine; S.L. is supported in part by R01 DK107682, R01 AA025208, U01 AA026917, UH2 AA026903, VA Merit Award 1I01CX000361, and Dean's Scholar in Medical Research Indiana University School of Medicine.
[a] Division of Gastroenterology and Hepatology, Department of Medicine, Indiana University School of Medicine, 702 Rotary Circle, Indianapolis, IN 46202, USA; [b] Key Laboratory of Carcinogenesis and Translational Research, Peking University Cancer Hospital, Beijing, China; [c] Department of Biochemistry and Molecular Biology, Indiana University School of Medicine, Indianapolis, IN, USA; [d] Roudebush Veterans Administration Medical Center, Indianapolis, IN, USA
* Corresponding author. Division of Gastroenterology and Hepatology, Department of Medicine, Indiana University School of Medicine, 702 Rotary Circle, Indianapolis, IN 46202.
E-mail address: sliangpu@iu.edu

2.3 billion people are current drinkers. Alcohol is consumed by more than half of the population in the Americas, Europe, and western Pacific.[2] Alcohol drinking is also a major problem in adolescents between 15 and 19 years old, and more than a quarter of the population (~155 million) in this age group are current drinkers.[2] Total per capita alcohol consumption in the world's population more than 15 years of age increased from 5.5 L of pure alcohol in 2005 to 6.4 L in 2016; the highest levels of per capita alcohol consumption are observed in WHO European region.[2] Taken together, alcohol is the most widely abused psychoactive substance, despite the knowledge of its potential adverse health and social outcomes.[3]

ALCOHOL CONSUMPTION AND ALCOHOL-ASSOCIATED LIVER DISEASE

Globally, alcohol use was the seventh leading risk factor for both deaths and disability-adjusted life-years (DALYs) in 2016, accounting for 2.2% of age-standardized female deaths and 6.8% of age-standardized male deaths.[4] For the population aged 15 to 49 years, female attributable DALYs were 2.3% and male attributable DALYs were 8.9%.[4] In 2016, of all deaths attributable to alcohol consumption worldwide, 28.7% were caused by injuries, 21.3% were caused by digestive diseases, 19% were caused by cardiovascular diseases, 12.9% were caused by infectious diseases, and 12.6% were caused by cancers. In contrast, about 49% of alcohol-attributable DALYs are caused by noncommunicable and mental health conditions, and about 40% are caused by injuries.[2]

Drinking becomes excessive when it causes or increases the risk for alcohol-related problems or complicates the management of other health problems. A standard drink is a measure of alcohol consumption in each type of alcoholic beverage, which contains a specific amount of pure alcohol. In the United States, 1 standard drink contains approximately 14 g of pure alcohol, which is equivalent to 355 mL (12 ounces) of regular beer, 150 mL (5 ounces) of wine, or 45 mL (1.5 ounces) of distilled spirits.[5] According to the National Institute on Alcohol Abuse and Alcoholism (NIAAA), excessive drinking is defined as men drinking more than 4 standard drinks in a day (or more than 14 per week) and women drinking more than 3 standard drinks in a day (or more than 7 per week).[6]

There is a direct relationship between the amount of alcohol consumed and the risk for alcohol-associated liver disease (ALD).[7,8] Early studies in France suggested that alcohol consumption of more than 80 g/d in men and 20 g/d in women significantly increased the risk of alcoholic cirrhosis.[9,10] The association between daily alcohol intake, type of alcoholic beverage consumed, drinking patterns, and ALD has been examined in 6534 subjects from 2 communities in northern Italy.[11] The risk threshold for developing either noncirrhotic alcohol-induced liver injury or alcoholic cirrhosis in both sexes was consuming 30 g of alcohol per day, and an increased risk of ALD was also found with increasing alcohol intake.[11] The relationship between self-reported alcohol intake and the risk of ALD was studied in 13,285 subjects with 12 years of follow-up. No liver injury was reported when the weekly alcohol intake was between 1 and 6 beverages; however, the risk was significantly increased when alcohol consumption was beyond this level: 7 to 13 beverages weekly for women and 14 to 27 beverages weekly for men.[12] The level of risky drinking for ALD differs from each study primarily because of the retrospective study designs with broad assumptions and estimation of alcohol consumed.[13]

There is a gender difference influencing the development of ALD. The greater vulnerability of women, and lower safe limits for consumption, have been recognized.[14] At any given level of alcohol intake, women had a significantly higher relative risk of developing ALD than men. In a large Danish population-based prospective study of 6152 subjects with a history of alcohol abuse, the alcoholic cirrhosis mortality was increased 27-fold and 35-fold in men and women, respectively, compared with that of the general population.[15] However, men had an overall higher incidence of alcohol-induced cirrhosis (0.2% annually) compared with women (0.03% annually).[10]

The types and patterns of alcohol intake also influence the development of ALD, independently of the level of alcohol consumption. For instance, the consumption of red wine may have a lower risk of ALD compared with other types of alcoholic beverages.[16] Drinking alcohol outside the mealtime and drinking multiple different alcoholic beverages both increase the risk of developing ALD.[11]

SPECTRUM OF ALCOHOL-ASSOCIATED LIVER DISEASE

ALD comprises a spectrum of histopathologic changes in patients with excessive alcohol use, ranging from simple alcoholic steatosis to steatohepatitis, alcoholic hepatitis (AH), fibrosis, and cirrhosis.[17–19] Alcoholic steatosis occurs in most of the excessive drinkers. A classic study reported that consumption of alcohol in sufficient quantities in the range of 120 to 150 g/d for a few weeks leads to the development of steatosis. The condition is reversible, with 4 weeks of abstinence leading to its resolution.[20] AH is a clinical syndrome and is characterized by an abrupt increase in serum bilirubin levels, fever, coagulopathy, and liver-related complications.[18,21] It occurs in a subset of patients with excessive alcohol use and is associated with significant morbidity and mortality.[18,22–24] Approximately 15% to 20% of excessive drinkers develop cirrhosis in their lifetimes.[25] Patients with alcoholic cirrhosis, in general, have clinical features similar to those with other chronic liver diseases. The liver test abnormalities in alcoholic cirrhosis are less pronounced than those in AH. The liver tests are nearly normal in patients with the compensated state. Complications from portal hypertension, such as ascites, hepatic encephalopathy, and esophageal varices, are common in decompensated patients.

EPIDEMIOLOGY OF ALCOHOL-ASSOCIATED LIVER DISEASE
Epidemiology of Alcoholic Steatosis

Although alcoholic steatosis is common among excessive drinkers, its prevalence in the general population is difficult to determine because most patients are asymptomatic and do not seek any medical attention. The estimated prevalence also depends on the diagnostic modalities being used to screen for steatosis. Ultrasonography is an acceptable initial screening tool for alcoholic steatosis because it is noninvasive, inexpensive, and widely available.[26] Steatosis normally appears as a diffuse hyperechogenicity caused by increased parenchymal reflectivity. Ultrasonography has a sensitivity around 60% to 90% and a specificity of approximately 90% to 95%, depending on the severity or degree of steatosis.[27] Magnetic resonance spectroscopy allows noninvasive studies into the molecular composition of tissues in vivo with high accuracy for measuring hepatic fat.[26,28] The controlled attenuation parameter is a noninvasive tool to assess alcoholic steatosis. The software is incorporated as part of liver stiffness measurement to enable it to measure the liver steatosis and fibrosis simultaneously.[29] Using the national health examination survey data from questionnaires, abdominal ultrasonography, and laboratory tests on US patients, the estimated prevalence of alcoholic steatosis was calculated.[30] Alcoholic steatosis was defined by alcohol consumption greater than 28 g/d in women and greater than 42 g/d in men, alanine aminotransferase (ALT) level greater than 25 U/L in women and greater than 35 U/L in men, and total bilirubin level less than 3 mg/dL, in the absence of viral hepatitis and metabolic syndrome. Hepatic fibrosis was determined with aspartate aminotransferase/platelet ratio and Fibrosis-4 score. Among approximately 34,000 respondents, 4.3% of the US population were identified with alcoholic steatosis. Over the 14-year study period, the prevalence of alcoholic steatosis remained stable at 4.3%; alcoholic steatosis with fibrosis stage 2 increased from 0.6% to 1.5% and with fibrosis stage 3 remained stable at 0.1% to 0.2%.[30] Although thought to be a benign condition previously, hepatic steatosis may trigger the development of advanced liver disease, with approximately 18% of patients progressing into fibrosis or cirrhosis in a decade.[31] This finding is supported by a recent meta-analysis finding that the annualized rate of progression from alcoholic steatosis to cirrhosis is approximately 3%, with annualized mortality around 6%. Of importance, patients with alcoholic steatosis also have higher nonliver (4% per year) mortality compared with liver-specific (1% per year) mortality.[32]

Prevalence of Alcoholic Hepatitis

The precise incidence and prevalence of AH are difficult to estimate because patients with AH may be completely asymptomatic and undiagnosed clinically.[21] In a nation-wide population-based estimate of AH incidence in Denmark between 1999 and 2008, the annual incidence increased from 37 million to 46 million in men and 24 million to 34 million in women, with a significant increase among middle-aged women.[33] The epidemiology of AH can also be examined by analyzing the hospitalization data, notably for patients with severe disease.[19,34] The authors reported an increase in total cases of AH-related hospitalization from 249,884 (0.66% of total admission in 2002) to 326,403 (0.83% of total admission in 2010) in the United States.[19] Hospitalized patients had a high prevalence of comorbidities, such as sepsis, acute renal insufficiency, and gastrointestinal bleeding.[19]

AH poses a significant financial burden in the health care system because of the high readmission rate, ranging from 20% to 25% at 30 days and around 37% at 90 days after discharge.[19,35–39] The data from a health care claims analysis of more than 15,000 commercially insured hospitalized patients with AH showed nearly 40,000 rehospitalizations, with more than 50% of the survivors rehospitalized within a year and nearly 75% through the second year, with the total health care cost of $2.2 billion over the 5-year study period.[37] The data from the National Readmissions Database showed the annual cost burden of $164 million and $321 million for 30-day and 90-day AH-related readmission, respectively.[39] The annualized rate of progression of AH to cirrhosis is around 10%, with annualized mortality from 5% to 15%.[32] Several clinical scoring systems predict patients with AH who are at high risk for mortality. The Maddrey discriminant function is used widely to predict 30-day mortality and identify a subset of patients who may benefit from treatment with corticosteroids.[40] The model for end-stage liver disease (MELD), using serum creatinine, serum bilirubin, and international normalized ratio, can accurately predict 30-day and 90-day mortality in patients with AH.[41,42] In addition, the Lille model, including an evolution of the bilirubin level in addition to the 3 baseline variables albumin, prothrombin time, and creatinine, can also predict mortality in AH.[43] A Lille score of more than 0.45 after 1 week of corticosteroid therapy is associated with 75% mortality in 6 months.[43] The combination of MELD and Lille score can better predict outcomes of patients with AH, compared with either model alone.[44]

Prevalence of Alcoholic Cirrhosis

Globally, ALD caused 23.6 million and 2.46 million cases of compensated and decompensated cirrhosis in 2017.[45] The age-standardized prevalence of decompensated alcoholic cirrhosis increased from 25.3 per 100,000 in 1990 to 30 per 100,000 in 2017, whereas the age-standardized prevalence of compensated alcoholic cirrhosis was stable from 290 per 100,000 to 288.1 per 100,000 in 1990 and 2017, respectively.[45] The overall prevalence of ALD in the US population is stable around 0.8% to 1% from 1988 to 2016[46] (**Fig. 1**). However, patients with stage 3 to 4 fibrosis increased from 2.2% in 2001 to 2002 to 6.6% in 2015 to 2016.[30] The number of hospitalizations among patients with alcoholic cirrhosis per 1000 increased by 32.8%, with the annualized mortality around 8%.[32,47] Patients aged 25 to 34 years experience the highest average annual percentage change in mortality from cirrhosis of any cause: 8.9% in 2009 to 12.2% in 2016. Increased death rates in this age group are driven primarily by alcoholic cirrhosis, with an average annual percentage change of 10.5% from 2009 to 2016.[48] During this period, the total number of patients with alcoholic cirrhosis listed for liver transplant increased by 63.4%.[47]

FACTORS INFLUENCING THE NATURAL HISTORY AND PROGRESSION OF ALCOHOL-ASSOCIATED LIVER DISEASE

In addition to alcohol consumption, multiple factors may influence the natural history and progression of ALD.

Obesity and Nonalcoholic Fatty Liver Disease

The obesity epidemic has led to an increase in the incidence of nonalcoholic fatty liver disease (NAFLD).[49,50] There seems to be a synergistic interaction between alcohol consumption and obesity and the development of liver disease.[51] The Dionysos study reveals that obese individuals with excessive drinking, defined as greater than 100 kg of alcohol consumed over a lifetime or greater than 60 g of alcohol daily, have a significantly higher prevalence of hepatic steatosis.[52] The data from a population-based study in the United States show a higher prevalence of abnormal ALT activity in overweight and obese individuals who consume alcohol compared with overweight and obese individuals with no alcohol consumption history.[53] Body mass index is an independent predictor for AH severity.[18] In our multicenter case-control study of 1293 patients with alcoholic cirrhosis compared with 754 heavy-drinking controls without liver disease, we found a significantly higher prevalence of diabetes (20.5% vs 6.5%) and

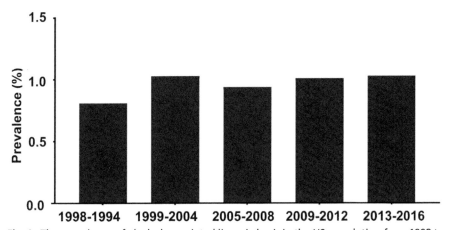

Fig. 1. The prevalence of alcohol-associated liver cirrhosis in the US population from 1998 to 2016 based on the National Health and Nutrition Examination Survey.[46]

body mass index (26.3 vs 24.2 kg/m^2) in patients with alcoholic cirrhosis compared with that in controls.[54] The specific mechanisms of liver injury caused by the combination of obesity and alcohol are not well understood; however, it is plausible that both conditions may augment hepatic oxidative stress through cytochrome P450 2E1 and proinflammatory cytokines leading to worsening liver injury from either condition alone.[51,55]

Genetic Factors

As previously mentioned, only a subset of excessive drinkers develop AH or alcoholic cirrhosis. Excessive drinkers with the gene variants in the patatinlike phospholipase domain–containing protein 3 (*PNPLA3*), transmembrane 6 superfamily 2 (*TM6SF2*), and membrane bound O-acyltransferase domain–containing 7 (*MBOAT7*) are susceptible to alcoholic cirrhosis.[56] The variants in hydroxysteroid 17-beta dehydrogenase 13 (*HSD17B13*) and Fas-associated Factor family member 2 (*FAF2*) are associated with a reduced risk of ALD.[57,58]

Coffee or Tea Consumption

The authors found that regular coffee consumption is associated with a lower risk of AH and alcoholic cirrhosis in heavy drinkers.[36,54,59] In our recent case-control study, we found that heavy drinkers without underlying liver disease are more likely to have been a coffee drinker during the period of excessive drinking and to have drunk more coffee per day compared with those with alcoholic cirrhosis.[54] We also found marginally significant protective effects of tea consumption when both tea and coffee were considered in the analysis.[54]

PERSPECTIVES AND CONCLUSION

The public health impact of ALD is growing, partly because of the increase in the incidence of AH and alcoholic cirrhosis.[17,60,61] In parallel, mortality and liver transplant rates for persons with ALD have increased substantially.[48,60,62] A recent modeling study using the Markov model showed a grim projection in the prevalence and mortality caused by ALD in the next 2 decades.[63] In a large study of more than 3000 patients with chronic liver diseases worldwide, only 3.8% of patients with ALD were seen at the early stages, defined as those without any signs of chronic liver disease or complications of portal hypertension, compared with ~17% to 30% for those with NAFLD or viral hepatitis.[64] Early detection of ALD among excessive drinkers is important because of the adverse impact on the survival of late diagnosis of ALD.[65] At the individual level, behavioral and pharmacologic interventions have been proved to reduce the harm of excessive alcohol use.[66] However, ALD is a population-level problem that requires broad policy-based solutions. Increased alcohol taxes may result in decreased alcohol sales and consumption and then reduced incidence of ALD.[67–69] One key measure of ALD's population-level burden is the number of patients evaluated and waitlisted for a liver transplant. The effect of alcohol tax on alcohol consumption and its influences on liver transplant listing for patients with ALD have been reported.[69] Future studies focusing on the efforts and strategies to decrease excessive alcohol use at the individual and population levels are urgently required to prevent adverse outcomes from ALD.

REFERENCES

1. McGovern PE, Zhang J, Tang J, et al. Fermented beverages of pre- and protohistoric China. Proc Natl Acad Sci U S A 2004;101:17593–8.

2. World Health Organization. Global status report on alcohol and health 2018. Available at: https://apps.who.int/iris/bitstream/handle/10665/274603/9789241565639-eng.pdf?ua=1. Accessed March 12, 2021.

3. Balakrishnan M, Pappas SC. Alcohol and the Law. Clin Liver Dis 2019;23:25–38.

4. Collaborators GBDA. Alcohol use and burden for 195 countries and territories, 1990-2016: a systematic analysis for the Global Burden of Disease Study 2016. Lancet 2018;392:1015–35.

5. Gmel G, Rehm J. Harmful alcohol use. National Institute on Alcohol Abuse and Alcoholism, National Institute of Health; 2003. Available at: http://pubs.niaaa.nih.gov/publications/arh27-1/52-62.htm.

6. Allen JP, Litten RZ. Recommendations on use of biomarkers in alcoholism treatment trials. Alcohol Clin Exp Res 2003;27:1667–70.

7. Ramstedt M. Per capita alcohol consumption and liver cirrhosis mortality in 14 European countries. Addiction 2001;96(Suppl 1):S19–33.

8. Cutright P, Fernquist RM. Predictors of per capita alcohol consumption and gender-specific liver cirrhosis mortality rates: thirteen European countries, circa 1970-1984 and 1995-2007. Omega (Westport) 2010;62:269–83.

9. Tuyns AJ, Pequignot G. Greater risk of ascitic cirrhosis in females in relation to alcohol consumption. Int J Epidemiol 1984;13:53–7.

10. Corrao G, Bagnardi V, Zambon A, et al. Exploring the dose-response relationship between alcohol consumption and the risk of several alcohol-related conditions: a meta-analysis. Addiction 1999;94:1551–73.

11. Bellentani S, Saccoccio G, Costa G, et al. Drinking habits as cofactors of risk for alcohol induced liver damage. The Dionysos Study Group. Gut 1997;41:845–50.

12. Becker U, Deis A, Sorensen TI, et al. Prediction of risk of liver disease by alcohol intake, sex, and age: a prospective population study. Hepatology 1996;23:1025–9.

13. Schwartz JM, Reinus JF. Prevalence and natural history of alcoholic liver disease. Clin Liver Dis 2012;16:659–66.

14. Frezza M, di PC, Pozzato G, et al. High blood alcohol levels in women. The role of decreased gastric alcohol dehydrogenase activity and first-pass metabolism. N Engl J Med 1990;322:95–9.

15. Kamper-Jorgensen M, Gronbaek M, Tolstrup J, et al. Alcohol and cirrhosis: dose–response or threshold effect? J Hepatol 2004;41:25–30.

16. Becker U, Gronbaek M, Johansen D, et al. Lower risk for alcohol-induced cirrhosis in wine drinkers. Hepatology 2002;35:868–75.

17. Liangpunsakul S, Haber P, McCaughan GW. Alcoholic liver disease in Asia, Europe, and North America. Gastroenterology 2016;150:1786–97.

18. Liangpunsakul S, Puri P, Shah VH, et al. Effects of age, sex, body weight, and quantity of alcohol consumption on occurrence and severity of alcoholic hepatitis. Clin Gastroenterol Hepatol 2016;14:1831–8.e3.

19. Jinjuvadia R, Liangpunsakul S. Trends in alcoholic hepatitis-related hospitalizations, financial burden, and mortality in the United States. J Clin Gastroenterol 2015;49:506–11.

20. Lieber CS, Jones DP, Decarli LM. Effects of prolonged ethanol intake: production of fatty liver despite adequate diets. J Clin Invest 1965;44:1009–21.

21. Crabb DW, Bataller R, Chalasani NP, et al. Standard definitions and common data elements for clinical trials in patients with alcoholic hepatitis: recommendation from the NIAAA alcoholic hepatitis consortia. Gastroenterology 2016;150:785–90.

22. Chayanupatkul M, Liangpunsakul S. Alcoholic hepatitis: a comprehensive review of pathogenesis and treatment. World J Gastroenterol 2014;20:6279–86.

23. Mandrekar P, Bataller R, Tsukamoto H, et al. Alcoholic hepatitis: translational approaches to develop targeted therapies. Hepatology 2016;64:1343–55.

24. Thursz MR, Richardson P, Allison M, et al. Prednisolone or pentoxifylline for alcoholic hepatitis. N Engl J Med 2015;372:1619–28.

25. Mills SJ, Harrison SA. Comparison of the natural history of alcoholic and nonalcoholic fatty liver disease. Curr Gastroenterol Rep 2005;7:32–6.

26. Moreno C, Mueller S, Szabo G. Non-invasive diagnosis and biomarkers in alcohol-related liver disease. J Hepatol 2019;70:273–83.

27. Lupsor-Platon M, Stefanescu H, Muresan D, et al. Noninvasive assessment of liver steatosis using ultrasound methods. Med Ultrason 2014;16:236–45.

28. Noureddin M, Lam J, Peterson MR, et al. Utility of magnetic resonance imaging versus histology for quantifying changes in liver fat in nonalcoholic fatty liver disease trials. Hepatology 2013;58:1930–40.

29. Thiele M, Rausch V, Fluhr G, et al. Controlled attenuation parameter and alcoholic hepatic steatosis: diagnostic accuracy and role of alcohol detoxification. J Hepatol 2018;68:1025–32.

30. Wong T, Dang K, Ladhani S, et al. Prevalence of alcoholic fatty liver disease among adults in the United States, 2001-2016. JAMA 2019;321:1723–5.

31. Teli MR, Day CP, Burt AD, et al. Determinants of progression to cirrhosis or fibrosis in pure alcoholic fatty liver. Lancet 1995;346:987–90.

32. Parker R, Aithal GP, Becker U, et al. Natural history of histologically proven alcohol-related liver disease: a systematic review. J Hepatol 2019;71:586–93.

33. Sandahl TD, Jepsen P, Thomsen KL, et al. Incidence and mortality of alcoholic hepatitis in Denmark 1999-2008: a nationwide population based cohort study. J Hepatol 2011;54:760–4.

34. Liangpunsakul S. Clinical characteristics and mortality of hospitalized alcoholic hepatitis patients in the United States. J Clin Gastroenterol 2011;45:714–9.

35. Comerford M, Lourens S, Liangpunsakul S, et al. Challenges in patient enrollment and retention in clinical studies for alcoholic hepatitis: experience of the TREAT consortium. Alcohol Clin Exp Res 2017;41:2000–6.

36. Lourens S, Sunjaya DB, Singal A, et al. Acute alcoholic hepatitis: natural history and predictors of mortality using a multicenter prospective study. Mayo Clin Proc Innov Qual Outcomes 2017;1:37–48.

37. Thompson JA, Martinson N, Martinson M. Mortality and costs associated with alcoholic hepatitis: a claims analysis of a commercially insured population. Alcohol 2018;71:57–63.

38. Peeraphatdit TB, Kamath PS, Karpyak VM, et al. Alcohol rehabilitation within 30 Days of hospital discharge is associated with reduced readmission, relapse, and death in patients with alcoholic hepatitis. Clin Gastroenterol Hepatol 2020; 18:477–85.e5.

39. Adejumo AC, Cholankeril G, Iqbal U, et al. Readmission rates and associated outcomes for alcoholic hepatitis: a nationwide cohort study. Dig Dis Sci 2020; 65:990–1002.

40. Maddrey WC, Boitnott JK, Bedine MS, et al. Corticosteroid therapy of alcoholic hepatitis. Gastroenterology 1978;75:193–9.

41. Dunn W, Jamil LH, Brown LS, et al. MELD accurately predicts mortality in patients with alcoholic hepatitis. Hepatology 2005;41:353–8.

42. Sheth M, Riggs M, Patel T. Utility of the Mayo End-Stage Liver Disease (MELD) score in assessing prognosis of patients with alcoholic hepatitis. BMC Gastroenterol 2002;2:2.

43. Louvet A, Naveau S, Abdelnour M, et al. The Lille model: a new tool for therapeutic strategy in patients with severe alcoholic hepatitis treated with steroids. Hepatology 2007;45:1348–54.

44. Louvet A, Labreuche J, Artru F, et al. Combining data from liver disease scoring systems better predicts outcomes of patients with alcoholic hepatitis. Gastroenterology 2015;149:398–406 e8 [quiz e16-7].

45. Collaborators GBDC. The global, regional, and national burden of cirrhosis by cause in 195 countries and territories, 1990-2017: a systematic analysis for the Global Burden of Disease Study 2017. Lancet Gastroenterol Hepatol 2020;5:245–66.

46. Younossi ZM, Stepanova M, Younossi Y, et al. Epidemiology of chronic liver diseases in the USA in the past three decades. Gut 2020;69:564–8.

47. Dang K, Hirode G, Singal AK, et al. Alcoholic liver disease epidemiology in the United States: a retrospective analysis of 3 US databases. Am J Gastroenterol 2020;115:96–104.

48. Tapper EB, Parikh ND. Mortality due to cirrhosis and liver cancer in the United States, 1999-2016: observational study. BMJ 2018;362:k2817.

49. Liangpunsakul S, Chalasani N. Lipid mediators of liver injury in nonalcoholic fatty liver disease. Am J Physiol Gastrointest Liver Physiol 2019;316:G75–81.

50. Li W, Alazawi W. Non-alcoholic fatty liver disease. Clin Med (Lond) 2020;20:509–12.

51. Idalsoaga F, Kulkarni AV, Mousa OY, et al. Non-alcoholic fatty liver disease and alcohol-related liver disease: two Intertwined entities. Front Med (Lausanne) 2020;7:448.

52. Bellentani S, Saccoccio G, Masutti F, et al. Prevalence of and risk factors for hepatic steatosis in Northern Italy. Ann Intern Med 2000;132:112–7.

53. Ruhl CE, Everhart JE. Joint effects of body weight and alcohol on elevated serum alanine aminotransferase in the United States population. Clin Gastroenterol Hepatol 2005;3:1260–8.

54. Whitfield JB, Masson S, Liangpunsakul S, et al. Obesity, diabetes, coffee, tea, and cannabis Use Alter risk for alcohol-related cirrhosis in 2 large cohorts of high-risk drinkers. Am J Gastroenterol 2021;116:106–15.

55. Liangpunsakul S, Kolwankar D, Pinto A, et al. Activity of CYP2E1 and CYP3A enzymes in adults with moderate alcohol consumption: a comparison with nonalcoholics. Hepatology 2005;41:1144–50.

56. Buch S, Stickel F, Trepo E, et al. A genome-wide association study confirms PNPLA3 and identifies TM6SF2 and MBOAT7 as risk loci for alcohol-related cirrhosis. Nat Genet 2015;47:1443–8.

57. Abul-Husn NS, Cheng X, Li AH, et al. A protein-truncating HSD17B13 variant and protection from chronic liver disease. N Engl J Med 2018;378:1096–106.

58. Schwantes-An TH, Darlay R, Mathurin P, et al. Genome-wide association study and meta-analysis on alcohol-related liver cirrhosis identifies novel genetic risk factors. Hepatology 2020.

59. Liangpunsakul S, Beaudoin JJ, Shah VH, et al. Interaction between the patatin-like phospholipase domain-containing protein 3 genotype and coffee drinking and the risk for acute alcoholic hepatitis. Hepatol Commun 2018;2:29–34.

60. Mellinger JL, Shedden K, Winder GS, et al. The high burden of alcoholic cirrhosis in privately insured persons in the United States. Hepatology 2018;68:872–82.

61. Flemming JA, Dewit Y, Mah JM, et al. Incidence of cirrhosis in young birth cohorts in Canada from 1997 to 2016: a retrospective population-based study. Lancet Gastroenterol Hepatol 2019;4:217–26.

62. Lee BP, Vittinghoff E, Dodge JL, et al. National trends and long-term outcomes of liver transplant for alcohol-associated liver disease in the United States. JAMA Intern Med 2019;179:340–8.

63. Julien J, Ayer T, Bethea ED, et al. Projected prevalence and mortality associated with alcohol-related liver disease in the USA, 2019-40: a modelling study. Lancet Public Health 2020;5:e316–23.

64. Shah ND, Ventura-Cots M, Abraldes JG, et al. Alcohol-related liver disease is rarely detected at early stages compared with liver diseases of other etiologies worldwide. Clin Gastroenterol Hepatol 2019;17:2320–9.e12.

65. Innes H, Morling JR, Aspinall EA, et al. Late diagnosis of chronic liver disease in a community cohort (UK biobank): determinants and impact on subsequent survival. Public Health 2020;187:165–71.

66. Peng JL, Patel MP, McGee B, et al. Management of alcohol misuse in patients with liver diseases. J Investig Med 2017;65:673–80.

67. Elder RW, Lawrence B, Ferguson A, et al. The effectiveness of tax policy interventions for reducing excessive alcohol consumption and related harms. Am J Prev Med 2010;38:217–29.

68. Aslam S, Buggs J, Melo S, et al. The association between alcoholic liver disease and alcohol tax. Am Surg 2021;87:92–6.

69. Shen NT, Bray J, Wahid NA, et al. Evaluation of alcohol taxes as a public health opportunity to reduce liver transplant listings for alcohol-related liver disease. Alcohol Clin Exp Res 2020;44:2307–15.

Current and Future Biomarkers in Alcoholic Hepatitis

Stephanie M. Rutledge, MD[a],*, Gene Y. Im, MD[b]

KEYWORDS

- Biomarker • Alcoholic hepatitis • Cytokines • Fibrosis • Maddrey's • microRNA
- Microbiome • Extracellular vesicles

KEY POINTS

- Alcoholic hepatitis (AH) is a clinical syndrome of jaundice, abdominal pain, and anorexia due to prolonged heavy alcohol intake, and is associated with alterations in gene expression, cytokines, immune response, and the gut microbiome.
- Although liver biopsy can confirm the diagnosis and rule out other causes of liver disease, it is neither safe nor cost-effective to perform a liver biopsy on all patients presenting with AH.
- Current validated prognostic scoring systems in AH include the model for end-stage liver disease score, the Maddrey modified discriminant function, Glasgow alcoholic hepatitis score, and Lille score, which help guide the clinician as to whether the patient should be treated with corticosteroids.
- There are novel biomarkers being studied that use changes in microRNA expression, alterations in the microbiome, and cytokine dysregulation, to diagnose and prognosticate in AH, but larger studies are needed before these biomarkers will become available in the clinical setting.
- It is important to determine whether there is underlying fibrosis in patients with alcohol-associated liver disease (ALD) and validated laboratory (FibroSure/FibroTest or Enhanced Liver Fibrosis test) and imaging (vibration-controlled transient elastography) methodologies can help quantify fibrosis in ALD.

The authors have no commercial or financial conflicts of interest or funding sources to declare.
[a] Division of Gastroenterology, Icahn School of Medicine at Mount Sinai, 1468 Madison Avenue, Annenberg Building Room 5-12, New York, NY 10029, USA; [b] Division of Liver Diseases, Icahn School of Medicine at Mount Sinai, Recanati/Miller Transplantation Institute, 5 East 98th Street, New York, NY 10029, USA
* Corresponding author.
E-mail address: stephanie.rutledge@mountsinai.org

INTRODUCTION

Alcoholic hepatitis (AH) is a uniquely severe clinical syndrome on the spectrum of alcohol-associated liver disease (ALD). It has a somewhat nonspecific and nebulous definition as a clinical syndrome of jaundice, anorexia, right upper quadrant pain with tenderness on examination, and features of the systemic inflammatory response syndrome (SIRS)[1,2] occurring after at least 6 months, but often decades, of heavy alcohol ingestion.[3] In an effort to create standardized diagnostic criteria, an expert consortia from the National Institute on Alcohol Abuse and Alcoholism (NIAAA) defined AH as definite (biopsy-proven), probable (clinically diagnosed without confounding factors), or possible (clinically diagnosed but confounding factors such as possible ischemic hepatitis, drug-induced liver injury [DILI], unclear alcohol use or atypical laboratory findings).[4]

It is challenging to establish reliable biomarkers in a disease with a variable presentation and nonspecific diagnostic criteria, especially as the global population's body mass index is increasing, which makes nonalcoholic steatohepatitis (NASH) a more common confounder. A recent study of 114 patients with ALD who underwent liver biopsy showed that the positive predictive value (PPV) of the NIAAA criteria for AH diagnosis was 81% with a false negative rate of 30%.[4,5] AH is a disease entity that badly needs biomarkers, as an accurate alcohol history can be notoriously difficult to obtain, and there are no clinical, laboratory, or radiographic features that are completely unique to AH. There is no equivalent of an anti–smooth muscle antibody to autoimmune hepatitis in AH, so a high level of clinical suspicion is required and thorough assessment for surreptitious alcohol use by patient interview and/or alcohol biomarkers.

Risk factors for AH include female sex, Caucasian race, obesity, binge drinking, and the patatinlike phospholipase domain–containing protein 3 (PNPLA3) genetic polymorphism.[6–8] There is a poorly understood relationship between the gut microbiome and development of AH: dysbiosis, increased gut permeability, and bacterial overgrowth seem to contribute to the pathogenesis.[9,10] The pathophysiology of AH involves translocation of bacterial lipopolysaccharide (LPS) via portal circulation into the liver, stimulation of Toll-like receptor 4 on hepatic macrophages and Kupffer cells, and initiation of an inflammatory cascade mediated by tumor necrosis factor-alpha.[11,12] Following this, proinflammatory cytokines (interleukin [IL]-1 and IL-6) and chemokines (such as IL-8) attract neutrophils to the liver[13] (**Fig. 1**). There is also direct toxicity of alcohol on hepatocytes, increased oxidative stress, suppressed hepatocyte proliferation, and activation of the adaptive immune system.[7,13,14]

Mortality related to AH can be as high as 30% to 50% at 3 months in those with a Maddrey discriminant function (DF) of greater than 32, and unfortunately there are few pharmacologic options available.[15] Improving short-term outcomes in AH depends on making the diagnosis early and risk-stratifying patients to determine who would benefit from corticosteroids, and who needs to be considered for early liver transplantation. Although liver biopsy can confirm the diagnosis and rule out other causes of liver disease, it is neither safe nor cost-effective to perform a liver biopsy on all patients presenting with AH.[16,17] One study of patients with suspected AH who underwent liver biopsy found that a white blood cell count greater than 11 and platelet count less than 148,000 was 85% to 90% accurate for a diagnosis of AH.[18]

As even moderate AH has significant associated mortality,[19] there is a need to develop reliable noninvasive biomarkers to confirm the diagnosis, risk-stratify patients, identify those benefiting from steroids, assess response to treatment, and ideally tailor treatment to the patient's metabolic or genomic profile, in so-called

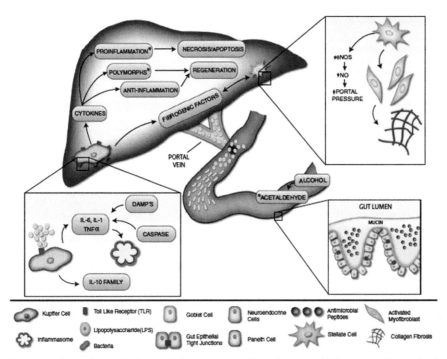

Fig. 1. Cytokine dysregulation and downstream effects in AH, which eventually results in hepatocyte necrosis. (*From* Singal AK, Kodali S, Vucovich LA, Darley-Usmar V, Schiano TD. Diagnosis and treatment of alcoholic hepatitis: a systematic review. *Alcoholism: Clinical and Experimental Research.* 2016;40(7):1390-1402.)

"precision" or "personalized" medicine. This review article discusses the existing bio-markers for AH and reviews biomarker candidates under development.

THE IDEAL BIOMARKER

As has been shown in other disease processes, the ideal biomarker is more likely a panel of molecules in combination, which increases sensitivity and specificity and can both diagnose and prognosticate.[20]

After an episode of AH, approximately 80% of patients will eventually progress to cirrhosis, but even patients who present with alcohol-associated end-stage liver disease at diagnosis have likely experienced years of "subclinical" AH and inflammation that eventually progressed with fibrosis.[21] An ideal biomarker would help to identify patients at risk for AH, fibrosis, and cirrhosis before a sentinel event. There exist simple biomarkers that suggest chronic alcohol use (such as mean corpuscular volume[22] and gamma glutamyltransferase[23]) and markers of recent alcohol ingestion (such as urine ethyl glucuronide [ETG][24] or serum phosphatidylethanol [Peth][25]). Cytokines (such as tumor necrosis factor [TNF]-alpha, IL-1, IL-6, and IL-8) have been proposed as markers of alcohol-induced tissue damage (and a TNF-alpha promoter polymorphism has been linked to susceptibility to AH),[26] but these cytokines are affected by a number of other factors (including nonalcoholic hepatitis) and may even normalize in alcohol-associated cirrhosis (AC).[27] Therefore, it has not yet been established whether dynamics in cytokine levels could be used to diagnose or prognosticate in AH.

When the diagnosis of AH is in question, due to atypical presentation or unclear alcohol history, we would ideally use a serum, plasma, stool, saliva, or urine biomarker with a rapid turnaround time and high accuracy. This biomarker would be specific for AH and would help to distinguish among ischemic hepatitis, DILI, and other causes of acute liver failure.

Perhaps even more useful than a diagnostic biomarker would be a prognostic biomarker, particularly a predictor of 28-day or 90-day mortality or response to treatment, when survival is mostly determined by liver-related events and infection.[4,28] Louvet and colleagues[29] have shown that continued heavy alcohol use ($\geq$30 g/d) is the best predictor of outcome at 6 to 12 months, so beyond 3 to 6 months from an index episode of AH, perhaps biomarkers for alcohol consumption (such as ETG or PEth) should be used instead.[30]

CLINICAL SETTINGS WHERE ALCOHOLIC HEPATITIS BIOMARKERS ARE NEEDED
Moderate Alcoholic Hepatitis

There exists a "moderate-severity" cohort with alcoholic steatohepatitis (ASH) on liver biopsy but without clinical symptoms, otherwise known as "walking ASH." This phenotype of patient may have underlying cirrhosis (up to 30%–40% of cases[31]) and may progress to clinical AH. This represents an ideal cohort to derive benefit from a risk-stratifying biomarker, fibrosis assessment, and early pharmacologic intervention before patients spiral into the inflammatory cascade of severe AH, which is difficult to reverse. One of the challenges is how to identify patients who are misusing alcohol and have "walking ASH" but have not yet reached medical attention. We do not know the true prevalence of "walking ASH," but ideally a noninvasive, low-cost biomarker could screen for and detect fibrosis or low-level inflammation in the primary care or alcohol rehabilitation setting.

A criticism of some of the interventional trials in AH is that these trials target a group with severe AH (modified Maddrey DF [mDF] >32), many of whom have irreversible multiorgan failure and in whom most medical treatments are ineffective. Furthermore, patients with nonsevere or moderate AH (mDF of <32 or model for end-stage liver disease [MELD] <20) have been shown to have unexpectedly high mortality rates of 6% at 28 days, 10% to 13% at 1 year, and 50% at 5 years, with the lack of alcohol abstinence associated with poorer outcomes.[19,32–35] Thus, this represents an ideal group for early pharmacologic and/or psychological intervention. Many patients who present with clinical AH and moderate MELD scores (12–19) are not treated pharmacologically and this is a group that may already have or go on to develop fibrosis and eventually cirrhosis[36] (Fig. 2). More studies are needed to better understand the natural history of moderate AH and "walking ASH," terms that have started to gain traction in the literature.[37]

SEVERE ALCOHOLIC HEPATITIS AND ACUTE-ON-CHRONIC LIVER FAILURE

Acute-on-chronic liver failure (ACLF) is a recently described syndrome characterized by acute decompensation of cirrhosis, often precipitated by infection or alcohol, and accompanied by failure of at least one other organ system with in-hospital mortality rates of at least 50%.[38] Alcohol is thought to be the etiology of approximately 25% of cases of ACLF.[39] A study by Sersté and colleagues[40] found that 48% of patients with severe AH met criteria for ACLF; this group had a poor response to steroids and a 28-day mortality rate of 54%, with mortality directly correlating with the number of organs in failure.

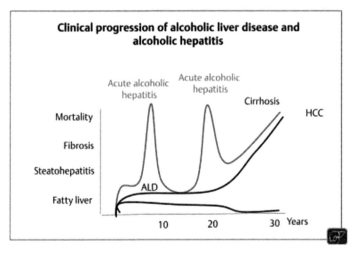

Fig. 2. Typical course of ALD. Chronic excess alcohol intake leads to steatohepatitis, fibrosis, and eventually cirrhosis. There may be superimposed episodes of AH or steatohepatitis can be subclinical without overt symptoms of inflammation, but eventual progresses to AC. (*From* Szabo G. Clinical trial design for alcoholic hepatitis. Paper presented at: Seminars in liver disease. Vol 37, Issue 4. Thieme NY. 2017; with permission.)

For patients with ACLF, the CLIF-C ACLF score (which includes surrogates for organ failure: creatinine, vasopressor use, bilirubin, encephalopathy, international normalized ratio [INR], and oxygenation parameters) is thought to be the best predictor of short-term mortality.[41] CLIF-C outperformed MELD-Na and Child-Turcotte-Pugh scores in a Portuguese cohort of 132 male patients, and a score of greater than 64 should trigger consideration for liver transplantation.[42] However, the CLIF-C score can have low accuracy, with the study by Sersté and colleagues[40] showing that both CLIF-C and mDF have low Harrel's C indices in predicting 28-day mortality in AH with ACLF (0.68 and 0.64, respectively, where 1 is perfectly accurate).

There are many gaps in knowledge relating to this cohort. It is unknown whether ACLF represents the most severe phenotype of AH associated with high levels of circulating LPS, SIRS, and multiorgan failure, or whether these are 2 distinct pathophysiologic processes. Does ACLF due to alcohol excess portend a worse prognosis compared with other causes of ACLF? Would biomarkers add prognostic information in this cohort, and should they be different biomarkers to those validated in non-ACLF severe AH? Perhaps this subgroup of patients with ACLF should be thought of as having different pathophysiology. It is remains to be seen how biomarkers and tailored therapies will be adopted for this cohort of patients with the most life-threatening ALD.

FIBROSIS

Biopsy-based studies have shown that among patients who consume heavy amounts of alcohol, only 10% will develop cirrhosis.[43] Thus, an important question is how to measure underlying fibrosis in patients who consume alcohol to try to predict who will develop AH or AC. We know that the presence of certain gene polymorphisms, such as the PNPLA3 gene,[8] and 11β-HSD1 gene induction and mRNA expression[44] increase the risk of and severity of ALD (**Table 1**). Genes involved in liver fibrogenesis, inflammation, and oxidative stress are upregulated in AH, and may represent targets for therapy.[45]

Table 1
List of genes with single nucleotide polymorphisms that are known to affect risk of alcohol-associated liver disease

Genetic Polymorphism	Effect on Risk of ALD	Year of Discovery of Association with ALD
PNPLA3 (patatinlike phospholipase domain–containing protein 3)	↑AC,[120] ↑AH,[8] ↑HCC[82]	2010
MBOAT7 (membrane bound O-acyltransferase domain–containing 6)	↑AC,[80] ↑HCC[121]	2015
TM6SF2 (transmembrane 6 superfamily member 2)	↑AC,[80] ↑HCC[82]	2015
HSD17B13 (hydroxysteroid 17-beta dehydrogenase 13)	↓risk of progression from steatosis to steatohepatitis,[86] ↓risk of severe AH[85]	2018
FAF2 (Fas Associated Factor family member 2)	↓AC[122]	2020
SERPINA1	↑AC[122]	2020

Abbreviations: ↑, increased risk; ↓, decreased risk; AC, alcohol-associated cirrhosis; AH, alcoholic hepatitis; ALD, alcohol-associated liver disease; HCC, hepatocellular carcinoma.

Thiele and colleagues[46] have shown that the Enhanced Liver Fibrosis (ELF) test (which uses serum biomarkers of extracellular matrix remodeling and fibrogenesis) and FibroTest (which uses age, gender, bilirubin, and several other serum biomarkers) can identify advanced liver fibrosis in patients with heavy alcohol consumption with an area under the receiver operating characteristic curve (AUROC) of more than 0.9 (using liver biopsy as the gold standard). They outperform the FIB-4 (based on age, platelet count, aspartate aminotransferase [AST] and alanine aminotransferase [ALT]) and APRI (AST-to-platelet ratio) scores.[47] These biomarkers may represent an ideal screening tool for the primary care or alcohol rehabilitation setting (which is where the patients in the study by Thiele and colleagues[46] were recruited from) who could benefit from early medical and/or psychiatric intervention.

Measuring liver stiffness with vibration-controlled transient elastography (VCTE) is advantageous over liver biopsy because of its excellent correlation with liver fibrosis, superior safety, and lower cost. VCTE assesses 1/5000 of liver volume compared with 1/50,000 with liver biopsy,[6,48] therefore reducing sampling error.[49] However, there are confounders of liver stiffness measurement in patients undergoing alcohol withdrawal. Acute liver inflammation results in falsely elevated liver stiffness scores and an overestimation of fibrosis. As AST elevation decreases, liver stiffness also decreases, and below an AST of 100 IU/L, liver stiffness measurement has been found to be accurate.[50] Early detection of fibrosis for VCTE, even in patients with ALD with concomitant liver diseases like hepatitis C, could improve health and motivation to change with appropriate linkage to care.

CURRENT ALGORITHMS TO PROGNOSTICATE IN ALCOHOLIC HEPATITIS

One of the earliest clinical tools to prognosticate in AH, which is still commonly used, is the mDF, which is based on the patient's prothrombin time (PT) compared with laboratory control PT, and serum bilirubin.[51] An mDF score of greater than 32 appears to identify those with 1-month mortality of 50% who may benefit from treatment with corticosteroids, but is less helpful at predicting intermediate and long-term outcomes.[51]

Some other disadvantages of the mDF include the control PT being poorly standardized and not reported by all laboratories; mDF is also based on patient cohorts from more than 4 decades ago, and supportive medical care has improved significantly since then.[52]

Studies have shown that using the MELD score to prognosticate in severe AH performs at least as well as mDF for prediction of 30-day and 90-day mortality.[52,53] A larger retrospective cohort study showed that an admission MELD of $\geq$18, first week MELD of $\geq$20, and first week change in MELD $\geq$2 were each independently associated with in-hospital mortality. A week 1 MELD cutoff of 20 had the best test characteristics, with 91% sensitivity and 85% specificity in predicting mortality, which significantly outperformed mDF.[54]

Other validated prognostic scores in AH include the Glasgow alcoholic hepatitis score (GAHS), which uses age, bilirubin, urea, PT, and white blood cell count,[55] and the age, serum bilirubin, INR, and creatinine (ABIC) score.[56] The GAHS is more specific than mDF and may avoid unnecessary treatment with steroids in certain patients.[57] A post hoc analysis of the STOPAH trial found that the MELD, GAHS, and ABIC scores all individually outperformed mDF.[58] Particularly useful appeared to be a baseline "static" score (based on variables at a single timepoint, such as MELD) on admission in combination with either the delta in the "static" score at day 7 or a "dynamic score" such as the Lille score.[58,59] As patients with AH present at different timepoints in their clinical trajectory, using this algorithm helps to inform the clinician when patients should start, stop, or avoid corticosteroids. Louvet and colleagues[60] showed that combining MELD plus Lille in a joint-effect model was a well-fitting prognostic model, helping to more accurately predict mortality at 2 and 6 months on a continuum from 0% to 100%, rather than crudely classifying patients into responders and nonresponders. This approach may be helpful in future early-phase clinical trials of pharmacologic treatment, whereby patients with low baseline static score could be enrolled into a trial and the intervention continued if the patient is not worsening at day 7.[60]

One of the key uses for biomarkers will be identifying patients who will not respond to and who should be excluded from receiving certain treatments, such as steroids.[61,62] Patients with the most severe AH often have comorbidities that preclude them from receiving steroids (such as gastrointestinal bleeding or sepsis). It is important to remember that the patients included in randomized controlled trials of treatment in AH were those who had none of the exclusionary comorbidities and were stable enough to wait for the prerequisite liver biopsy in some trials. This makes obtaining real-world data and finding effective therapies for severe disease more difficult.

There remain many gaps in knowledge relating to how drinking pattern, and host genetic, microbiome, infectious, immunologic, and liver regenerative factors affect outcomes in AH.[7] Understanding this will be key to risk-stratifying patients and developing tailored treatments.

FUTURE BIOMARKERS IN ALCOHOLIC HEPATITIS
Diagnostic Biomarkers

Alcohol-associated liver disease/nonalcoholic fatty liver disease score
Dunn and colleagues[63] developed the ALD/nonalcoholic fatty liver disease (NAFLD) Index (ANI score). The ANI score uses a number of variables (body mass index, gender, mean corpuscular volume, and AST:ALT ratio) to distinguish between alcoholic and nonalcoholic steatohepatitis (ASH vs NASH), independent of recent alcohol consumption. Gamma-glutamyl transferase (GGT) also showed promise in

differentiating between ASH and NASH, but GGT values were available for only 31% of patients in this study.[63]

AshTest

The AshTest uses a panel of serum biomarkers to diagnose ASH in a cohort of patients with heavy alcohol use (alcohol intake of >50 g/d). At a cutoff of 0.50, it could identify ASH with a sensitivity of 0.80 and a specificity of 0.84.[64] The AshTest correlated strongly with histologic grade of AH, with particularly high predictive values in severe histologic cases, and is proposed as an alternative to mDF for determining which patients would benefit from corticosteroids.[64] In 2015, the test was validated in a cohort of 123 patients. It correlated better with histologic grade of AH than MELD or mDF, identified patients who should be treated with steroids with accuracy similar to liver biopsy, but did not have any prognostic value.[65] The AshTest is still not widely used in clinical practice, perhaps because of limited commercial availability of the test and lack of fully independent validation (**Table 2**).

Breathprints

A new development in diagnostic AH biomarkers was the discovery of a unique "breathprint" in patients with AH, characterized by high levels of trimethylamine (TMA), acetone, and pentane, described as the TAP score. Using a cutoff of 36 distinguishes patients with AH compared with healthy controls or patients with decompensated AC with 90% sensitivity and 80% specificity.[66] The initial discovery of elevated TMA in levels in the breath and urine of patients with ALD was in the 1950s when it was observed that these patients had a characteristic unpleasant smell from their breath and urine.[67] It is believed that elevated TMA levels may be due to decreased ability of the liver to convert TMA to trimethylamine oxide (TMAO) in liver disease,[67] and it has been shown that TMA levels correlate with MELD score.[66] Another theory is that alcohol-induced intestinal bacteria overgrowth, increased gut permeability, and translocation of LPS to the liver results in increased TMA levels.[68] It is unknown whether TMA represents a therapeutic target in AH, or whether it is just an innocent bystander and marker of damage. The "breathprint" is an attractive noninvasive marker, but larger studies are needed to validate and determine its prognostic value.

Prognostic Biomarkers and Therapeutic Targets

Cytokeratin-18

Cytokeratin-18 (CK-18) is an intermediate filament protein, present in simple epithelial tissues, the main component of Mallory bodies, and previously used as a tumor marker.[69] More than 20 years ago, circulating cytokeratin-18 levels were shown to correlate with liver cell necrosis and hyaline degeneration on biopsy in AH.[70,71] The theory is that excess serum CK fragments are derived from hepatocyte necrosis.[72] Bissonnette and colleagues[73] used a test cohort of 151 consecutive patients undergoing transjugular liver biopsy for clinical suspicion of AH: n = 83 in the test cohort with median MELD of 20 and mDF of 46, and n = 68 in the validation cohort. They showed that specific circulating fragments of CK-18, M30, and M65 epitopes, could be a very useful noninvasive diagnostic tool in AH. M65 was particularly valuable marker, where a cutoff of more than 2000 IU/L had a PPV of 91% and less than 641 IU/L had a negative predictive value (NPV) of 88% for the diagnosis of AH. Using their proposed algorithm with the aforementioned cutoffs could obviate the need for liver biopsy in two-thirds of cases.[73] A study of 87 patients who underwent liver biopsy for suspicion of AH showed that a specific plasma N-glycomic profile (log NA3Fb/NG1A2F) combined with CK-18 M65 had a diagnostic accuracy for AH of 97% and could avoid liver biopsy in 55% of patients with ABIC $\geq$6.71.[74]

Table 2
A list of some of the currently available and in-development biomarkers in alcoholic hepatitis, divided into diagnostic and prognostic categories

Biomarker	Human/Mouse Study	Available in Clinical Practice	Sensitivity/Specificity if Available	Study
Diagnostic biomarkers				
PNPLA3 gene polymorphism	Human	Yes	N/a	Salameh et al,[8] 2015
White blood count > 11K and platelets <148K	Human	Yes	Sensitivity = 44%, specificity = 100% for diagnosis of AH (PPV 100%, NPV 38%)	Hardy et al,[18] 2013
ANI score	Human	Yes	Sensitivity = 93.5%, specificity of 92% to distinguish AH from NASH	Dunn et al,[63] 2006
Breath trimethylamine, acetone and pentane	Human	No	Sensitivity = 90%, specificity = 80% to distinguish AH from healthy control or alcohol-associated cirrhosis	Hanouneh et al,[66] 2014
AshTest	Human	No	Sensitivity = 80%, specificity of 84% for diagnosis of AH	Thabut et al,[64] 2006; Rudler et al,[65] 2015
Cytokeratin-18 M65 level: ALT ratio	Human	No	Sensitivity = 97.1%, specificity = 82.9% to distinguish AH from NASH	Vatsalya et al,[76] 2019
Cytokeratin-18 M65 level	Human	No	M65 > 2000 IU/L: sensitivity = 67%, specificity = 92% (PPV of 91%) M65 < 641 IU/L: sensitivity = 93%, specificity = 62% (NPV of 88%) for diagnosis of AH	Bissonnette et al,[73] 2017
Cytokeratin-18 M65 and M30 levels	Human	No	N/a	Woolbright et al,[75] 2017
Fibroblast growth factor (FGF) 21	Mouse	No	N/a	Grigorios et al,[123] 2020

(continued on next page)

Table 2 (continued)				
Biomarker	Human/Mouse Study	Available in Clinical Practice	Sensitivity/Specificity if Available	Study
miRNA-192, miRNA-122, miRNA-30a	Mouse	No	miR-192 AUC = 0.96, miRNA-122 AUC = 0.92, miRNA-30a AUC = 0.85 to distinguish alcohol-fed mice from controls	Momen-Heravi et al,[90] 2015
miRNA-192, miRNA-30a	Human	No	miRNA-192 AUC = 0.95, miRNA-30a AUC = 0.58 for diagnosis of AH (vs control)	Momen-Heravi et al,[90] 2015
miRNA-155 in Kupffer cells	Mouse	No	Higher in alcohol-fed vs control mice and correlates with TNF-alpha induction	Bala et al,[99] 2011
Biomarkers to prognosticate and assess response to treatment				
Cytokeratin-18 M30/M65 ratio (cutoff of 0.3884)	Human	No	Sensitivity = 90%, specificity = 86% for 30-d mortality	Woolbright et al,[75] 2017
Cytokeratin-18 M65 levels (cutoff of 8403 U/L)	Human	No	Sensitivity = 80%, specificity = 79% for 30-d mortality	Woolbright et al,[75] 2017
Cytokeratin-18 M65 & M30 levels	Human	No	AUC 0.652 for M65, AUC 0.744 for M30 for 90-d mortality	Vatsalya et al,[76] 2019
Cytokeratin-18 M30 level (cutoff of >5000 U/L)	Human	No	Predicts patients who will benefit from prednisolone at 90 d	Atkinson et al,[77] 2020
ASCA levels	Human	Yes	Sensitivity = 97%, specificity = 47%. PPV = 49%, NPV = 97% for 90-d mortality	Lang et al,[107] 2020

ASCA levels + MELD score	Human	Yes	Sensitivity = 74%, specificity = 81%, PPV = 67%, NPV = 86% for 90-d mortality	Lang et al,[107] 2020
MicroRNA-182 expression in the liver	Human	No	Sensitivity = 79%, specificity = 74% for 90-d mortality	Blaya et al,[92] 2016
MELD cutoff of 11	Human	Yes	Sensitivity = 81%, specificity = 86% for 30-d mortality	Sheth et al,[53] 2002
Week 1 MELD cutoff of 20	Human	Yes	Sensitivity = 91%, specificity = 85% for in-hospital mortality	Srikureja et al,[54] 2005
ABIC score cutoff of 8.555	Human	Yes	Sensitivity = 80%, specificity = 79% for 30-d mortality (AUC = 0.8)	Woolbright et al,[75] 2017
Maddrey modified DF cutoff of 32	Human	Yes	Sensitivity = 83%, specificity = 60% for in-hospital mortality; AUC of 0.673 and 0.670 for 28-d and 90-d mortality respectively	Srikureja et al,[54] 2005 Forrest et al,[58] 2018
Dynamic score of baseline MELD and Lille score	Human	Yes	Akaike Information Criterion score (measure derived from the likelihood model) of 1305, c-statistic of 0.75 for 2- and 6-mo mortality	Louvet et al,[60] 2015
Total and conjugated bile acids	Human	Yes	Correlates with MELD score	Brandl et al, et al,[124] 2018
Bile acid profile	Human	No	Increase in C4 from healthy controls to moderate AH to severe AH (P<.005 for both); decrease in intestinal microbial metabolite isoursodeoxycholic acid also correlates with severity	Muthiah et al,[125] 2020

(continued on next page)

Table 2
(continued)

Biomarker	Human/Mouse Study	Available in Clinical Practice	Sensitivity/Specificity if Available	Study
Serum FGF 19	Human	Yes	Correlates with fibrosis stage and in patients with MELD $\geq$29, correlates with 30-d mortality[126]	Brandl et al,[124] 2018
Enterococcus faecalis cytolysin	Human	No	AUC of 0.81 for 90-d mortality	Duan et al,[104] 2019
Plasma metabolome signatures	Human	No	Baseline levels of L-kynurenine, indole acrylic acid, lecithin & prostaglandin B1 are predictors of non-response to steroids and non- survival (AUROC >0.80; $P<.05$)	Maras et al,[126] 2020

Abbreviations: ABIC, age, bilirubin, urea, PT, and white blood cell count,[55] and the age, serum bilirubin, INR, and creatinine; AH, alcoholic hepatitis; ALT, alanine aminotransferase; ANI, alcohol-associated liver disease/nonalcoholic fatty liver disease index; ASCA, anti–*Saccharomyces cerevisiae* antibodies; AUC, area under the curve; DF, discriminant function; FGF, fibroblast growth factor; MELD, model for end-stage liver disease; miRNA, microRNA; N/a, not available; NASH, nonalcoholic steatohepatitis; NPV, negative predictive value; PNPLA3, patatinlike phospholipase domain-containing protein 3; PPV, positive predictive value; TNF, tumor necrosis factor.

Woolbright and colleagues[75] found that levels of M30 and M65 could differentiate AH from AC, and that M65 levels and the M30-M65 ratio were predictive of 30-day mortality in AH, with the M30-M65 ratio outperforming MELD and ABIC scores. Another study showed that M30 and M65 outperformed 4 biomarkers (mDF, MELD, ABIC, GAHS) in predicting 90-day mortality.[76] A more recent post hoc analysis of 824 patients from the STOPAH trial showed that using CK-18 fragments could have rendered diagnostic biopsy unnecessary in 84% of all AH cases, and that CK-18 strongly predicted 90-day mortality and responsiveness to steroids.[77] In those with M30 greater than 5000 U/L, prednisolone was associated with a significant reduction in mortality at 90 days (odds ratio 0.43, 95% confidence interval [CI] 0.19–0.95, $P = .040$).[77] This suggests that M30 may be able to identify a subset of patients with significant inflammation who will benefit from steroids.

Of note, CK-18 levels are also elevated in NASH, where levels seem to correlate with fibrosis.[78] The M65-ALT ratio may help differentiate patients with AH from those with NASH.[76]

Genetics (patatinlike phospholipase domain–containing protein 3)
There are significant genetic factors relating to prognosis in AH. The gene signature MELD (gs-MELD) score used the expression pattern of 123 genes on liver biopsy plus MELD score to predict 90-day survival in AH with an area under the curve (AUC) of 0.86.[79] Variants in genes such as PNPLA3, transmembrane 6 superfamily member 2 (TM6SF2), and membrane bound O-acyltransferase domain–containing 7 (MBOAT7) have been shown to increase the risk of ALD (PNPLA3 more associated with steatosis and inflammation; MBOAT7 more with fibrosis and cirrhosis).[8,80,81] Polymorphisms in PNPLA3 and TM6SF2 are associated with higher risk of hepatocellular carcinoma in persons with AC.[82] Persons of Hispanic ethnicity are at higher risk for ALD, including AH, than non-Hispanic white and African American persons, which is at least partially related to genetics.[83] Polymorphisms in the alcohol-metabolizing genes (alcohol dehydrogenases) have been associated with increased risk of alcohol-use disorder but do not correlate with risk of liver disease.[84] Recently, a polymorphism encoding for the hepatic lipid droplet protein hydroxysteroid 17-beta dehydrogenase 13 (HSD17B13) was shown to be protective against ALD, AH, AC, and non-ALD.[85] Interestingly, the HSD17B13 variant mitigated the risk of liver injury associated with the PNPLA3 variant.[86]

PNPLA3 increases predisposition to developing ALD and is associated with more severe disease.[7] A genome-wide association study using the STOPAH cohort found that homozygosity for rs738409:G in PNPLA3 independently conferred significant additional risk of medium-term mortality in patients with severe AH with hazard ratio of 1.69.[8,87] Clearly, there is a strong genetic component to ALD and AH, and the discovery of PNPLA3 may just be scratching the surface. Hopefully in the future, we will be able to use a patient's genomics to prognosticate, predict response to therapy, and eventually tailor therapy.

MicroRNAs
MicroRNAs (miRNAs) are small noncoding RNAs of ~22 nucleotides, found in circulating extracellular vesicles (EVs) or exosomes, and regulate a significant portion of the human genome. MiRNAs, such as miRNA-155, regulate genes involved in TNF-alpha regulation, inflammatory response to endotoxin, and various other immune responses, as well as LPS and oxidative stress signaling pathways.[88,89] Alcohol-fed mice demonstrate increased levels of EVs, and human subjects with AH have been shown to have higher levels of miRNA-192 and miRNA-30a, compared with healthy individuals.[90]

Animal models suggest that miRNA-182 is associated with cholangiocyte damage and ductular reaction, both of which are poor prognostic factors in AH.[91] In vivo human studies show that miRNA-182 is highly expressed in AH, and that its expression on liver biopsy but not in the serum correlates with disease severity and short-term mortality, so it may not be a practical biomarker.[92] Alcohol affects the expression of other miRNAs, such as miRNA-212, which regulates gut permeability and sensitizes macrophages to LPS-driven proinflammatory response,[93,94] and miRNA-199, which upregulates endothelin-1 and hypoxia-inducible factor-1α, thus increasing inflammation and steatosis.[95] Circulating miRNAs, together with cytokines or other biomarkers, may eventually compose a powerful prognostication tool and possible therapeutic target, but the studies remain preliminary and small in size.

Extracellular vesicles as tailored treatment

As described previously, EVs that originate from hepatocytes have the ability to modulate liver macrophages and regulate liver regeneration.[96] EVs present an exciting opportunity for drug delivery, having the ability to deliver tissue-targeted miRNA, which can regulate gene expression in the host target cell, and early studies have shown promise in using EVs to deliver therapy in liver disease.[97,98] For example, Bala and colleagues found that EVs could deliver a miRNA-155 inhibitor in vivo resulting in decreased TNF-alpha levels in alcohol-fed mice.[99] The eventual hope is that miRNA manipulation in human subjects with AH could downregulate the inflammatory pathways. EVs can be extracted and stored for years, so potentially stem-cell–derived EVs could be isolated from patients with early-stage liver disease and manipulated for future "personalized medicine" if the patient develops more advanced liver disease.[100] Although a very attractive concept, it is important to remember that the safety of EVs is not fully known, particularly relating to carcinogenesis, and regulation standards still need to be established.[101]

The microbiome as a biomarker

Jiang and colleagues performed a transcriptome and metabolomic analysis of chronic and binge ethanol-fed mice and found that ethanol upregulated and downregulated genes that controlled immune response, inflammation, fatty acid oxidation, apoptosis, and glucose, triglyceride, and bile acid metabolism. They found that the *Prok2* gene, which encodes for prokineticin 2, an inflammatory cytokinelike molecule, was downregulated in ethanol-fed mice. *Prok2* correlated negatively with abundance of the bacteria *Allobaculum* in the gut, which opens up exciting possibilities of manipulating *Prok2* expression in patients with ALD, as a method of controlling inflammation and/or the gut microbiome.[102]

The gut microbiome is significantly altered in AH, and the microbiome contributes to susceptibility to and severity of AH (**Fig. 3**).[103] Specifically, cytolytic *Enterococcus faecalis* is increased and correlates directly with mortality in AH.[104] A mouse study found that bacteriophages that target and reduce cytolytic *E faecalis* in the gut could abolish ethanol-induced liver disease in mice, presenting an exciting future therapeutic target.[104] In addition, a pilot study in humans has shown that fecal microbiota transplant in AH is safe and may improve clinical outcomes.[105] The intestinal virome is also significantly altered in AH, with certain viral taxa associated with higher MELD scores and decreased 90-day mortality.[106]

Patients with ALD have decreased gut fungal diversity with overgrowth of *Candida* species. Serum anti–*Saccharomyces cerevisiae* antibodies (ASCA) can be used as a surrogate of systemic immune response to fungi. Patients with AH have higher ASCA levels compared with controls or patients with alcohol use

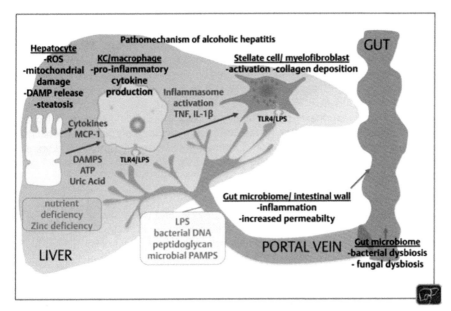

Fig. 3. Pathophysiology of AH, showing how changes in the gut microbiome mediates liver inflammation. (*From* Szabo G. Clinical trial design for alcoholic hepatitis. Paper presented at: Seminars in liver disease. Vol 37, Issue 4. Thieme NY. 2017; with permission.)

disorder without AH, and higher ASCA levels were associated with lower 90-day survival in AH.[107]

Cytokines

Cytokines are mediators of cellular communication, which are produced by many cells in the liver. It has been shown that abnormal cytokine metabolism is a key feature of AH, and that cytokines contribute to inflammation (such as IL-6 and IL-8), increase oxidative stress (TNF-alpha), regulate liver regeneration (IL-6, TNF-alpha, hepatocyte growth factor, tissue growth factor-alpha), control fibrinogenesis transforming growth factor beta 1 or TGF-β1) and induce hepatocyte death.[108] Levels of TNF-alpha and proinflammatory cytokines seem to correlate with clinical outcomes in ALD so cytokine manipulation presents an ideal therapeutic target.[109] Steroids work in AH by inhibiting the proinflammatory cytokine production. Ideally, future pharmacologic therapies could neutralize circulating cytokines or cytokine receptors, administer anti-inflammatory cytokines, or inhibit cytokine production.[108] Initially, there was hope that anti-TNF agents, used commonly in autoimmune conditions, could reduce liver inflammation and mortality in AH. However, early studies of high-dose infliximab with prednisone[110] and of etanercept[111] showed increased rates of infection and gastrointestinal bleeding, resulting in early discontinuation. Cytokines remain an attractive pharmacologic target in AH, but may require specific patient selection, and perhaps measurement of cytokine levels to identify the patients who could benefit.

Other emerging biomarkers

Lipidomics have begun to emerge as a promising class of biomarkers in many disease entities, and ALD is no exception. Thiele and colleagues[112] showed that sphingomyelins decrease significantly in the peripheral circulation and the liver, and negatively correlate with fibrosis stage. Lipid metabolites (plasma oxylipin levels) have been shown to differ among severe AH, moderate AH, and socially drinking healthy controls, which may represent future therapeutic targets.[113] Another new biomarker showing promise is the bromodeoxyuridine incorporation in lymphocyte steroid sensitivity (BLISS) assay, which was able to differentiate between AH survivors and nonsurvivors with AUROC of 0.95 (95% CI 0.84–1.0) and a sensitivity of 90% in identifying steroid responsive patients with an NPV of 86%.[114] Molecular ellipticity of the albumin-bilirubin complex (measured using circular dichroism spectroscopy) may be correlated with short-term and intermediate-term outcomes in severe AH, but the study only evaluated men who were treated with steroids, and has not been externally validated.[115,116]

Practical biomarkers

Although clinical scores such as MELD, Maddrey DF, and Lille scores are widely used in clinical practice, many of the novel biomarkers we have discussed remain available only in research settings, with few biomarkers available for routine clinical use. At the time of writing this article, biomarkers available for commercial use include PNPLA3 gene testing (via ARUP Laboratories, Salt Lake City, UT), which is associated with increased predisposition to and severity of ALD. For determination of fibrosis, available biomarkers include the blood tests FibroTest (FibroSure in the United States) or the ELF test, and imaging with VCTE (FibroScan in the United States). FibroSure can be sent via Laboratory Corporation of America Holdings (labcorp) but it must be specified whether the patient's diagnosis is that of ASH, NASH, or hepatitis C, and in real-world patients these diagnoses may coexist. FibroMeter uses liver stiffness measured via FibroScan combined with age, gender, and 5 blood parameters (platelets, GGT, PT ratio, alpha-2-macroglobulin, and AST), and is validated in viral hepatitides,[117] NAFLD,[118] and ALD.[119]

We believe that CK-18 fragments (specifically M30 and M65) represent some of the most exciting biomarkers in development. If given access to any biomarker, this would be the one we would opt for, given its excellent PPV and NPV for the diagnosis of AH (M65 > 2000 IU/L has 91% PPV and <642 IU/L has 88% NPV), and its superiority over MELD and ABIC scores at predicting 30-day mortality in AH.[73,75] In a setting with unlimited resources, a combined model of multidisciplinary patient interview, CK-18 with PNPLA3 gene testing and a fibrosis assessment could be a comprehensive evaluation to determine a patient's individual likelihood of AH, as well as severity and risk of progression of disease.

SUMMARY

AH is a severe manifestation of ALD, which can occur in young people, is associated with significant morbidity and mortality, and often is superimposed on undiagnosed liver fibrosis due to years of excess alcohol use. Over the past 2 decades, studies have revealed more about the pathophysiology of AH, and we now understand that it is associated with cytokine dysregulation, alterations in gene expression, immune response, and the gut microbiome.

However, risk-stratification and treatment for AH remain in the infant stages. We still use a clinical risk calculator tool from the 1980s (mDF) to decide which patients receive the only proven treatment for AH, corticosteroids, which have limited benefit, multiple contraindications, and a suboptimal risk profile in a tenuous population at risk for bleeding and infection. There is a need to develop reliable, noninvasive biomarkers with rapid turnaround times to prognosticate at a molecular level and develop a "precision medicine" approach, in which the specific treatment is tailored to a patient's individual metabolomics, genomics, and microbiomics. To achieve this lofty goal, large multicenter studies will be needed with a diverse population of well-characterized patients who range the full spectrum of severity in AH.

CLINICS CARE POINTS

- Alcoholic hepatitis (AH) is a clinical diagnosis, however there are laboratory markers that can help guide the clinician in making the diagnosis (leucocytosis, AST:ALT ratio of greater than 2:1) and clinical scores to prognosticate in AH (Maddrey modified discriminant function, Lille score, Glasgow alcoholic hepatitis score). These scores help to guide whether to start, stop or continue treatment with corticosteroids.
- Acute inflammation tends to cause over-estimation of liver stiffness on vibration-controlled transient elastography (FibroScan), therefore it has been suggested that we adjust the liver stiffness result for the elevation in liver enzymes at the time of fibrosis testing.
- There are novel biomarkers in the pipeline to help diagnose and prognosticate in alcoholic hepatitis but most of these remain under development and are not commercially available for clinical use.

REFERENCES

1. Michelena J, Altamirano J, Abraldes JG, et al. Systemic inflammatory response and serum lipopolysaccharide levels predict multiple organ failure and death in alcoholic hepatitis. Hepatology 2015;62(3):762–72.
2. Mendenhall C. Alcoholic hepatitis. Clin Gastroenterol 1981;10(2):417–41.
3. Naveau S, Giraud V, Borotto E, et al. Excess weight risk factor for alcoholic liver disease. Hepatology 1997;25(1):108–11.
4. Crabb DW, Bataller R, Chalasani NP, et al. Standard definitions and common data elements for clinical trials in patients with alcoholic hepatitis: recommendation from the NIAAA Alcoholic Hepatitis Consortia. Gastroenterology 2016; 150(4):785–90.
5. Avitabile E, Pose E, Graupera I, et al. Non-invasive criteria for diagnosis of alcoholic hepatitis: use in clinical practice and correlation with prognosis. J Hepatol 2020;73:S173.
6. Singal AK, Kodali S, Vucovich LA, et al. Diagnosis and treatment of alcoholic hepatitis: a systematic review. Alcohol Clin Exp Res 2016;40(7):1390–402.
7. Sanyal AJ, Gao B, Szabo G. Gaps in knowledge and research priorities for alcoholic hepatitis. Gastroenterology 2015;149(1):4–9.
8. Salameh H, Raff E, Erwin A, et al. PNPLA3 gene polymorphism is associated with predisposition to and severity of alcoholic liver disease. Am J Gastroenterol 2015;110(6):846–56.
9. Lowe PP, Gyongyosi B, Satishchandran A, et al. Alcohol-related changes in the intestinal microbiome influence neutrophil infiltration, inflammation and steatosis in early alcoholic hepatitis in mice. PLoS One 2017;12(3):e0174544.
10. Bajaj JS. Alcohol, liver disease and the gut microbiota. Nat Rev Gastroenterol Hepatol 2019;16(4):235–46.
11. McClain CJ, Cohen DA. Increased tumor necrosis factor production by monocytes in alcoholic hepatitis. Hepatology 1989;9(3):349–51.
12. Keshavarzian A, Farhadi A, Forsyth CB, et al. Evidence that chronic alcohol exposure promotes intestinal oxidative stress, intestinal hyperpermeability and

endotoxemia prior to development of alcoholic steatohepatitis in rats. J Hepatol 2009;50(3):538–47.

13. Gao B, Bataller R. Alcoholic liver disease: pathogenesis and new therapeutic targets. Gastroenterology 2011;141(5):1572–85.

14. Albano E. Role of adaptive immunity in alcoholic liver disease. Int J Hepatol 2012;2012:893026.

15. Maddrey WC, Boitnott JK, Bedine MS, et al. Corticosteroid therapy of alcoholic hepatitis. Gastroenterology 1978;75(2):193–9.

16. Singal AK, Bailey SM. Cellular abnormalities and emerging biomarkers in alcohol-associated liver disease. Gene Expr 2018;19(1):49–60.

17. Kalambokis G, Manousou P, Vibhakorn S, et al. Transjugular liver biopsy–indications, adequacy, quality of specimens, and complications–a systematic review. J Hepatol 2007;47(2):284–94.

18. Hardy T, Wells C, Kendrick S, et al. White cell count and platelet count associate with histological alcoholic hepatitis in jaundiced harmful drinkers. BMC Gastroenterol 2013;13(1):55.

19. Degré D, Stauber RE, Englebert G, et al. Long-term outcomes in patients with decompensated alcohol-related liver disease, steatohepatitis and Maddrey's discriminant function< 32. J Hepatol 2020;72(4):636–42.

20. Rinck D, Frieling H, Freitag A, et al. Combinations of carbohydrate-deficient transferrin, mean corpuscular erythrocyte volume, gamma-glutamyltransferase, homocysteine and folate increase the significance of biological markers in alcohol dependent patients. Drug Alcohol Depend 2007; 89(1):60–5.

21. Schwartz JM, Reinus JF. Prevalence and natural history of alcoholic liver disease. Clin Liver Dis 2012;16(4):659.

22. Koch H, Meerkerk G-J, Zaat JO, et al. Accuracy of carbohydrate-deficient transferrin in the detection of excessive alcohol consumption: a systematic review. Alcohol Alcohol 2004;39(2):75–85.

23. Taracha E, Habrat B, Woźiak P, et al. The activity of β-Hexosaminidase (uHex) and γ-glutamyl-transferase (uGGT) in urine as non-invasive markers of chronic alcohol abuse: I. Alcohol-dependent subjects. World J Biol Psychiatry 2001; 2(4):184–9.

24. Kissack JC, Bishop J, Roper AL. Ethylglucuronide as a biomarker for ethanol detection. Pharmacotherapy 2008;28(6):769–81.

25. Comasco E, Nordquist N, Leppert J, et al. Adolescent alcohol consumption: biomarkers PEth and FAEE in relation to interview and questionnaire data. J Stud Alcohol Drugs 2009;70(5):797–804.

26. Grove J, Daly AK, Bassendine MF, et al. Association of a tumor necrosis factor promoter polymorphism with susceptibility to alcoholic steatohepatitis. Hepatology 1997;26(1):143–6.

27. Achur RN, Freeman WM, Vrana KE. Circulating cytokines as biomarkers of alcohol abuse and alcoholism. J Neuroimmune Pharmacol 2010;5(1):83–91.

28. Orntoft NW, Sandahl TD, Jepsen P, et al. Short-term and long-term causes of death in patients with alcoholic hepatitis in Denmark. Clin Gastroenterol Hepatol 2014;12(10):1739–44.e1.

29. Louvet A, Labreuche J, Artru F, et al. Main drivers of outcome differ between short term and long term in severe alcoholic hepatitis: a prospective study. Hepatology 2017;66(5):1464–73.

30. Helander A, Böttcher M, Fehr C, et al. Detection times for urinary ethyl glucuronide and ethyl Sulfate in heavy drinkers during alcohol detoxification. Alcohol Alcohol 2008;44(1):55–61.
31. Naveau S, Montembault S, Balian A, et al. Biological diagnosis of the type of liver disease in alcoholic patients with abnormal liver function tests. Gastroenterol Clin Biol 1999;23(11):1215–24.
32. Potts J, Goubet S, Heneghan M, et al. Determinants of long-term outcome in severe alcoholic hepatitis. Aliment Pharmacol Ther 2013;38(6):584–95.
33. Samala N, Gawrieh S, Tang Q, et al. Clinical characteristics and outcomes of mild to moderate alcoholic hepatitis. Gastro Hep 2019;1(4):161–5.
34. Bennett K, Enki DG, Thursz M, et al. Systematic review with meta-analysis: high mortality in patients with non-severe alcoholic hepatitis. Aliment Pharmacol Ther 2019;50(3):249–57.
35. Delphine D, Stauber RE, Gaël E, et al. Long-term outcome of symptomatic alcoholic hepatitis with a Maddrey discriminant function< 32. J Hepatol 2020;73: S175.
36. Szabo G. Clinical trial design for alcoholic hepatitis. Semin Liver Dis 2017;37(4): 332–42.
37. Crabb DW, Im GY, Szabo G, et al. Diagnosis and treatment of alcohol-associated liver diseases: 2019 practice guidance from the American Association for the Study of Liver Diseases. Hepatology 2020;71(1):306–33.
38. Jalan R, Gines P, Olson JC, et al. Acute-on chronic liver failure. J Hepatol 2012; 57(6):1336–48.
39. Moreau R, Jalan R, Gines P, et al. Acute-on-chronic liver failure is a distinct syndrome that develops in patients with acute decompensation of cirrhosis. Gastroenterology 2013;144(7):1426–37, 1437.e1-9.
40. Sersté T, Cornillie A, Njimi H, et al. The prognostic value of acute-on-chronic liver failure during the course of severe alcoholic hepatitis. J Hepatol 2018;69(2): 318–24.
41. Jalan R, Saliba F, Pavesi M, et al. Development and validation of a prognostic score to predict mortality in patients with acute-on-chronic liver failure. J Hepatol 2014;61(5):1038–47.
42. Barosa R, Roque-Ramos L, Patita M, et al. CLIF-C ACLF score is a better mortality predictor than MELD, MELD-Na and CTP in patients with Acute on chronic liver failure admitted to the ward. Rev Esp Enferm Dig 2017;109(6):399–405.
43. Bellentani S, Saccoccio G, Costa G, et al. Drinking habits as cofactors of risk for alcohol induced liver damage. Gut 1997;41(6):845–50.
44. Ahmed A, Saksena S, Sherlock M, et al. Induction of hepatic 11β-hydroxysteroid dehydrogenase type 1 in patients with alcoholic liver disease. Clin Endocrinol (Oxf) 2008;68(6):898–903.
45. Colmenero J, Bataller R, Sancho–Bru P, et al. Hepatic expression of candidate genes in patients with alcoholic hepatitis: correlation with disease severity. Gastroenterology 2007;132(2):687–97.
46. Thiele M, Madsen BS, Hansen JF, et al. Accuracy of the enhanced liver fibrosis test vs FibroTest, elastography, and indirect markers in detection of advanced fibrosis in patients with alcoholic liver disease. Gastroenterology 2018;154(5): 1369–79.
47. Xie Q, Zhou X, Huang P, et al. The performance of enhanced liver fibrosis (ELF) test for the staging of liver fibrosis: a meta-analysis. PLoS One 2014;9(4): e92772.

48. Sandrin L, Fourquet B, Hasquenoph J-M, et al. Transient elastography: a new noninvasive method for assessment of hepatic fibrosis. Ultrasound Med Biol 2003;29(12):1705–13.

49. Regev A, Berho M, Jeffers LJ, et al. Sampling error and intraobserver variation in liver biopsy in patients with chronic HCV infection. Am J Gastroenterol 2002; 97(10):2614–8.

50. Mueller S, Sandrin L. Liver stiffness: a novel parameter for the diagnosis of liver disease. Hepat Med 2010;2:49.

51. Carithers RL Jr, Herlong HF, Diehl AM, et al. Methylprednisolone therapy in patients with severe alcoholic hepatitis: a randomized multicenter trial. Ann Intern Med 1989;110(9):685–90.

52. Dunn W, Jamil LH, Brown LS, et al. MELD accurately predicts mortality in patients with alcoholic hepatitis. Hepatology 2005;41(2):353–8.

53. Sheth M, Riggs M, Patel T. Utility of the Mayo End-Stage Liver Disease (MELD) score in assessing prognosis of patients with alcoholic hepatitis. BMC Gastroenterol 2002;2(1):1–5.

54. Srikureja W, Kyulo NL, Runyon BA, et al. MELD score is a better prognostic model than Child-Turcotte-Pugh score or Discriminant Function score in patients with alcoholic hepatitis. J Hepatol 2005;42(5):700–6.

55. Forrest EH, Evans CDJ, Stewart S, et al. Analysis of factors predictive of mortality in alcoholic hepatitis and derivation and validation of the Glasgow alcoholic hepatitis score. Gut 2005;54(8):1174–9.

56. Dominguez M, Rincón D, Abraldes JG, et al. A new scoring system for prognostic stratification of patients with alcoholic hepatitis. Am J Gastroenterol 2008;103(11):2747–56.

57. Forrest EH, Morris A, Stewart S, et al. The Glasgow alcoholic hepatitis score identifies patients who may benefit from corticosteroids. Gut 2007;56(12): 1743–6.

58. Forrest EH, Atkinson SR, Richardson P, et al. Application of prognostic scores in the STOPAH trial: discriminant function is no longer the optimal scoring system in alcoholic hepatitis. J Hepatol 2018;68(3):511–8.

59. Louvet A, Naveau S, Abdelnour M, et al. The Lille model: a new tool for therapeutic strategy in patients with severe alcoholic hepatitis treated with steroids. Hepatology 2007;45(6):1348–54.

60. Louvet A, Labreuche J, Artru F, et al. Combining data from liver disease scoring systems better predicts outcomes of patients with alcoholic hepatitis. Gastroenterology 2015;149(2):398–406.e8.

61. Vergis N, Atkinson SR, Knapp S, et al. In patients with severe alcoholic hepatitis, prednisolone increases susceptibility to infection and infection-related mortality, and is associated with high circulating levels of bacterial DNA. Gastroenterology 2017;152(5):1068–77.e4.

62. Thursz MR, Richardson P, Allison M, et al. Prednisolone or pentoxifylline for alcoholic hepatitis. N Engl J Med 2015;372(17):1619–28.

63. Dunn W, Angulo P, Sanderson S, et al. Utility of a new model to diagnose an alcohol basis for steatohepatitis. Gastroenterology 2006;131(4):1057–63.

64. Thabut D, Naveau S, Charlotte F, et al. The diagnostic value of biomarkers (AshTest) for the prediction of alcoholic steato-hepatitis in patients with chronic alcoholic liver disease. J Hepatol 2006;44(6):1175–85.

65. Rudler M, Mouri S, Charlotte F, et al. Validation of AshTest as a non-invasive alternative to transjugular liver biopsy in patients with suspected severe acute alcoholic hepatitis. PLoS One 2015;10(8):e0134302.

66. Hanouneh IA, Zein NN, Cikach F, et al. The breathprints in patients with liver disease identify novel breath biomarkers in alcoholic hepatitis. Clin Gastroenterol Hepatol 2014;12(3):516–23.
67. Wranne L. Urinary excretion of trimethylamine and trimethylamine oxide following trimethylamine-administration to normals and to patients with liver disease. Acta Med Scand 1955;153(6):433–41.
68. Rao R. Endotoxemia and gut barrier dysfunction in alcoholic liver disease. Hepatology 2009;50(2):638.
69. Omary MB, Ku N-O, Strnad P, et al. Toward unraveling the complexity of simple epithelial keratins in human disease. J Clin Invest 2009;119(7):1794–805.
70. Gonzalez-Quintela A, Mella C, Perez L, et al. Increased serum tissue polypeptide specific antigen (TPS) in alcoholics: a possible marker of alcoholic hepatitis. Alcohol Clin Exp Res 2000;24(8):1222–6.
71. Gonzalez-Quintela A, Garcia J, Campos J, et al. Serum cytokeratins in alcoholic liver disease: contrasting levels of cytokeratin-18 and cytokeratin-19. Alcohol 2006;38(1):45–9.
72. Kramer G, Erdal H, Mertens HJ, et al. Differentiation between cell death modes using measurements of different soluble forms of extracellular cytokeratin 18. Cancer Res 2004;64(5):1751–6.
73. Bissonnette J, Altamirano J, Devue C, et al. A prospective study of the utility of plasma biomarkers to diagnose alcoholic hepatitis. Hepatology 2017;66(2): 555–63.
74. Xavier V, Geerts A, Meuris L, et al. Plasma protein glycomics combined with circulating fragments of cytokeratin-18 are reliable biomarkers to diagnose alcoholic hepatitis. J Hepatol 2020;73:S193–4.
75. Woolbright BL, Bridges BW, Dunn W, et al. Cell death and prognosis of mortality in alcoholic hepatitis patients using plasma keratin-18. Gene Expr 2017;17(4): 301–12.
76. Vatsalya V, Cave MC, Kong M, et al. Keratin 18 is a diagnostic and prognostic factor for acute alcoholic hepatitis. Clin Gastroenterol Hepatol 2019;18(9): 2046–54.
77. Atkinson SR, Grove JI, Liebig S, et al. In severe alcoholic hepatitis, serum cytokeratin-18 fragments are diagnostic, prognostic and theragnostic biomarkers. Am J Gastroenterol 2020;115(11):1857–68.
78. Feldstein AE, Wieckowska A, Lopez AR, et al. Cytokeratin-18 fragment levels as noninvasive biomarkers for nonalcoholic steatohepatitis: a multicenter validation study. Hepatology 2009;50(4):1072–8.
79. Trépo E, Goossens N, Fujiwara N, et al. Combination of gene expression signature and model for end-stage liver disease score predicts survival of patients with severe alcoholic hepatitis. Gastroenterology 2018;154(4):965–75.
80. Buch S, Stickel F, Trépo E, et al. A genome-wide association study confirms PNPLA3 and identifies TM6SF2 and MBOAT7 as risk loci for alcohol-related cirrhosis. Nat Genet 2015;47(12):1443–8.
81. Mueller J, Rausch V, Peccerella T, et al. The role of PNPLA3, MBOAT7 and TM6SF2 during alcohol detoxification: different mechanisms of fibrosis and steatosis development. J Hepatol 2020;73:S182.
82. Stickel F, Buch S, Nischalke HD, et al. Genetic variants in PNPLA3 and TM6SF2 predispose to the development of hepatocellular carcinoma in individuals with alcohol-related cirrhosis. Am J Gastroenterol 2018;113(10):1475–83.
83. Levy RE, Catana AM, Durbin-Johnson B, et al. Ethnic differences in presentation and severity of alcoholic liver disease. Alcohol Clin Exp Res 2015;39(3):566–74.

84. Crabb DW, Matsumoto M, Chang D, et al. Overview of the role of alcohol dehydrogenase and aldehyde dehydrogenase and their variants in the genesis of alcohol-related pathology. Proc Nutr Soc 2004;63(1):49–63.

85. Atkinson S, Buckley T, Strnad P, et al. Genetic variation in HSD17B3 reduces the risk for developing severe alcoholic hepatitis. J Hepatol 2020;73:S61–2.

86. Abul-Husn NS, Cheng X, Li AH, et al. A protein-truncating HSD17B13 variant and protection from chronic liver disease. N Engl J Med 2018;378(12): 1096–106.

87. Atkinson SR, Way MJ, McQuillin A, et al. Homozygosity for rs738409: G in PNPLA3 is associated with increased mortality following an episode of severe alcoholic hepatitis. J Hepatol 2017;67(1):120–7.

88. Bala S, Szabo G. MicroRNA signature in alcoholic liver disease. Int J Hepatol 2012;2012:498232.

89. Alexander M, Hu R, Runtsch MC, et al. Exosome-delivered microRNAs modulate the inflammatory response to endotoxin. Nat Commun 2015;6(1):1–16.

90. Momen-Heravi F, Saha B, Kodys K, et al. Increased number of circulating exosomes and their microRNA cargos are potential novel biomarkers in alcoholic hepatitis. J Transl Med 2015;13(1):261.

91. Sancho-Bru P, Altamirano J, Rodrigo-Torres D, et al. Liver progenitor cell markers correlate with liver damage and predict short-term mortality in patients with alcoholic hepatitis. Hepatology 2012;55(6):1931–41.

92. Blaya D, Coll M, Rodrigo-Torres D, et al. Integrative microRNA profiling in alcoholic hepatitis reveals a role for microRNA-182 in liver injury and inflammation. Gut 2016;65(9):1535–45.

93. Tang Y, Banan A, Forsyth CB, et al. Effect of alcohol on miR-212 expression in intestinal epithelial cells and its potential role in alcoholic liver disease. Alcohol Clin Exp Res 2008;32(2):355–64.

94. Momen-Heravi F, Bala S, Kodys K, et al. Exosomes derived from alcohol-treated hepatocytes horizontally transfer liver specific miRNA-122 and sensitize monocytes to LPS. Sci Rep 2015;5:9991.

95. Yeligar S, Tsukamoto H, Kalra VK. Ethanol-induced expression of ET-1 and ET-BR in liver sinusoidal endothelial cells and human endothelial cells involves hypoxia-inducible factor-1α and microRNA-199. J Immunol 2009;183(8): 5232–43.

96. Yáñez-Mó M, Siljander PR-M, Andreu Z, et al. Biological properties of extracellular vesicles and their physiological functions. J extracellular vesicles 2015; 4(1):27066.

97. Bala S, Csak T, Momen-Heravi F, et al. Biodistribution and function of extracellular miRNA-155 in mice. Sci Rep 2015;5(1):1–12.

98. Momen-Heravi F, Bala S, Bukong T, et al. Exosome-mediated delivery of functionally active miRNA-155 inhibitor to macrophages. Nanomed Nanotechnol Biol Med 2014;10(7):1517–27.

99. Bala S, Marcos M, Kodys K, et al. Up-regulation of microRNA-155 in macrophages contributes to increased tumor necrosis factor α (TNFα) production via increased mRNA half-life in alcoholic liver disease. J Biol Chem 2011; 286(2):1436–44.

100. Fleury A, Martinez MC, Le Lay S. Extracellular vesicles as therapeutic tools in cardiovascular diseases. Front Immunol 2014;5:370.

101. Szabo G, Momen-Heravi F. Extracellular vesicles in liver disease and potential as biomarkers and therapeutic targets. Nat Rev Gastroenterol Hepatol 2017; 14(8):455.

102. Jiang L, Chu H, Gao B, et al. Transcriptomic profiling identifies novel hepatic and intestinal genes following chronic plus binge ethanol feeding in mice. Dig Dis Sci 2020;65(12):3592–604.

103. Llopis M, Cassard A, Wrzosek L, et al. Intestinal microbiota contributes to individual susceptibility to alcoholic liver disease. Gut 2016;65(5):830–9.

104. Duan Y, Llorente C, Lang S, et al. Bacteriophage targeting of gut bacterium attenuates alcoholic liver disease. Nature 2019;575(7783):505–11.

105. Philips CA, Pande A, Shasthry SM, et al. Healthy donor fecal microbiota transplantation in steroid-ineligible severe alcoholic hepatitis: a pilot study. Clin Gastroenterol Hepatol 2017;15(4):600–2.

106. Jiang L, Lang S, Duan Y, et al. Intestinal virome in patients with alcoholic hepatitis. Hepatology 2020;72(6):2182–96.

107. Lang S, Duan Y, Liu J, et al. Intestinal fungal dysbiosis and systemic immune response to fungi in patients with alcoholic hepatitis. Hepatology 2020;71(2): 522–38.

108. McClain CJ, Song Z, Barve SS, et al. Recent advances in alcoholic liver disease IV. Dysregulated cytokine metabolism in alcoholic liver disease. Am J Physiol Gastrointestinal Liver Physiol 2004;287(3):G497–502.

109. McClain CJ, Barve S, Deaciuc I, Kugelmas M, Hill D. Cytokines in alcoholic liver disease. Paper presented at: Seminars in liver disease1999.

110. Naveau S, Chollet-Martin S, Dharancy S, et al. A double-blind randomized controlled trial of infliximab associated with prednisolone in acute alcoholic hepatitis. Hepatology 2004;39(5):1390–7.

111. Menon KN, Stadheim L, Kamath PS, et al. A pilot study of the safety and tolerability of etanercept in patients with alcoholic hepatitis. Am J Gastroenterol 2004;99(2):255–60.

112. Thiele M, Trost K, Suvitaival T, et al. Lipidomics profiling reveals a distinct pattern of selective lipid depletion in the circulation and liver tissue in patients with progressive alcohol-associated liver fibrosis: a biopsy-controlled study in 400 people. J Hepatol 2020;73:S58.

113. Warner J, Zirnheld K, Vatsalya V, et al. Alterations and role of bioactive lipid metabolites (oxylipins) in human and experimental ALD: associations with disease severity. J Hepatol 2020;73:S181.

114. Yates E, Tan H, Dhanda A. A novel lymphocyte proliferation assay accurately predicts 90-day survival in severe alcoholic hepatitis patients. J Hepatol 2020; 73:S176.

115. Das S, Maras JS, Maiwall R, et al. Molecular ellipticity of circulating albumin-bilirubin complex associates with mortality in patients with severe alcoholic hepatitis. Clin Gastroenterol Hepatol 2018;16(8):1322–32.e4.

116. Calmet F, Martin P. A new marker for severity of alcoholic hepatitis. Clin Gastroenterol Hepatol 2018;16(8):1207–8.

117. Calès P, De Ledinghen V, Halfon P, et al. Evaluating the accuracy and increasing the reliable diagnosis rate of blood tests for liver fibrosis in chronic hepatitis C. Liver Int 2008;28(10):1352–62.

118. Dincses E, Yilmaz Y. Diagnostic usefulness of FibroMeter VCTE for hepatic fibrosis in patients with nonalcoholic fatty liver disease. Eur J Gastroenterol Hepatol 2015;27(10):1149–53.

119. Calès P, Boursier J, Oberti F, et al. FibroMeters: a family of blood tests for liver fibrosis. Gastroenterol Clin Biol 2008;32(6):40–51.

120. Stickel F, Buch S, Lau K, et al. Genetic variation in the PNPLA3 gene is associated with alcoholic liver injury in Caucasians. Hepatology 2011;53(1):86–95.

121. Donati B, Dongiovanni P, Romeo S, et al. MBOAT7 rs641738 variant and hepatocellular carcinoma in non-cirrhotic individuals. Sci Rep 2017;7(1):1–10.
122. Schwantes-An TH, Darlay R, Mathurin P, et al. Genome-wide association study and meta-analysis on alcohol-related liver cirrhosis identifies novel genetic risk factors. Hepatology 2020. https://doi.org/10.1002/hep.31535.
123. Grigorios C, Karatayli E, Hall R, et al. Fibroblast growth factor 21 response in a preclinical model of alcohol induced acute-on-chronic liver injury. J Hepatol 2020;73:S177–8.
124. Brandl K, Hartmann P, Jih LJ, et al. Dysregulation of serum bile acids and FGF19 in alcoholic hepatitis. J Hepatol 2018;69(2):396–405.
125. Muthiah M, Smirnova E, Puri P, et al. The development and severity of alcoholic hepatitis is associated with decreased intestinal microbiome-derived secondary bile acid isoursodeoxycholic acid. J Hepatol 2020;73:S187.
126. Maras J, Bhat A, Yadav G, et al. Temporal change in the plasma metabolome profile is indicative of outcome in severe alcoholic hepatitis. J Hepatol 2020;73:S180.

Genetic and Environmental Susceptibility to Alcoholic Hepatitis

Marsha Y. Morgan, MD[a],*, Moksh Sharma, BSc[a],
Stephen R. Atkinson, MD, PhD[b]

KEYWORDS

- Alcoholic hepatitis • Alcohol-related cirrhosis • Alcohol-related liver disease
- Alcohol-related steatohepatitis • Environmental risk factors • Genetic risk factors
- Host susceptibility

KEY POINTS

- Prolonged alcohol misuse is associated with the development of a spectrum of liver injury, ranging from steatosis through steatohepatitis, fibrosis, and cirrhosis, to hepatocellular carcinoma.
- Cirrhosis only develops in the minority of excessive drinkers and its clinical course is usually insidious, often presenting only with the onset of hepatic decompensation.
- A small proportion of patients with evolving or established alcohol-related liver disease develop the clinical syndrome of alcoholic hepatitis, which manifests as the comparatively rapid onset of often profound liver failure.
- A number of constitutional, environmental, and genetic factors have been identified as associated with the risk for developing alcohol-related cirrhosis.
- The same risk factors may play a role in the development of alcoholic hepatitis, but the possibility that additional more specific risk factors exist remains to be delineated.

INTRODUCTION

The development of advanced liver injury in patients who misuse alcohol, even those who consume the greatest quantities, is not inevitable. Indeed, only a comparative minority of heavy drinkers develop significant liver disease. Furthermore, the rate of progression shows significant heterogeneity. Considerable effort has been invested in trying to determine the environmental and genetic factors that influence the development of advanced alcohol-related liver disease, especially the risk factors that predispose to the clinical syndrome of alcoholic hepatitis.

[a] UCL Institute for Liver & Digestive Health, Division of Medicine, Royal Free Campus, University College, Rowland Hill Street, Hampstead, London NW3 2PF, UK; [b] Department of Metabolism, Digestion and Reproduction, Imperial College London, South Kensington Campus, London SW7 2AZ, UK
* Corresponding author.
E-mail address: marsha.morgan@ucl.ac.uk

Clin Liver Dis 25 (2021) 517–535
https://doi.org/10.1016/j.cld.2021.04.001
1089-3261/21/© 2021 Elsevier Inc. All rights reserved.
liver.theclinics.com

STEATOHEPATITIS AND ALCOHOLIC HEPATITIS: NOMENCLATURE

There is considerable confusion over the nomenclature of alcohol-related liver disease and in particular, the terms steatohepatitis and alcoholic hepatitis. The recent definitions provided by the European Association for the Study of the Liver (EASL) will be adopted here (**Table 1**).[1]

The vast majority of people who develop alcohol-related cirrhosis progress through the stages of steatosis, steatohepatitis, and fibrosis to reach this end point. Most do so silently and often do not present until their liver disease finally decompensates. However, a comparatively small number of people with a history of prolonged heavy and ongoing alcohol misuse develop the clinical syndrome of alcoholic hepatitis, which manifests as the recent onset of jaundice, frequently accompanied by other features of liver failure such as hepatic encephalopathy, coagulopathy, and ascites.[2] These people show histological features of a steatohepatitis, often florid, and a high proportion have established cirrhosis. This condition has a high associated mortality of 15% to 30% in the first month and upwards of 50% within 1 year of presentation.[3]

The presence of steatohepatitis is considered a necessary prerequisite for the development of progressive liver disease leading to cirrhosis. However, it is only infrequently accompanied by the clinical syndrome of alcoholic hepatitis, and this distinction is extremely important. Thus, exploring the environmental and genetic risk factors for the development of alcoholic hepatitis is a 2-step process as the majority of people with this syndrome already have established cirrhosis, indicating phenotypic overlap. In consequence, the risk factors that predispose to the development of alcohol-related liver disease *per se* must first be delineated and then factors that may be additionally or specifically associated with the risk for developing the clinical syndrome of alcoholic hepatitis can be explored.

NATURAL HISTORY OF ALCOHOL-RELATED LIVER DISEASE

Excess alcohol consumption is associated with the development of liver injury. Early liver biopsy studies identified a spectrum of change associated with sustained alcohol ingestion progressing from steatosis to steatohepatitis, fibrosis, cirrhosis, and hepatocellular carcinoma (HCC) (**Fig. 1**). These stages are not mutually exclusive and often coexist. The prevalence of biopsy-proven liver disease among drinkers is largely unknown although a recent meta-analysis reported that within cohorts of hazardous drinkers, approximately 15% had normal liver histology, 27% had hepatic steatosis, 24% had steatohepatitis, while 26% had cirrhosis.[4] The annualized rates of progression of precirrhotic disease to cirrhosis were 1% (0%–8%) for patients with normal histology, 3% (2%–4%) for hepatic steatosis, 10% (6%–17%) for steatohepatitis, and 8% (3%–19%) for fibrosis.[4]

Overall, it is estimated that only 15% to 20% of people drinking excessively will develop cirrhosis, no matter how much they drink or for how long.[5,6] The prevalence of cirrhosis among individuals abusing alcohol varies from 9% to 18% in autopsy studies and from 12% to 31% based on liver biopsy series.[6–8] In a recent meta-analysis based on 38 observational studies, the incidence of alcohol-related cirrhosis in cohorts with alcohol problems ranged from 7% to 16% after 8 to 12 years.[9]

Modulating effects of drinking behavior

The effects of drinking behaviour on the evolution of alcohol-related liver disease are substantial (**Fig. 2**). Steatosis usually resolves within 2 to 4 weeks of cessation of alcohol consumption.[10] Steatohepatitis develops in only a proportion of drinkers

Table 1
Nomenclature of alcohol-related liver disease

Term	Definition	Old Nomenclature
Alcohol-related liver disease	Any form of liver disease, irrespective of severity, attributable to excess alcohol consumption. Comprises the entire spectrum of disease from steatosis through to cirrhosis	Alcoholic liver disease
Alcohol-related cirrhosis	End-stage liver disease attributable to excess alcohol consumption	Alcoholic cirrhosis
Steatohepatitis due to alcohol-related liver disease	A histologically defined lesion typified by the presence of features including steatosis, ballooning degeneration of hepatocytes, inflammatory infiltrates, Mallory–Denk bodies and megamitochondria	Alcoholic steatohepatitis
Alcoholic hepatitis	A clinical syndrome typified by the recent onset of progressive and typically profound jaundice, often with additional clinical features of liver failure, in patients with a history of chronic, excess alcohol use	Alcoholic hepatitis

Adapted from EASL Clinical Practice Guidelines: Management of alcohol-related liver disease. J Hepatol 2018;69:154-181; with permission.

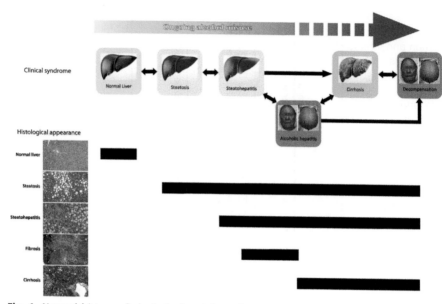

Fig. 1. Natural history of alcohol-related liver disease. (*Top*) The development of alcohol-related cirrhosis progress through the stages of steatosis, steatohepatitis, and fibrosis. The majority of patients do not present until their liver disease finally decompensates. A comparatively small number of people develop the clinical syndrome of alcoholic hepatitis, which manifests as the recent onset of often profound liver failure. (*Bottom*) Although the histological stages of alcohol-related liver disease are described separately, they often coexist. Thus, patients with alcohol-related cirrhosis may also have steatosis while patients with alcoholic hepatitis have a steatohepatitis, often florid, but may also have established cirrhosis.

even after decades of alcohol abuse and is assumed to be a precirrhotic lesion, although its natural history is not well-understood. Thus, Galambos[11] in a serial liver biopsy study in individuals with steatohepatitis showed that 38% developed cirrhosis, 52% retained the hepatitic lesion, whereas in 10% the liver lesion regressed despite continued alcohol use. Abstinence did not guarantee regression of the lesion; of those who maintained abstinence 27% had normal histology, 55% retained the hepatitic lesion and 18% developed cirrhosis.[11]

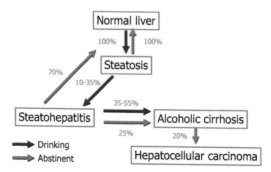

Fig. 2. Effects of continued drinking and abstinence from alcohol on the evolution of alcohol-related liver disease.

Parés and colleagues[12] showed that in men with mild to moderate steatohepatitis, subsequent drinking behavior is the major factor influencing outcome, whereas in women and in individuals with severe steatohepatitis, of both sexes, progression to cirrhosis is more likely to occur and is less influenced by subsequent drinking behavior. Data from 2 long-term serial biopsy studies confirmed that the effects of abstinence from alcohol on the progression of steatohepatitis are not entirely predictable and provided evidence that, over a given threshold, the risk of developing cirrhosis was unrelated to the average daily intake of alcohol.[13,14] In addition, they confirmed that progression to cirrhosis was more likely in women and in individuals with severe steatohepatitis, irrespective of subsequent drinking behavior.[14] Although cirrhosis is an irreversible lesion, abstinence from alcohol can have a significant beneficial effect on outcome even in patients with established disease.[15]

RISK FACTORS FOR THE DEVELOPMENT OF ALCOHOL-RELATED CIRRHOSIS

Environmental and Host-Related Factors

Drinking behavior

Excessive alcohol consumption is the major epidemiologic factor determining the risk for developing alcohol-related cirrhosis.[16] However, the precise nature of the relationship between alcohol consumption and cirrhosis risk is debated.[17] Results from early seminal studies[18–23] and a later meta-analysis of 15 studies[24] showed that the risk for developing cirrhosis was significantly increased with alcohol intakes of approximately 25 to 30 g/d and that thereafter the risk increased, almost exponentially, with greater daily as well as cumulative alcohol consumption. However, a Danish group reported that there was a risk threshold at approximately 60 g/d, beyond which there was no further dose–response relationship and no additional risk with drinking greater amounts of alcohol.[17,25] Conversely, a more recent Danish study reported a clear dose-dependent association between the level of alcohol intake and the risk for developing cirrhosis among both men and women drinking more than 24 g/d.[26] A recent meta-analysis of 7 studies reported a steadily increasing dose–response relationship in women from as little as 12 g/d and some evidence for a threshold effect in men with alcohol intakes or more than 84 g/d.[27]

A number of studies have reported that daily drinking is associated with a higher cirrhosis risk than binge drinking.[13,22,25–28] However, failing to take account of the total amount of alcohol consumed when comparing regular and binge drinkers may confound these findings.[28,29] There is some evidence that drinking wine, as opposed to other beverage types, is associated with a lower cirrhosis risk.[26,30] However, it is the amount of contained alcohol that is the key factor[31]; apparent differences in cirrhosis risk, by beverage, are likely confounded by variations in dietary and lifestyle factors.[32,33] Consuming alcohol together with food may decrease the cirrhosis risk,[23] whereas regular consumption of a diet high in fat but low in carbohydrate and protein may increase the risk.[32]

Sex

Men consume significantly more alcohol than women and consequently have higher alcohol-related cirrhosis rates.[20,34] However, women have a significantly higher relative risk for developing alcohol-related liver disease than men for a given level of alcohol consumption.[34] This difference has been consistently reported across individual studies[20,24,34,35] and in a meta-analysis involving 1,477,887 individuals (**Fig. 3**).[36] The thresholds above which alcohol consumption should be considered harmful are, accordingly, lower in women at 20 to 40 g/d than in men at more than 60 g/d.[31] The difference in susceptibility primarily relates to sex-related differences in body

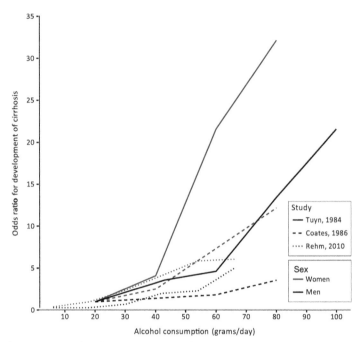

Fig. 3. Odd ratios (ORs) for the development of cirrhosis at different levels of alcohol consumption, by sex. Data are drawn from 2 case-control studies[20,35] and a meta-analysis.[36] Although the ORs vary between studies, potentially as a function of the estimation of alcohol consumption and case acquisition, within studies the risk of cirrhosis for a given level of alcohol consumption is consistently higher in women than in men.

composition which result in a smaller apparent volume of distribution of alcohol in women and consequently higher blood alcohol concentration, for a given weight-adjusted ingested dose, and greater tissue levels of exposure.[37]

Ethnicity

There are notable interethnic differences in alcohol-related cirrhosis risk. A study in the UK reported that non-Muslim men of south Asian descent present with alcohol-related cirrhosis at a younger age and with a higher than expected frequency, compared to their white British counterparts, whereas Afro-Caribbean men were significantly underrepresented in this patient group.[38] In the United States, white men and women of Hispanic, predominantly Mexican ancestry, have a higher risk for cirrhosis mortality compared with black and white non-Hispanic men and women.[39] Individuals of Hispanic origin have also been shown to present with alcohol-related cirrhosis up to 10 years earlier than their white Caucasian counterparts.[40] However, these differences could represent constitutional differences in alcohol metabolism or differences relating to the amounts and types of alcohol consumed, dietary intake, socioeconomic status, and access to health care.

An interesting paradox is the indirect protection against the development of alcohol-related cirrhosis afforded to individuals of east Asian ancestry who carry the single nucleotide polymorphism rs671 in *ALDH2* and, as a consequence, develop high concentrations of circulating acetaldehyde following alcohol ingestion and so tend to avoid alcohol. A meta-analysis of published studies identified a significant and robust association between possession of this variant and the development of alcohol-related physical harm, including cirrhosis.[41] There is, however, no evidence that this finding is anything other than an indirect effect.

Body weight and composition

Both alcohol misuse and obesity are independent risk factors for the development of cirrhosis. Whether obesity is an independent risk factor for the development of alcohol-related cirrhosis is debated. Overweight or obese white, middle-aged women in the UK who consume low to moderate amounts of alcohol are at increased risk for developing cirrhosis compared with women with a body mass index (BMI) of 22.5 to 25.0; the risk increases by about 28% for each 5-unit increase in BMI.[42] The absolute increase in cirrhosis rates with increasing BMI is substantially greater in women drinking 150 g or more of alcohol per week than those drinking 70 g a week (**Table 2**). However, compared with the other known risk factors for cirrhosis, the effect of obesity in this study was moderate but none of the participants drank excessively with only a small proportion consuming more than 3 drinks a day. The resultant liver injury likely represents the combined insults of both alcohol and obesity.

However, Naveau and colleagues[43] undertook a detailed study of patients with a history of prolonged harmful use of alcohol, in whom the degree of liver injury was confirmed histologically. They reported that those who had been overweight for at least 10 years, defined as a BMI of 25 or higher for women and 27 or higher for men, were 2.15 times more likely to have cirrhosis than their counterparts who were not overweight. In a later study, the same group reported that the visceral abdominal fat level, assessed using abdominal height in the supine position, is an independent risk factor for the development of fibrosis in patients with a history of prolonged harmful use of alcohol, regardless of total body fat content assessed using the BMI.[44]

Tobacco and cannabis

The prevalence of tobacco smoking among individuals who drink excessively is high.[45] Cigarette smoking is independently associated with the risk for developing alcohol-related cirrhosis with smokers of a pack or more per day at treble the risk of non-smokers.[46] This risk is particularly high among women.[45] Thus, in a very large Danish population-based study, with a mean follow-up time of 21 years, approximately 26% of cases of alcohol-related cirrhosis in women and 8% of cases in men could be attributed to smoking, after adjustment for alcohol intake.[45] Conversely, the GenomALC consortium recently reported a lower prevalence of smoking in cases with alcohol-related cirrhosis than in controls drinking excessively with no liver disease.[47]

In a large and complex analysis of the 2014 Healthcare Cost and Utilization Project-Nationwide Inpatient Sample, involving 319,514 participants with a past or current history of alcohol abuse, Adejumo and colleagues[48] reported that additional cannabis use was associated with a 55% decrease in the likelihood of developing alcohol-related cirrhosis; the greater the intake of cannabis, the greater the decrease

Table 2
Cirrhosis risk in women drinking low to moderate amounts of alcohol, by Body Mass Index

Alcohol Intake (g/wk)	<70		≥150	
Body Mass Index	22.5–25.0	≥30.0	22.5–25.0	≥30.0
Absolute risk (95% confidence interval) of cirrhosis/1000 women over 5 y	0.8 (0.7–0.9)	1.0 (0.9–1.2)	2.7 (2.1–3.4)	5.0 (3.8–6.6)

Adapted from Liu B, Balkwill A, Reeves G, et al. Body mass index and risk of liver cirrhosis in middle aged UK women: prospective study. BMJ 2010; 340:c912; with permission.

in the likelihood of cirrhosis development.[48] The GenomALC consortium reported that in individuals with a history of alcohol abuse prolonged regular cannabis use was 3 times commoner in controls with no liver disease (27%) than in cases with alcohol-related cirrhosis (9%); the prevalence differences in cannabis use between cases and controls were highly significant up to the age of 60 years.[47]

Coffee drinking

Coffee drinking is inversely related to alcohol-related cirrhosis risk, suggesting a protective effect[46]; people drinking 4 or more cups a day have one-fifth the risk of developing cirrhosis of noncoffee drinkers.[46] Kennedy and colleagues[49] undertook a meta-analysis of 9 studies to further characterize the relationship between coffee consumption and cirrhosis risk. They confirmed the protective effect of coffee on cirrhosis risk and the dose-related effect. They concluded that an increase in coffee consumption of 2 cups per day is associated with a near halving of the cirrhosis risk. In the GenomALC study controls with no liver disease were more likely than cases with alcohol-related cirrhosis to have been coffee drinkers during the time they were drinking alcohol heavily and to have drunk more coffee per day.[47]

Comorbid liver disease

Alcohol may act synergistically with other injurious agents to increase the risk for developing significant liver injury. Thus, individuals who drink heavily and have features of the metabolic syndrome,[43,50] chronic hepatitis B and C viral infections,[51,52] or HIV infection[53] display accelerated rates of hepatic fibrosis. People with chronic hepatitis C virus infection whose alcohol intake exceeds 50 g/d have a significantly higher risk of advanced fibrosis than those who drink less or not at all.[54] Patients with hereditary hemochromatosis who drink more than 60 g of alcohol per day are approximately 9 times more likely to develop cirrhosis than those who drink less than this amount.[55]

GENETIC RISK FACTORS

Familiarity and Heritability

There are very few epidemiologic studies relating to the familiarity and heritability of alcohol-related cirrhosis.

No formal family studies have been conducted in people with alcohol-related liver disease. However, in the GenomALC study cirrhosis risk was significantly increased in individuals with a history of prolonged excessive alcohol consumption if their father also drank excessively and died of liver disease.[47,56] These findings are potentially supportive of a genetic contribution, but the effects of a shared environment or of inherited epigenetic changes, such as imprinting or other mechanisms of selective transmission, cannot be excluded.

Available estimates of the heritability of alcohol-related cirrhosis are available from a single study of 15,924 male twin pairs.[57] The concordance for alcohol-related cirrhosis was 3 times higher in monozygotic than in dizygotic twins and this finding was confirmed in a second analysis undertaken more than a decade later.[58] The heritability estimates for alcohol-related cirrhosis ranged from 21% to 67%. There was some disagreement between the 2 reports in relation to the proportion of the genetic variance that was independent of the heritability of alcohol dependence.[58]

Candidate Gene Studies

The selection of candidates for genetic studies in alcohol-related liver disease has, in the main, been based on assumptions relating to the mechanisms of the liver injury. Thus, associations have been sought, in case-control studies, between the development of alcohol-related liver injury and functional variants in loci implicated in alcohol and lipid metabolism, endotoxin-mediated inflammation and cytokines, immune responses, and oxidative stress and fibrogenesis, among others.[59–61]

These studies have, with few exceptions, shown no evidence of association between the genetic variants of interest and the risk for developing alcohol-related cirrhosis.[59–61] However, meta-analyses of the association studies involving *tumor necrosis factor-α (TNFA)* and *glutathione s-transferase 1 (GSTM1)* suggest that variants at these loci may be associated with an increased risk for developing alcohol-related liver disease.[62,63] However, no significant associations with these loci have been identified in genome-wide association studies (GWAS).[64–66]

In 2008, Romeo and colleagues[67] reported that rs738409:G in *patatin-like phospholipase domain-containing protein 3 (PNPLA3)* was strongly associated with the risk for developing non–alcohol-related fatty liver disease. The evaluation of this locus, using a candidate gene approach, identified and validated robust associations between this variant in *PNPLA3* and the risk for developing alcohol-related cirrhosis, both in individual studies and meta-analyses.[68–72] The effect sizes were in the range expected for a relatively frequent single nucleotide polymorphism in a complex disease while the population-attributable risk for progression to alcohol-related cirrhosis conferred by carriage of *PNPLA3* rs738409:G was 26.6%, suggesting that other modifiers are likely to exist.[73] Studies have also shown that carriers of *PNPLA3:* rs738409:G (1) present with cirrhosis after a shorter drinking history,[74] (2) develop decompensated cirrhosis at an earlier stage of their disease history,[75] and (3) are more likely to die of their liver disease.[76]

In 2018, Abul-Husn and colleagues[77] identified a splice variant rs72613567 in *hydroxysteroid 17-beta dehydrogenase13 (HSD17B13)* that appeared to protect against the development of alcohol-related cirrhosis in people of European decent, although the total number of cases was very small. This variant also appeared to attenuate the risk for developing progressive liver injury associated with carriage of rs738409:G in *PNPLA3*. A case-control study, undertaken by Stickel and colleagues,[78] involving 6171 participants, found that carriage of *HSD17B13* rs72613567:TA was associated with a lower risk for developing both alcohol-related cirrhosis (odds ratio [OR], 0.79; 95% confidence interval [CI], 0.72–0.88; $P = 8.13 \times 10^{-6}$) and HCC (OR, 0.77; 95% CI, 0.68–0.89; $P = 2.27 \times 10^{-4}$). They further reported that carriage of *HSD17B13* rs72613567:TA attenuated the risk for developing alcohol-related cirrhosis associated with *PNPLA3* rs738409:G in both men and women, but the protective effect against the subsequent development of HCC was observed only in men.[78]

Finally, in 2019, Strnad and coworkers[79] identified a significant association between heterozygous carriage of the Pi*Z (rs28929474) variant in *serpin family A member 1 (SERPINA1)* and the risk for developing alcohol-related cirrhosis (adjusted OR, 5.8; 95% CI. 2.9–11.7). Homozygous carriage of Pi*Z is associated with severe alpha 1 antitrypsin deficiency, which results in damage to the lungs and liver.

Thus, case-control studies have identified variants in *PNPLA3*, *HSD17B13*, and *SERPINA1*, which differentially affect the risk for developing advanced alcohol-related liver disease.

Genome-wide Association Studies

Three GWAS in alcohol-related cirrhosis have been undertaken to date.[64–66] These studies have confirmed the associations between cirrhosis risk and variants at loci encoding *PNPLA3*, *HSD17B13*, and *SERPINA1* at genome-wide significance.

Additionally, they have identified several novel variants, also at genome-wide significance, that are associated with either an increased risk for developing advanced alcohol-related liver disease, for example, rs58542926 in *transmembrane 6 superfamily member 2* (*TM6SF2*); rs641738 in *membrane-bound O-acyltransferase domain containing 7* (MBOAT7), and rs15052 in *heterogeneous nuclear ribonucleoprotein U like 1* (*HNRNPUL1*) or else provide protection against its development, for example, rs2642438 in *mitochondrial amidoxime reducing component 1* (*MARC1*) and rs374702773 in *fas associated factor family member 2* (*FAF2*) (**Table 3**).

It is highly likely that larger studies and further meta-analyses will identify additional risk and protective factors associated with the development of alcohol-related cirrhosis.

Epigenetics

Epigenetic modifications are hereditable changes that impact on gene expression without altering the nucleotide sequence. Examples include: DNA methylation, histone modifications and RNA silencing by microRNAs. Epigenetic mechanisms that are deregulated by alcohol in the liver may contribute to the pathogenesis and progression of alcohol-related liver disease, but their role as possible risk factors for the development of alcohol-related liver disease needs further exploration.

SPECIFIC RISK FACTORS FOR THE CLINICAL SYNDROME OF ALCOHOLIC HEPATITIS

Very little information is available on possible environmental and genetic risk factors, additionally or specifically associated with the risk for developing the clinical syndrome of alcoholic hepatitis.

Drinking Behavior

There does not seem to be a direct relationship between the amount or pattern of drinking and the development of alcoholic hepatitis beyond the generally accepted threshold of more than 40 g/d for women and more than 60 g/d for men for a minimum of 6 months.[80–82]

Anecdotally, many patients with alcoholic hepatitis report a decrease in food intake in the weeks or months before presentation, together with an increase in alcohol intake or additional binge drinking. This observation is supported by data in mice showing that chronic ethanol feeding plus a single binge dose of ethanol exacerbates hepatic steatosis and neutrophilic inflammation over and above the effects of chronic or binge ethanol feeding alone.[83] However, it is not supported by available observational data, albeit limited, from the Translational Research and Evolving Alcoholic Hepatitis Treatment (TREAT) consortium; they reported that the total amount of alcohol consumed in the 30 days before presentation and the rates of binge drinking in cases with alcoholic hepatitis were significantly lower than in heavy drinking controls with no liver disease.[81]

Case definition in this study was based largely on clinical evaluation and on laboratory findings of a serum bilirubin or more than 2 mg/dL (34 μmol/L) and a serum aspartate aminotransferase activity of more than 50 U/L, but the mean (± 1 standard deviation) MELD score of 22 ± 7.1 and the mean Maddrey discriminant function of 41.6 ± 29.1 would indicate that a high proportion of the included cases did not have severe disease. Thus, the relationship between the recency and nature of alcohol consumption and the risk for developing alcoholic hepatitis remains unclear.

Demographic and Lifestyle Factors

Older patients recruited by the TREAT consortium were less likely to present with severe alcoholic hepatitis; indeed, age at presentation was significantly and inversely

Table 3
Genes identified in GWAS which associate with the risk for developing alcohol-related cirrhosis at genome-wide significance

Study	Phenotypes	Gene	Lead Single Nucleotide Polymorphism[a]
Buch et al,[64] 2015	Alcohol-related cirrhosis (n = 712)	PNPLA3	rs738409:G (OR, 2.03, $P = 1.54 \times 10^{-48}$)[b]
	Heavy drinking controls (n = 1426)	SUGP1	rs10401969:C (OR, 1.57, $P = 7.89 \times 10^{-10}$)[d,f]
		MBOAT7	rs626283:C (OR, 1.33, $P = 1.03 \times 10^{-9}$)[d]
Innes et al,[65] 2020	APRI, FIB-4, Forns index, serum alanine aminotransferase and aspartate aminotransferase in hazardous drinkers from UK Biobank (n = 35,839)	PNPLA3	rs738408:T ($\beta = 0.803$, $P = 2.21 \times 10^{-51}$)[b,e]
		SUGP1	rs10401969:C ($\beta = 0.660$, $P = 1.21 \times 10^{-15}$)[b,f]
		HNF1A	rs11065384:T ($\beta = 0.199$, $P = 1.01 \times 10^{-4}$)[b]
		ARHGEF3	rs11925835:T ($\beta = -0.134$, $P = 6.64 \times 10^{-3}$)[b]
		SERPINA1	rs28929474:T ($\beta = 0.717$, $P = 2.77 \times 10^{-5}$)[b]
		TRIB1	rs2954038:C ($\beta = 0.140$, $P = 8.75 \times 10^{-3}$)[b]
		HNRNPUL1	rs15052:C ($\beta = 0.220$, $P = 1.06 \times 10^{-3}$)[b]
		MARC1	rs2642438:A ($\beta = -0.223$, $P = 4.51 \times 10^{-5}$)[b]
		HSD17B13	rs72613567:TA ($\beta = -0.237$, 1.38×10^{-5})[b]
Schwantes-An et al,[66] 2021	Alcohol-related cirrhosis (n = 1128)	PNPLA3	rs2294915:T (OR, 2.07, $P = 1.28 \times 10^{-53}$)[b,e]
	Heavy drinking controls (n = 614)	HSD17B13	rs10433937:G (OR, 0.78, $P = 2.85 \times 10^{-9}$)[b,a]
		FAF2	rs11134977:C (OR, = 0.79, $P = 1.56 \times 10^{-8}$)[c]
		SERPINA1	rs28929474:T (OR, 1.90, $P = 1.99 \times 10^{-8}$)[d]
		SUGP1	rs10401969:C (OR, 1.49, $P = 2.40 \times 10^{-9}$)[d,f]

a The most significantly associated single nucleotide polymorphism at a given locus reported by the study authors.
Single nucleotide polymorphisms, risk alleles, ORs, β estimates and P values are based on the final reported meta-analyses of study results.
b Genome-wide significance reported in the primary analysis.
c Genome-wide significance reported in a conditional analysis.
d Genome-wide significance reported in meta-analysis with replication or additional cohorts.
e In strong linkage disequilibrium with PNPLA3:rs738409.
f In strong linkage disequilibrium with TM6SF2:rs5854926.

associated with the severity of the disease.[81,82] Female sex has also been reported to be an independent risk factor for the development of alcoholic hepatitis.[43]

Excess weight is a risk factor for the development of alcohol-related liver disease per se and has also been shown to be an independent risk factor for the development of steatohepatitis on liver biopsy.[43] Thus, people drinking excessively who have been overweight for at least 10 years, defined by a BMI of 25 or greater in women and 27 or greater in men, are 3 times more likely to develop biopsy-proven steatohepatitis than those who are not overweight, even after adjusting for age, sex, and drinking behavior.[43] A report from the TREAT consortium also confirmed that BMI is an independent predictor of severe alcoholic hepatitis.[81]

In contrast, coffee consumption may be protective.[82] Thus, the TREAT consortium found that regular coffee consumption was associated independently with a significantly lower risk for developing severe alcoholic hepatitis (OR, 0.26; 95% CI, 0.15–0.46); only 20% of patients with this syndrome drank coffee regularly compared with 44% of heavy drinkers with no liver disease ($P<.001$).[82]

Genetic Factors

Patients with alcoholic hepatitis often have a background of cirrhosis or else rapidly progress toward cirrhosis irrespective of their subsequent drinking behavior. This finding suggests that both presentations have a similar genetic background, but as severe alcoholic hepatitis only develops in a minority of patients with alcohol-related liver injury there may be additional genetic variants that are exclusively associated with the risk for developing this syndrome.

A small candidate gene study, published in 2011, identified rs738409:G in *PNPLA3* as a risk factor for developing severe alcoholic hepatitis.[84] This finding was confirmed in a much larger study involving the STOPAH cohort.[85] A later reanalysis of the STOPAH data identified a significant interaction between the rs738409 genotype and sex in relation to medium-term mortality, which was independent of the return to drinking.[86] Thus, men who were homozygous for *PNPLA3* rs738409:G had a significantly reduced medium term mortality if they remained abstinent from alcohol whereas their female counterparts had a significantly improved medium-term survival even if they continued to drink.[86]

Carriage of *HSD17B13*:rs72613567:TA decreases the risk for developing alcohol-related cirrhosis and HCC and attenuates the disease risks associated with carriage of *PNPLA3*:rs738409:G. A recent candidate gene study reported that carriage of rs72613567:TA was also associated with a decreased risk for developing severe alcoholic hepatitis and likewise attenuated the risk associated with carriage of *PNPLA3*:rs738409:G.[87] In addition, carriage of rs72613567:TA was associate with less severe liver dysfunction, lower disease severity scores, and a decrease in serum markers of hepatocellular injury.[87]

In 2017, the TREAT consortium reported the result of an preliminary GWAS designed to explore the genetic variability between heavy drinkers with and without alcoholic hepatitis.[88] Their study cohort was of European decent and comprised of 90 cases with alcoholic hepatitis and 93 controls drinking excessively but had no evidence of liver disease. No single genetic marker was associated with the risk for developing alcoholic hepatitis at genome-wide significance; an association signal was observed for *PNPLA3* rs738409 ($P = 0.01$; OR, 1.9; 95% CI, 1.1–3.1). A variety of bioinformatics techniques were used to identify gene sets and pathways that might be of importance in the development of this syndrome; several of the identified pathways were involved in lymphocyte activation, chemokine signaling, and ethanol degradation. This study had significant limitations in terms of statistical power; thus these preliminary findings need further exploration in much larger population cohorts.[88]

The results of a more recent GWAS support the concept that the development of severe alcoholic hepatitis may be associated with additional genetic risk factors.[89] The study population was of white British/Irish descent and comprised of 812 cases with severe alcoholic hepatitis from the STOPAH trial and 936 controls with a history of alcohol dependence but without evidence of significant liver injury. The results confirmed the previously described pivotal role of *PNPLA3*:rs738409 in determining the risk for developing severe alcoholic hepatitis.[85] In addition, potential risk loci were identified in *ATP2C2* (*ATPase secretory pathway Ca2+ transporter*), which encodes a Mn^+/Ca^{2+} transporter and is highly expressed in the gastrointestinal tract; *PHYH* (*phytanoyl-CoA 2-hydroxylase*), which is implicated in phytanic acid metabolism; phytanic acid binds to and/or activates the transcription factors peroxisome proliferator-activated receptors-α and retinoid X receptor; and *ANGPT1* (*angiopoietin 1*), which encodes the angiogenic promoter angiopoietin 1. A gene set enrichment analysis delineated significant associations between the susceptibility to develop severe alcoholic hepatitis and pathways involved in lipid metabolism and inflammation, particularly gene groups involved in sterol regulator element binding protein signaling, IL-17 secretion, and the regulation of natural killer T-cell proliferation. These findings will need further validation.

Clinical Implications of Genetic Testing

There is some evidence that knowledge of the genetic risk factors for advanced alcohol-related liver disease might facilitate the management of individuals misusing alcohol. Thus, carriage of *PNPLA3* rs738409 and *TM6SF2* rs58542926 accounts for one-half of the attributable risk for HCC in patients with alcohol-related cirrhosis and it has been suggested that genotyping these 2 single nucleotide polymorphisms would facilitate HCC risk stratification in this population.[90] Similarly a genetic risk

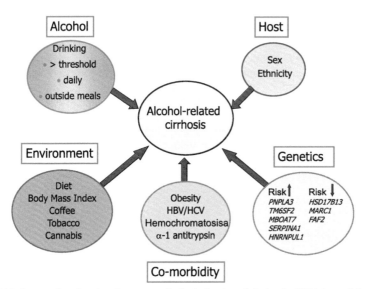

Fig. 4. Risk factors for the development of alcohol-related cirrhosis. HBV, hepatitis B virus; HCV, hepatitis C virus.

score based on allelic variants in *PNPLA3*, *TM6SF2*, and *HSD17B13* has been shown to be useful in identifying individuals in the general population at greater risk for cirrhosis and HCC.[91] Nevertheless, it is unlikely that genetic testing will play a role in the management of people drinking harmfully or those with alcohol-related liver disease at the present time. However, an increased understanding of the genetic basis of alcohol-related liver disease may provide insights into it pathogenesis and help identify potential therapeutic targets.

SUMMARY

The development of advanced alcohol-related liver disease is associated with a complex interplay between constitutional, environmental, and genetic risk factors (**Fig. 4**). The duration and quantity of alcohol consumption are clear determinants of advanced disease, with female sex increasing the risk of liver disease for any given level of consumption; the role of ethnicity is less clear. Lifestyle factors such as diet, body weight, and tobacco and cannabis use play a role, as does the presence of other risk factors for liver disease such as obesity and chronic infection with hepatitis B and C. Recent large-scale GWAS have now identified several genetic loci consistently associated with the risk for developing alcohol-related cirrhosis. Of particular interest is the fact that genes at these loci seem to be predominantly related to lipid metabolism and many are also risk loci for the development of non–alcohol-related fatty liver disease. However, the precise biological mechanisms resulting in the development of alcohol-related liver disease remain to be elucidated. The association between these factors and alcohol-related cirrhosis is taken as a proxy indicator for their association with the development of alcoholic steatohepatitis in the absence of studies evaluating this histologic phenotype. There is some evidence that demographic, lifestyle, and genetic factors may play a role in the development of the clinical syndrome of alcoholic hepatitis, but further delineation of these risk factors is required.

CLINICS CARE POINTS

- Only a minority of individuals who drink heavily will develop significant alcohol-related liver disease but susceptible individuals can not be identified, with any certainty, at the present time.
- The main management goal in people drinking at hazardous and harmful levels is to significantly reduce their alcohol consumption.
- Additional attention should be paid to the other modifiable risk factors for the development of advanced liver disease; thus, encouraging weight loss, smoking cessation and increasing coffee consumption may also confer benefit.
- The popularity of genetics home testing may prompt enquires from patients about their personal risk for developing alcohol-related liver disease; this may provide an opportunity to advise modification of any identifiable risk factors.

DISCLOSURE

The authors have nothing to disclose.

REFERENCES

1. European Association for the Study of the Liver. EASL clinical practice guidelines: management of alcohol-related liver disease. J Hepatol 2018;69:154–81.

2. Sandahl TD, Jepsen P, Thomsen KL, et al. Incidence and mortality of alcoholic hepatitis in Denmark 1999-2008: a nationwide population based cohort study. J Hepatol 2011;54:760–4.

3. Thursz MR, Richardson P, Allison M, et al. Prednisolone or pentoxifylline for alcoholic hepatitis. N Engl J Med 2015;372:1619–28.

4. Parker R, Aithal G, Becker U, et al. Natural history of histologically proven alcohol-related liver disease: a systematic review. J Hepatol 2019;71:586–93.

5. Lelbach WK. [Liver damage in chronic alcoholism. Results of a clinical, clinical-chemical and bioptic-histological study in 526 alcoholic patients during a low-calorie diet in an open drinking sanatorium]. Acta Hepatosplenol 1966;13:321–49.

6. Leevy CM. Cirrhosis in alcoholics. Med Clin North Am 1968;52:1445–51.

7. Lelbach WK. Leberschaden bei chronischem Alcoholismuss I-III. Acta Hepatosplenologica 1966;13:321–49.

8. Cirrhosis: Major Problems in Internal Medicine. In: Galambos JT, editor. Volume XV11. Philadelphia: WB Saunders; 1979.

9. Askgaard G, Kjær MS, Tolstrup JS. Opportunities to prevent alcoholic liver cirrhosis in high-risk populations: a systematic review with meta-analysis. Am J Gastroenterol 2019;114:221–32.

10. Leevy CM. Fatty liver: a study of 270 patients with biopsy proven fatty liver and a review of literature. Medicine 1962;41:249–76.

11. Galambos JT. Natural history of alcoholic hepatitis. 3. Histological changes. Gastroenterology 1972;63:1026–35.

12. Parés A, Caballería J, Bruguera M, et al. Histological course of alcoholic hepatitis. Influence of abstinence, sex and extent of hepatic damage. J Hepatol 1986;2:33–42.

13. Sørensen TI, Orholm M, Bentsen KD, et al. Prospective evaluation of alcohol abuse and alcoholic liver injury in men as predictors of development of cirrhosis. Lancet 1984;2:241–4.

14. Marbet UA, Bianchi L, Meury U, et al. Long-term histological evaluation of the natural history and prognostic factors of alcoholic liver disease. J Hepatol 1987;4:364–72.

15. Saunders JB, Walters JR, Davies AP, et al. A 20-year prospective study of cirrhosis. Br Med J 1981;282:263–6.

16. Lelbach WK. [Dose-effect relation in alcoholic liver lesions]. Dtsch Med Wochenschr 1972;97:1435–6.

17. Sørensen TI. Alcohol and liver injury: dose-related or permissive effect? Liver 1989;9:189–97.

18. Péquignot G. [The role of alcohol in the aetiology of liver cirrhoses in France; results and significance of a systematic survey]. Munch Med Wochenschr 1961;103:1464–8.

19. Péquignot G, Tuyns AJ, Berta JL. Ascitic cirrhosis in relation to alcohol consumption. Int J Epidemiol 1978;7:113–20.

20. Tuyns AJ, Péquignot G. Greater risk of ascitic cirrhosis in females in relation to alcohol consumption. Int J Epidemiol 1984;13:53–7.

21. Lelbach WK. Cirrhosis in the alcoholic and its relation to the volume of alcohol abuse. Ann N Y Acad Sci 1975;252:85–105.

22. Lelbach WK. Epidemiology of alcoholic liver disease. Prog Liver Dis 1976;5:494–515.

23. Bellentani S, Saccoccio G, Costa G, et al. Drinking habits as cofactors of risk for alcohol induced liver damage. Gut 1997;41:845–50.

24. Corrao G, Bagnardi V, Zambon A, et al. A metaanalysis of alcohol consumption and the risk of 15 diseases. Prev Med 2004;38:613–9.

25. Kamper-Jørgensen M, Grønbæk M, Tolstrup J, et al. Alcohol and cirrhosis: dose-response or threshold effect? J Hepatol 2004;41:25–30.

26. Askgaard G, Grønbæk M, Kjær MS, et al. Alcohol drinking pattern and risk of alcoholic liver cirrhosis: a prospective cohort study. J Hepatol 2015;62:1061–7.

27. Roerecke M, Vafaei A, Hasan OSM, et al. Alcohol consumption and risk of liver cirrhosis: a systematic review and meta-analysis. Am J Gastroenterol 2019;114:1574–86.

28. Rehm J, Roerecke M. Patterns of drinking and liver cirrhosis - what do we know and where do we go? J Hepatol 2015;62:1000–1.

29. Aberg F, Helenius-Hietala J, Puukka P, et al. Binge drinking and the risk of liver events: a population-based cohort study. Liver Int 2017;37:1373–81.

30. Becker U, Gronbaek M, Johansen D, et al. Lower risk of alcohol induced cirrhosis in wine drinkers. Hepatology 2002;35:868–75.

31. Tuyns AJ, Estève J, Péquignot G. Ethanol is cirrhogenic, whatever the beverage. Br J Addict 1984;79:389–93.

32. Rotily M, Durbec JP, Berthezene P, et al. Diet and alcohol in liver cirrhosis: a case-control study. Eur J Clin Nutr 1990;44:595–603.

33. Johansen D, Friis K, Skovenborg E, et al. Food buying habits of people who buy wine or beer: cross sectional study. Br Med J 2006;332:519–22.

34. Becker U, Deis A, Sørensen TI, et al. Prediction of risk of liver disease by alcohol intake, sex, and age: a prospective population study. Hepatology 1996;23:1025–9.

35. Coates RA, Halliday ML, Rankin JG, et al. Risk of fatty infiltration or cirrhosis of the liver in relation to ethanol consumption: a case-control study. Clin Invest Med 1986;9:26–32.

36. Rehm J, Taylor B, Mohapatra S, et al. Alcohol as a risk factor for liver cirrhosis: a systematic review and meta-analysis. Drug Alcohol Rev 2010;29:437–45.

37. Marshall AW, Kingstone D, Boss M, et al. Ethanol elimination in males and females: relationship to menstrual cycle and body composition. Hepatology 1983;3:701–6.

38. Douds AC, Cox MA, Iqbal TH, et al. Ethnic differences in cirrhosis of the liver in a British city: alcoholic cirrhosis in South Asian men. Alcohol Alcohol 2003;38:148–50.

39. Stinson FS, Grant BF, Dufour MC. The critical dimension of ethnicity in liver cirrhosis mortality statistics. Alcohol Clin Exp Res 2001;25:1181–7.

40. Levy RE, Catana AM, Durbin-Johnson B, et al. Ethnic differences in presentation and severity of alcoholic liver disease. Alcohol Clin Exp Res 2015;39:566–74.

41. Li D, Zhao H, Gelernter J. Strong association of the alcohol dehydrogenase 1B gene (ADH1B) with alcohol dependence and alcohol-induced medical diseases. Biol Psychiatry 2011;70:504–12.

42. Liu B, Balkwill A, Reeves G, et al. Body mass index and risk of liver cirrhosis in middle aged UK women: prospective study. Br Med J 2010;340:c912.

43. Naveau S, Giraud V, Borotto E, et al. Excess weight risk factor for alcoholic liver disease. Hepatology 1997;25:108–11.

44. Naveau S, Dobrin AS, Balian A, et al. Body fat distribution and risk factors for fibrosis in patients with alcoholic liver disease. Alcohol Clin Exp Res 2013;37:332–8.

45. Dam MK, Flensborg-Madsen T, Eliasen M, et al. Smoking and risk of liver cirrhosis: a population-based cohort study. Scand J Gastroenterol 2013;48: 585–91.

46. Klatsky AL, Armstrong MA. Alcohol, smoking, coffee, and cirrhosis. Am J Epidemiol 1992;136:1248–57.

47. Whitfield JB, Masson S, Liangpunsakul S, et al. Obesity, diabetes, coffee, tea, and cannabis use alter risk for alcohol-related cirrhosis in 2 large cohorts of high-risk drinkers. Am J Gastroenterol 2021;116:106–15.

48. Adejumo AC, Ajayi TO, Adegbala OM, et al. Cannabis use is associated with reduced prevalence of progressive stages of alcoholic liver disease. Liver Int 2018;38:1475–86.

49. Kennedy OJ, Roderick P, Buchanan R, et al. Systematic review with meta-analysis: coffee consumption and the risk of cirrhosis. Aliment Pharmacol Ther 2016;43:562–74.

50. Aberg F, Helenius-Hietala J, Puukka P, et al. Interaction between alcohol consumption and metabolic syndrome in predicting severe liver disease in the general population. Hepatology 2018;67:2141–9.

51. Noda K, Yoshihara H, Suzuki K, et al. Progression of type C chronic hepatitis to liver cirrhosis and hepatocellular carcinoma–its relationship to alcohol drinking and the age of transfusion. Alcohol Clin Exp Res 1996;20:95a–100a.

52. Serfaty L, Poujol-Robert A, Carbonell N, et al. Effect of the interaction between steatosis and alcohol intake on liver fibrosis progression in chronic hepatitis C. Am J Gastroenterol 2002;97:1807–12.

53. Canan CE, Lau B, McCaul ME, et al. Effect of alcohol consumption on all-cause and liver-related mortality among HIV-infected individuals. HIV Med 2017;18: 332–41.

54. Monto A, Patel K, Bostrom A, et al. Risks of a range of alcohol intake on hepatitis C-related fibrosis. Hepatology 2004;39:826–34.

55. Fletcher LM, Dixon JL, Purdie DM, et al. Excess alcohol greatly increases the prevalence of cirrhosis in hereditary hemochromatosis. Gastroenterology 2002; 122:281–9.

56. Whitfield JB, Rahman K, Haber PS, et al. Brief report: genetics of alcoholic cirrhosis-GenomALC multinational study. Alcohol Clin Exp Res 2015;39:836–42.

57. Hrubec Z, Omenn GS. Evidence of genetic predisposition to alcoholic cirrhosis and psychosis - twin concordances for alcoholism and its biological end-points by zygosity among male veterans. Alcohol Clin Exp Res 1981;5:207–15.

58. Reed T, Page WF, Viken RJ, et al. Genetic predisposition to organs specific end-points of alcoholism. Alcohol Clin Exp Res 1996;20:1528–33.

59. Anstee QM, Daly AK, Day CP. Genetics of alcoholic liver disease. Semin Liver Dis 2015;35:361–74.

60. Stickel F, Moreno C, Hampe J, et al. The genetics of alcohol dependence and alcohol-related liver disease. J Hepatol 2017;66:195–211.

61. Meroni M, Longo M, Rametta R, et al. Genetic and epigenetic modifiers of alcoholic liver disease. Int J Mol Sci 2018;19:3857–78.

62. Marcos M, Gomez-Munuera M, Pastor I, et al. Tumor necrosis factor polymorphisms and alcoholic liver disease: a HuGE review and meta-analysis. Am J Epidemiol 2009;170:948–56.

63. Marcos M, Pastor I, Chamorro AJ, et al. Meta-analysis: glutathione-S-transferase allelic variants are associated with alcoholic liver disease. Aliment Pharmacol Ther 2011;34:1159–72.

64. Buch S, Stickel F, Trépo E, et al. A genome-wide association study confirms *PNPLA3* and identifies *TM6SF2* and *MBOAT7* as risk loci for alcohol-related cirrhosis. Nat Genet 2015;47:1443–8.

65. Innes H, Buch S, Hutchinson S, et al. Genome-wide association study for alcohol-related cirrhosis identifies risk loci in *MARC1* and *HNRNPUL1*. Gastroenterology 2020;159:1276–89.

66. Schwantes-An TH, Darlay R, Mathurin P, et al. Genome-wide association study and meta-analysis on alcohol-related liver cirrhosis identifies novel genetic risk factors. Hepatology 2021;73:1920–31.

67. Romeo S, Kozlitina J, Xing C, et al. Genetic variation in *PNPLA3* confers susceptibility to nonalcoholic fatty liver disease. Nat Genet 2008;40:1461–5.

68. Chamorro AJ, Torres JL, Miron-Canelo JA, et al. Systematic review with meta-analysis: the I148M variant of patatin-like phospholipase domain-containing 3 gene (*PNPLA3*) is significantly associated with alcoholic liver cirrhosis. Aliment Pharmacol Ther 2014;40:571–81.

69. Singal AG, Manjunath H, Yopp AC, et al. The effect of *PNPLA3* on fibrosis progression and development of hepatocellular carcinoma: a meta-analysis. Am J Gastroenterol 2014;109:325–34.

70. Trépo E, Nahon P, Bontempi G, et al. Association between the *PNPLA3* (rs738409 C>G) variant and hepatocellular carcinoma: evidence from a meta-analysis of individual participant data. Hepatology 2014;59:2170–7.

71. Salameh H, Raff E, Erwin A, et al. *PNPLA3* gene polymorphism Is associated with predisposition to and severity of alcoholic liver disease. Am J Gastroenterol 2015; 110:846–56.

72. Li JF, Zheng EQ, Xie M. Association between rs738409 polymorphism in *patatin-like phospholipase domain-containing protein 3* (*PNPLA3*) gene and hepatocellular carcinoma susceptibility: evidence from case-control studies. Gene 2019;685:143–8.

73. Stickel F, Buch S, Lau K, et al. Genetic variation in the *PNPLA3* gene is associated with alcoholic liver injury in Caucasians. Hepatology 2011;53:86–95.

74. Burza MA, Molinaro A, Attilia ML, et al. *PNPLA3* I148M (rs738409) genetic variant and age at onset of at-risk alcohol consumption are independent risk factors for alcoholic cirrhosis. Liver Int 2014;34:514–20.

75. Friedrich K, Wannhoff A, Kattner S, et al. *PNPLA3* in end-stage liver disease: alcohol consumption, hepatocellular carcinoma development, and transplantation-free survival. J Gastroenterol Hepatol 2014;29:1477–84.

76. Valenti L, Motta BM, Soardo G, et al. *PNPLA3* I148M polymorphism, clinical presentation, and survival in patients with hepatocellular carcinoma. PLoS One 2013; 8:e75982.

77. Abul-Husn NS, Cheng X, Li AH, et al. A protein-truncating *HSD17B13* variant and protection from chronic liver disease. N Engl J Med 2018;378:1096–106.

78. Stickel F, Lutz P, Buch S, et al. Genetic variation in *HSD17B13* reduces the risk of developing cirrhosis and hepatocellular carcinoma in alcohol misusers. Hepatology 2020;72:88–102.

79. Strnad P, Buch S, Hamesch K, et al. Heterozygous carriage of the alpha1-antitrypsin Pi*Z variant increases the risk to develop liver cirrhosis. Gut 2019; 68:1099–107.

80. Crabb DW, Bataller R, Chalasani NP, et al. Standard definitions and common data elements for clinical trials in patients with alcoholic hepatitis: recommendation from the NIAAA Alcoholic Hepatitis Consortia. Gastroenterology 2016;150: 785–90.

81. Liangpunsakul S, Puri P, Shah VH, et al. Effects of age, sex, body weight, and quantity of alcohol consumption on occurrence and severity of alcoholic hepatitis. Clin Gastroenterol Hepatol 2016;14:1831–8.
82. Lourens S, Sunjaya DB, Singal A, et al. Acute alcoholic hepatitis: natural history and predictors of mortality using a multicenter prospective study. Mayo Clin Proc Innov Qual Outcomes 2017;1:37–48.
83. Bertola A, Park O, Gao B. Chronic plus binge ethanol feeding synergistically induces neutrophil infiltration and liver injury in mice: a critical role for E-selectin. Hepatology 2013;58:1814–23.
84. Nguyen-Khac E, Houchi H, Dreher M-L, et al. Is *PNPLA3* polymorphism involved in severe acute alcoholic hepatitis. Hepatology 2011;54(S1):976A.
85. Atkinson SR, Way MJ, McQuillin A, et al. Homozygosity for rs738409:G in *PNPLA3* is associated with increased mortality following an episode of severe alcoholic hepatitis. J Hepatol 2017;67:120–7.
86. Atkinson SR, Way MJ, McQuillin A, et al. Reply to: "The *PNPLA3* SNP rs738409:G allele is associated with increased liver disease-associated mortality but reduced overall mortality in a population-based cohort. ' J Hepatol 2018;68:840–66.
87. Atkinson SR, Buckley T, Strnad P, et al. Genetic variation in *HSD17B13* reduces the risk for developing severe alcoholic hepatitis. J Hepatol 2020;73(Suppl1): S61–2.
88. Beaudoin JJ, Long N, Liangpunsakul S, et al. An exploratory genome-wide analysis of genetic risk for alcoholic hepatitis. Scand J Gastroenterol 2017;52:1263–9.
89. Sharma M, Atkinson S, McQuillin A, et al. A genome-wide association study of severe alcoholic hepatitis. Gut 2020;69(Suppl 1):A4–5. O8.
90. Stickel F, Buch S, Nischalke HD, et al. Genetic variants in *PNPLA3* and *TM6SF2* predispose to the development of hepatocellular carcinoma in individuals with alcohol-related cirrhosis. Am J Gastroenterol 2018;113:1475–83.
91. Gellert-Kristensen H, Richardson TG, Davey Smith G, et al. Combined effect of *PNPLA3*, *TM6SF2*, and *HSD17B13* variants on risk of cirrhosis and hepatocellular carcinoma in the general population. Hepatology 2020;72:845–56.

Moderate Alcoholic Hepatitis

Ana Clemente-Sánchez, MD[a,b], Aline Oliveira-Mello, PhD[a], Ramón Bataller, MD, PhD[c],*

KEYWORDS

• Alcoholic hepatitis • Moderate • Nonsevere • MELD • Survival • Abstinence

KEY POINTS

• Moderate alcoholic hepatitis (AH) is a frequent disease with a probable underestimated incidence compared with its severe form.
• A homogeneous definition of severity according to the different available prognostic scores is lacking. MELD score seems to be most accurate score.
• Patients with moderate AH have a mortality in the short to medium term up to 3% to 7% and as high as 13% to 20% at 1 year.
• Long-term abstinence is the main goal of the treatment because it is an independent predictor of long-term survival in these patients.
• Pathophysiologically oriented therapies aimed at improving the outcomes in this population are needed.

INTRODUCTION

Alcohol-related liver disease (ALD) represents one of the leading causes of chronic liver disease in Europe and the United States. According to the Global Status Report on Alcohol and Health 2018 from the World Health Organization, ALD accounts for 50% of cirrhosis cases and 50% of liver-related deaths worldwide.[1–3] ALD encompasses a range of disorders, including simple liver steatosis, alcoholic steatohepatitis (ASH), fibrosis, cirrhosis, and hepatocellular carcinoma (HCC)[4] (**Fig. 1**). In addition, patients with underlying ALD and active heavy drinking can develop an episode of acute-on-chronic liver injury characterized by the rapid onset of jaundice, infiltration of polymorphonuclear leukocytes, hepatocellular damage, and liver-related complications called "alcoholic hepatitis" (AH), which portends a poor

[a] Division of Gastroenterology, Hepatology and Nutrition, Department of Medicine, University of Pittsburgh Medical Center (UPMC), BST West 11th Floor, Suite 1116-17, 200 Lothrop Street, Pittsburgh, PA 15213, USA; [b] CIBERehd, Instituto de Salud Carlos III, Avenida Monforte de Lemos, 3-5, Pavilion 11th, Floor 0, Madrid 28029, Spain; [c] Division of Gastroenterology, Hepatology and Nutrition, University of Pittsburgh, Kaufmann Medical Building, 3471 Fifth Avenue, Suite 201.19, Pittsburgh, PA 15213, USA
* Corresponding author.
E-mail address: bataller@pitt.edu

Clin Liver Dis 25 (2021) 537–555
https://doi.org/10.1016/j.cld.2021.03.001
1089-3261/21/© 2021 Elsevier Inc. All rights reserved.
liver.theclinics.com

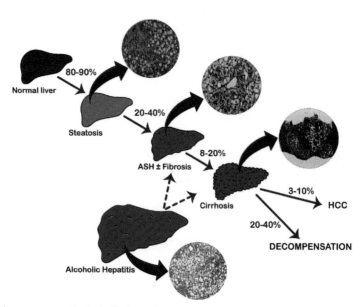

Fig. 1. The spectrum of alcoholic liver disease.

prognosis. The severe form of this disease is associated with a high short-term mortality up to 30% at 28 days and a long-term mortality exceeding 50% at 1 year.[5] The initial attempts to assess the severity of this disease were performed by Maddrey and colleagues[6] in 1978. Patients with higher prothrombin time and serum bilirubin at admission showed increased mortality. Therefore, a scoring system including these 2 parameters named discriminant function (DF) was developed. The initial threshold to consider the disease as severe was set at 93 and subsequently adjusted to 32 to overcome disparities secondary to interlaboratory variations.[7] Thus, patients with a DF score less than 32 have been traditionally considered as having a "nonsevere" or a "moderate" AH. Nevertheless, other clinical, histologic, and hemodynamic scores aimed at better characterizing the prognosis of patients with AH have been developed in recent years.[8–12] Among the clinical scores, the Model for End-Stage Liver Disease (MELD) has emerged as one of the most accurate at establishing the prognosis of the disease with a threshold set at ≥21 for those with severe AH.[8] Therefore, a MELD score less than 21 is increasingly accepted as the best scoring system to define a moderate AH.

The natural history of moderate AH is not well known but involves significant morbidity and mortality. Most observational studies and clinical trials have focused on severe AH, whereas only few original studies have recently delineated the natural history of the moderate form. In particular, a recent systematic review and meta-analysis along with a couple of observational studies have specifically focused on patients with moderate AH. These studies show a nonnegligible mortality up to 6% and 13% at 28 days and 1 year, respectively, challenging the "nonsevere" nomenclature.[13–15] Finally, there is a gap in knowledge regarding the specific therapeutic strategies for patients with less severe forms of the disease because they have been traditionally excluded from clinical trials. This review is aimed at summarizing the available evidence concerning the natural history, diagnosis, and management options in patients with moderate AH.

NATURAL HISTORY
Epidemiology

Patients with underlying ALD (with or without cirrhosis) and sustained alcohol abuse are at risk of developing AH. The incidence of AH in patients with underlying liver injury at less advanced stages of the disease is not well known. In patients with established cirrhosis, it may occur in up to 40% of cases.[5] The incidence of moderate AH is probably underestimated given that some of these patients may present with mild symptoms, such as jaundice. Nonetheless, data from the STOPAH trial[16] suggest that it might be even more common than the severe form. Specifically, a total of 2006 patients out of the 3109 that were evaluated for the trial were considered screen failures because they did not fulfill the inclusion criteria (DF < 32 or bilirubin <4.68 mg/dL), which represents nearly 65% of the entire population screened.[14] Similarly, a recent study that included patients with AH from the TREAT Consortium showed that the incidence of moderate AH in this cohort, defined as MELD score ≤20 at presentation, was 39% (100 patients with moderate AH out of 255 patients recruited with diagnosis of AH).[13] Thus, it is very likely that this is an underestimated entity in terms of incidence.

The demographic characteristics of patients with moderate AH are not well described. Only inconclusive information regarding age and gender can be extracted from previous observational studies and clinical trials. In only 6 out of 25 studies included in a recent review, gender and age ranges were reported.[14] However, a recent study aimed at describing the clinical characteristics and outcomes of patients with mild to moderate AH showed that they are more likely to be men (68% vs 55%) and older (49 vs 44 years) as compared with patients with severe AH. In addition, these patients seem to have a lower body mass index compared with those with severe AH (27 vs 31 kg/m^2), which is in accordance with previous information showing that obesity is independently associated with mortality at 3 months in patients with AH. No differences were found regarding the amount and duration of alcohol consumption between the groups, suggesting that other involved factors, such as demographic, genetic, and environmental, may play an important role in disease severity. Actually, because of the differences seen in coffee consumption and PNPLA3 genotype between patients with moderate and severe AH in this study, the investigators hypothesized that there might be an interaction between this environmental and genetic factor that impacts severity.[13,17] Similar results regarding gender and age have been reported in a series of 121 patients with acutely decompensated ALD, with histologic steatohepatitis and DF less than 32. Interestingly, up to 84% of the patients in this series had underlying histologically proven cirrhosis, a higher prevalence than that described for the whole spectrum of AH.[5,15]

Prognostic Scores to Define Moderate Alcoholic Hepatitis

Stratification of patients according to the severity of the disease is crucial to identifying those with the highest risk of death in the short term that could benefit from therapies beyond the general management and supportive care, such as corticosteroids, investigational drugs from clinical trials, or liver transplantation.

To date, 4 different scores are available to predict short-term mortality in patients with AH with reasonable accuracy, that is, Maddrey's DF,[6] MELD score,[8] age, serum bilirubin, international normalized ratio (INR), and serum creatinine (ABIC) score,[11] and Glasgow alcoholic hepatitis score (GAHS).[9] Each score was generated from different variables independently associated with survival in each cohort. Lille score[18] is a dynamic score developed to evaluate the response to corticosteroid therapy and is associated with a particular risk of 1-month mortality according to that response.

Thus, it is only applicable in patients with severe AH who are candidates to receive prednisolone.

As previously addressed, patients with a DF score less than 32 are considered as having a "nonsevere" or a "moderate" AH. Patients with a DF less than 32 have a 30-day survival greater than 90% with supportive care.[19] MELD score, which was initially developed to predict survival following transjugular intrahepatic portosystemic shunt for refractory variceal bleeding or refractory ascites,[20] has shown to be useful for predicting 90-day mortality in patients with AH. It has both a sensitivity and a specificity of 75% using a threshold of 21 points. The overall accuracy of GAHS in its original description was 81% and 75% to predict 28-day and 84-day outcome. A cutoff of 9 was selected to optimize the specificity to predict mortality at 28 days (89%) and 84 days (90%). That threshold showed a mortality in patients with AH and GAHS less than 9 of 13% and 21% at 28 days and 84 days, respectively. Finally, the ABIC score can identify patients with low (<6.71), intermediate (6.71–8.99), and high risk (≥9.0) of death. Patients with an ABIC score less than 6.71 had an excellent short- and long-term prognosis in the original cohort with survival rates of 100% and 97.1% at 90 days and 1 year, respectively.

The accuracy of these scores to predict short-term mortality has been previously explored and validated in external cohorts without significant differences among them,[21–23] except for a poor performance of DF in severe AH patients recruited to the STOPAH trial compared with MELD, ABIC, and GAHS scores.[24] Nevertheless, in a large worldwide cohort (Morales Arraez D, Ventura Cots M, Altamirano J, et al, abstract presented in AASLD 2020, unpublished data, 2021), the authors showed that MELD score has the best performance in predicting short-term mortality compared with other scores. A total of 2581 patients from 85 centers were included in this study aimed at assessing the accuracy of the different scores to predict short-term mortality in AH at a worldwide scale. In this cohort, the performance of GAHS and ABIC was inferior to MELD score but significantly better than Maddrey's DF, which had the worst accuracy to predict death, with significant differences between all scores and DF. The sample size along with the inclusion of AH patients of different severity and from different geographic regions confers robustness to the authors' results compared with previous validation series. These results suggest that MELD score should be the elective prognostic score to stratify the severity of the disease. **Table 1** shows a summary of the main characteristics of the static prognostic scores and observed mortality according to their severity cutoffs.

Besides the clinical scores based mainly on laboratory parameters associated with mortality in patients with AH, the histologic features of the disease have been shown to be a complementary prognostic tool in patients who undergo liver biopsy to confirm the diagnosis. The Alcoholic Hepatitis Histologic Score (AHHS) was developed in a series of 121 patients with histologically proven AH and further validated in an independent cohort of 109 patients. AHHS adequately stratifies patients with a low (0–3 points), moderate (4–5 points), and high (6–9 points) risk of death at 90 days (100%, 83%, and 64% survival, respectively).[12]

Mortality Associated with Moderate Alcoholic Hepatitis

The mortality associated with moderate AH has been described in a recent systematic review and meta-analysis, and 2 observational studies specifically focused on this phenotype. Bennet and colleagues[14] compiled the data from 25 studies (n = 1372 patients), including prospective and retrospective observational studies and clinical trials available in literature that reported mortality of patients with nonsevere AH at either 28 days, 90 days, or 1 year. The definition used for nonsevere AH was based on

Table 1
Static prognostic scores in alcoholic hepatitis

Score	Variables	Significance	Severity Cut-Off	Mortality Observed
Maddrey's DF	Bilirubin, PT	Evaluates risk of mortality at 30 d	<32: nonsevere	≥32: severe	At 30 d: • DF < 32: <10% • DF ≥ 32: >20%–30%
MELD	Bilirubin, INR, creatinine	Evaluates risk of mortality at 90 d	<21: nonsevere	≥21: severe	At 90 d: • MELD <21: <20% • MELD ≥21: ≥20% The probability of 90-d mortality according to MELD score can be calculated with the next formula: $P = e^{(-4.3+0.16\times MELD)}/[1 + e^{(-4.3+0.16\times MELD)}]$
GAHS	Bilirubin, INR, urea, WBC, age	Evaluates risk of mortality at 28 d and 84 d	<9: nonsevere	≥9: severe	At 28 d: • GAHS <9: 13% • GAHS ≥9: 54% At 84 d: • GAHS <9: 21% • GAHS ≥9: 60%
ABIC	Bilirubin, INR, creatinine, age	Evaluates risk of mortality at 90 d and 1 y	<6.71: low risk	6.71–8.99: intermediate risk	≥9: high risk	At 90 d: • ABIC <6.71: 0% • ABIC 6.71–8.99: 30% • ABIC ≥9: 75% At 1 y: • ABIC <6.71: 2.9% • ABIC 6.71–8.99: 35.7% • ABIC ≥9: 66.7%

Abbreviations: PT, prothrombin time; WBC, white blood cell count.

previously accepted cutoffs of the available prognostic scores as follows: DF less than 32, MELD score less than 21,[8] ABIC less than 6.71,[11] or bilirubin less than 4.97 mg/dL with histologic confirmation. Even if there was substantial heterogeneity in their primary analysis because of differences in study design, inclusion criteria, or severity definitions, the results showed a nonnegligible mortality of 6% at 28 days (n = 993 patients), 7% at 90 days (n = 775 patients), and 13% at 1 year (n = 224 patients). A similar mortality of 2%, 3%, and 10.3% at 30 days, 90 days, and 1 year, respectively, has been recently reported in patients with moderate AH defined as MELD score ≤20 at presentation.[13] There are few pieces of data available regarding the prognosis of moderate AH patients at long term beyond 12 months. In a recently published series of patients with ASH and acutely decompensated ALD with a DF less than 32, the mortality at 2 and 5 years was up to 30% and 49%, respectively. Similar long-term survival data have been previously reported in patients that survived a first episode of AH with a median MELD score of 16 at presentation in whom the overall mortality was 38% with a median follow-up of 55 months.[25] As consistently reported in all these studies, the cause of death in patients with moderate AH was secondary to liver-related complications, including severe infections in up to 80% of cases.[13–15,25] These mortalities strongly suggest that the so-called nonsevere AH should no longer be considered a benign form of the disease because it entails a short-term mortality comparable to other acute life-threatening diseases (ie, acute myocardial infarction) and a 1-year mortality similar to that of cirrhotic patients with moderately impaired liver function.[26] **Table 2** summarizes the reported short- and long-term mortalities in patients with moderate AH available in literature.

Interestingly, a sensitivity analysis comparing the estimated mortality between studies published in or before 2010 and those published after 2010 showed no differences.[14] This analysis is in agreement with previous meta-analysis of mortality in all spectrums of AH that did not show a change in mortality at 28 and 90 days over time with a small but statistically significant increase in 180-day mortality.[27] These data points support that despite the improvement in the management of the disease over the last decades, there is still a dire need for the development of new therapies for AH patients, including for those with less severe forms.

The main factors likely to impact the long-term prognosis of patients with moderate AH that present with jaundice at admission are alcohol abstinence (hazard ratio [HR], 0.39) and overt hepatic encephalopathy at the moment of presentation (HR, 3.84). Patients with encephalopathy at presentation have a significantly reduced survival at 5 years compared with those without (21.4% ± 9.3% and 62.8% ± 7.5%, respectively). Similarly, those patients that do not remain completely abstinent during follow-up after an episode of moderate AH have a notably reduced survival compared with those with total cessation of alcohol use without any relapse episode (39.2% ± 7.4% and 71.7% ± 10.9%, respectively).[15]

DIAGNOSIS

Regardless of the severity, AH should be suspected in individuals with history of sustained (>6 months) heavy alcohol use considered as 3 drinks (~40 g) per day for women and 4 drinks (~50–60 g) per day for men and acute onset of jaundice that can be accompanied by other signs and symptoms, such as malaise, tender hepatomegaly, and liver-related complications (ascites, encephalopathy, bacterial infection, and variceal bleeding), especially in patients with underlying cirrhosis. History of heavy and sustained alcohol use is mandatory to suspect an AH episode; nevertheless, it is important to bear in mind that some patients may be intermittently abstinent (up to

Table 2
Reported short- and long-term mortality in published studies focused on moderate alcoholic hepatitis

Study	Definition of Moderate AH	28- or 30-d Mortality, %	90-d Mortality, %	1-y Mortality, %	2-y Mortality, %	5-y Mortality, %
Samala et al[13]	MELD score ≤20 at presentation	2	3	10.3	—	—
Bennett at al[14]	DF < 32, MELD < 21, ABIC < 6.7 or bilirubin < 4.97 mg/dL with histologic confirmation	6	7	13	—	—
Degre et al[15]	Acutely decompensated ALD with histologically proven ASH and Maddrey's DF < 32	3.3	5.8	20	30	49

8 weeks before the jaundice onset), and alcohol consumption underreporting is frequent.[19]

Serum bilirubin is usually elevated (>3 mg/dL), as well as the aspartate aminotransferase (AST) (>50 IU/mL) and AST to alanine aminotransferase (ALT) ratio of greater than 1.5 (usually >2). It is important to take into consideration that the AST and ALT do not typically exceed 400 IU/mL, and when that is the case, an alternative cause with similar clinical presentation, such as drug-induced liver injury (DILI) and ischemic hepatitis, should be considered. Screening of other potential causes of jaundice should be part of the general differential diagnosis workup (biliary obstruction, HCC, viral hepatitis, severe autoimmune liver disease, Wilson disease). A histologic confirmation is recommended in those cases in which other confounding factors or concomitant diseases cannot be excluded by clinical criteria, laboratory findings, and imaging procedures.[19] Typical histologic findings include macrovesicular steatosis, neutrophil infiltration, hepatocyte ballooning, and Mallory-Denk bodies. Fibrosis is always present with pericellular or perisinusoidal distribution showing a classic chicken-wire fence pattern as it extends outward, sometimes all the way to the portal tract.[28] Most patients have underlying cirrhosis.[12,15] Other common findings include the presence of megamitochondria and bilirubinostasis, which along with fibrosis and polymorphonuclear neutrophils infiltration are associated with prognosis.[12]

In 2016, a panel of experts from the National Institute on Alcohol Abuse and Alcoholism (NIAAA) Alcoholic Hepatitis Consortia proposed a set of standard definitions to address diagnostic criteria of AH and practical issues to homogenize the research in the AH scenario. In summary, a "definite" AH is that with compatible clinical diagnosis and histologic confirmation. In the absence of histologic assessment, the diagnosis of AH should be considered as "probable" if no other confounding factors are present (ie, autoimmune markers, metabolic liver diseases, sepsis, shock, cocaine use, DILI). In the presence of potential confounding factors, even if the clinical picture is compatible with AH, the diagnosis should be considered as "possible" and histologic confirmation is strongly advised.[19]

Finally, there is an interesting question that arises from recent literature in patients with moderate AH in which 2 different phenotypes of patients that fulfilled the selected criteria to consider the disease as nonsevere or moderate were described. Patients with jaundice and a clinical diagnosis of AH and patients with histologic ASH that may not have had jaundice admitted to the hospital and with similar mortality rates.[14,15] Even if they have similar outcomes in terms of survival, it is difficult to determine in those patients with compatible histology but without jaundice, if mortality is actually driven by an AH episode or, what seems more likely, by the underlying liver disease. These two clinically and histologically overlapped entities represent a diagnostic challenge in clinical practice.

Fig. 2 depicts an algorithm with the general diagnostic approach of AH.

MANAGEMENT OPTIONS

The management of moderate AH has not evolved in the last few decades because most studies assessing specific therapies are performed in patients with severe forms. Corticosteroids, because of their nonselective systemic anti-inflammatory effect, have been traditionally used to treat severe AH patients when there are no contraindications. Nevertheless, there is robust evidence showing that the benefit of corticosteroids is modest, improving the mortality only in the short term, with a considerable proportion of adverse events, mainly serious infections.[16,29] Whether corticosteroids could be effective in patients with moderate AH is unknown, and in most centers, these patients do not receive any specific therapy.

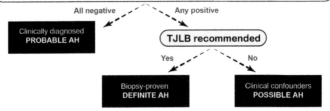

CLINICAL PICTURE

- Patient with sustained heavy **alcohol intake**: 3 drinks (~ 40 g) per day for women and 4 drinks (~ 50–60 g) per day for men > 6 months. In some patients last drink up to 8 weeks before admission. Underreporting is common: suspect if stigmata of alcoholism, compatible laboratory findings, positive alcohol test, other alcohol-induced organ damage (polyneuropathy, chronic pancreatitis).

- **Clinical presentation**: recent onset jaundice, malaise, ascites, edema, itching, fever, shortness of breath due to massive ascites, confusion/lethargy/agitation (Differential diagnosis: Portosystemic encephalopathy, withdrawal syndrome, alcohol-induced cognitive dysfunction, Wernicke-Korsakoff, seizures).

- **Physical exam findings**: signs of alcohol abuse (facial erythema, rhinophyma, Dupuytren, muscle wasting), stigmata cirrhosis, ascites, tender hepatomegaly, splenomegaly, peripheral edema, asterixis, altered mental status, signs of cerebellar dysfunction/peripheral neuropathy.

- **Laboratory findings**: abrupt rise in bilirubin >3 mg/dL (usually >5 mg/dL), Elevation AST (AST/ALT usually >2, both <400 U/L). Other potential findings: GGT>100 U/mL, alkaline phosphatase mildly elevated, Albumin <3.0 g/L, INR>1.5, Platelet count <150,000, Hemoglobin <12 g/L, elevated mean corpuscular volume.

SCREENING CAUSES OF JAUNDICE

- Rule out biliary obstruction, metastases or HCC (CT scan and if indicated, MRI or MRCP).
- Rule out drug-induced liver injury (DILI)
- Rule out acute viral hepatitis (A, B and C) if first episode and/or clinical suspicion.
- Rule out severe autoimmune hepatitis if first episode and/or clinical suspicion (ANA, ASMA, IgG).
- Rule out metabolic liver disease with acute onset such as Wilson disease

WHEN TO PERFORM A TJLB

- Suspicion ischemic hepatitis: hypotension/massive bleeding or recent cocaine.
- Sepsis at admission (clinical diagnosis or positive culture plus SIRS).
- Suspicion of malignant liver disease based on clinical and/or imaging criteria.
- Atypical laboratory findings (eg, AST or ALT >500 U/L, alkaline phosphatase >400 U/L).
- Uncertain alcohol assessment including under-reporting.
- Use of any potential hepatotoxic substance in the last 3 months.
- Possible indication of a salvage liver transplantation.

All negative   Any positive

Clinically diagnosed **PROBABLE AH**   (**TJLB recommended**)

Yes   No

Biopsy-proven **DEFINITE AH**   Clinical confounders **POSSIBLE AH**

Fig. 2. Algorithm of the general diagnostic approach in AH. ANA, antinuclear antibody; ASMA, anti–smooth-muscle antibody; CT, computed tomography; GGT, gamma-glutamyl transferase; MRCP, magnetic resonance cholangiopancreatography; TJLB, transjugular liver biopsy. (Data from Refs.[19,51–53])

There is intense research activity aimed at developing new therapies that specifically target different pathways involved in the pathophysiology of the disease and, as a result, several clinical trials are underway. Unfortunately, patients with moderate AH have usually been excluded from clinical trials because they have more favorable outcomes when alcohol abstinence and conservative general measures are implemented. As previously discussed, recent data have shown that mortality in this subgroup of patients should not be underestimated, and the paradigm of systematically excluding them from clinical trials should be reconsidered. Some ongoing clinical trials are recruiting patients with MELD scores within the current definition of moderate AH.[30]

To date, the cornerstones in the treatment of moderate AH are long-term abstinence, nutritional support, and management of the underlying liver disease. In this review, the authors provide a summary of the evidence related to these therapeutic modalities as well as some information regarding the ongoing clinical trials, including patients with less severe forms of the disease.

Alcohol Abstinence

Alcohol abstinence is the main goal of management because, in the long term, it increases survival in patients with AH. Conversely, a return to alcohol consumption after an episode of AH has a dose-dependent effect on mortality.[25,31,32] Recent studies focused on identifying predictors of long-term survival in patients with AH have shown that alcohol abstinence is independently associated with long-term survival in patients with moderate AH.[15] Besides being the most important risk factor for ALD progression and precluding patient eligibility for an eventual liver transplant,[33–35] patients that continue drinking after an episode of AH are at high risk of developing recurrent episodes. Such episodes have a more severe clinical course and higher morbidity and mortality (60%).[36] Therefore, alcohol abstinence must be closely monitored in all patients after discharge of an AH episode regardless of the severity, because approximately up to two-thirds of patients who survive the episode will relapse in the long term.[25,37–39] Abstinence treatment should be based on an integrated approach involving not only the patients and their relatives but also a multidisciplinary team of health care professionals, including hepatologists, addiction specialists, counselors, dietitians, specialized nurses, and social workers, to provide and to closely monitor psychosocial and pharmacologic interventions as well as to refer to rehabilitation programs.[4,5,40] In fact, there are data that suggest that an early intervention within 30 days after discharge of an episode of AH is associated with a lower risk of hospital readmissions, alcohol relapse, and death.[41] Inpatient detoxification is strongly advised in those patients with heavy active drinking or those who have experienced previous alcohol withdrawal syndrome.[5,42] Regarding pharmacologic interventions, several drugs have been shown to prevent alcohol relapse in patients with alcohol use disorder, but most of them either have not been tested in patients with underlying ALD or have known potential of hepatotoxicity, which may preclude their use in this population. Among them, the ones with a safer profile seem to be acamprosate,[42] because of the absence of hepatic metabolism, and baclofen, which is the only drug that has been studied in a randomized double-blind placebo-controlled trial in patients with decompensated ALD[43] and even in a small series of AH patients.[44] However, data from a large pharmacoepidemiologic study in France have recently raised some concerns about baclofen safety.[45] The pharmaceutical therapies for maintaining alcohol abstinence in patients with ALD have been further reviewed elsewhere.[30,40,42] The use of biomarkers for monitoring alcohol use may be a valuable complementary tool to detect early alcohol relapse episodes because owing to the stigma associated with this disease, many patients underreport their alcohol consumption.[40,46]

Nutritional Support

Malnutrition is a common feature in patients with ALD, and it is especially relevant in patients with AH in whom decreased oral intake and underlying hypermetabolic state can lead to nutritional deficiencies. Therefore, a thorough nutritional assessment in patients with an AH episode is mandatory. Current recommendations are based on ensuring an oral intake of 30 to 35 kcal/kg per day and 1.5 g/kg per day of protein split into 3 to 5 meals, including a late-evening snack, which may contribute to ameliorate catabolism adverse effects and muscle mass loss.[30,40,47] Evaluation and empirical supplementation of micronutrients and vitamins might also be recommended because deficiencies are common in these patients. Special attention should be paid to group B vitamins, like thiamine, to prevent Wernicke encephalopathy, liposoluble vitamins, such as vitamin D, because its deficiency has been associated with increased liver damage and mortality in ALD,[48] and zinc, which seems to improve in combination with lactulose mild hepatic encephalopathy manifestations.[49] Intensive supplemental enteral nutrition via a nasogastric tube has only been tested in severe cases, and even if it could improve liver function, it has not proven beneficial in survival and should be cautiously considered because of the risk of aspiration pneumonia.[50]

Management of the Underlying Liver Disease

Up to 70% of patients with ALD that develop an episode of AH will have underlying cirrhosis.[5] In a recent retrospective study in patients with moderate AH with histologic assessment, an even higher prevalence of cirrhosis (84%) has been reported.[15] As previously discussed, the cause of death in patients with moderate AH is secondary to liver-related complications, including severe infections in up to 80% of patients.[13–15,25] Therefore, assessing the severity of the underlying liver disease at presentation of an AH episode with prognostic purposes and to establish the most appropriate follow-up strategy should be part of the general management in all patients regardless of the severity. Patients with less severe forms of AH may also present or develop complications related to the underlying liver disease, such as ascites, portal hypertensive bleeding, acute kidney injury, or hepatic encephalopathy, that should be managed according to the current recommendations.[51–54] Special attention should be paid to infections. In patients with severe AH, the prevalence of infection within 90 days of diagnosis is as high as 42% with an increased risk in those who receive corticosteroids.[55,56] The prevalence of infection in patients with less severe forms of AH is not well described, but represents one of main causes of death in this population, as is the case with other liver-related complications. Distinguishing between infection and systemic inflammatory response syndrome (SIRS) in the absence of infection can be challenging. In a series of AH patients with histologic confirmation and a mean MELD score at presentation of 21 (48.1% of patients had MELD >21), the prevalence of SIRS without infection was 32%. SIRS has been shown as a major determinant of multiorgan failure and mortality in patients within the whole severity spectrum of AH.[55] Besides the treatment of acute liver-related complications, prophylactic therapies, to prevent either new decompensations or the recurrence of current complications, such as antibiotics for spontaneous bacterial peritonitis or β-blockers for variceal bleeding, should be initiated during admission when indicated.[54] Those patients with underlying cirrhosis or advanced fibrosis, especially with continued alcohol consumption after the episode, should be enrolled in screening programs for the early detection of gastroesophageal varices[54,57] and HCC[58,59] following the current guidelines.

Early liver transplantation for AH is restricted to highly selected patients with severe forms who do not respond to medical therapy. Nevertheless, patients with less severe forms are at risk for developing life-threatening liver-related complications during follow-up secondary to the underlying advanced liver disease, even after maintaining alcohol abstinence. When indicated, liver transplantation should be considered as part of the management of ALD on a case-by-case basis after a sobriety period (usually 6 months) in patients with a prior episode of moderate AH according to the latest evidence.[60]

Fig. 3 depicts a suggested algorithm for the management of moderate AH.

Novel Therapies

Many new therapies for AH have been evaluated in recent decades in different clinical trials; however, most of them were in patients with severe AH. Nevertheless, patients with less severe forms of the disease have recently become the target population of a few ongoing clinical trials, which represents an encouraging turnaround in the research activity of the field. Pathophysiologically oriented therapies aimed at

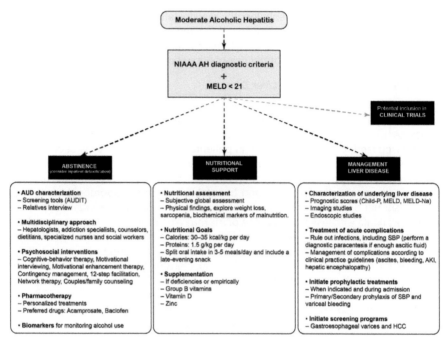

Fig. 3. Suggested algorithm for the management of moderate AH. AKI, acute kidney injury; AUD, alcohol use disorder; AUDIT, Alcohol Use Disorders Inventory Test; Child-P, Child-Pugh; SBP, spontaneous bacterial peritonitis. (Data from Refs.[40,42,54])

improving the outcomes in this population are urgently needed given the mortality associated with the so-called nonsevere or moderate AH, as recently shown.[13–15]

Gut-liver dysfunction has become one of the most attractive and studied pathophysiological mechanisms of ALD in the last few years. Bacterial translocation as a result of the gut barrier dysfunction, among other mechanisms, may play a relevant role in the progression of the disease, including in patients with AH. An open-label single-arm trial aimed at investigating the effect of gut sterilization on macrophage activation in patients with AH with a combination of orally formulated antibiotics (vancomycin, gentamycin, and meropenem) has recently concluded the recruitment (NCT03157388). According to the available information, patients with AH without any specific cutoff of severity have been included; however, there are no published data available at the moment. A different approach to target the gut-liver axis via administration probiotic supplements containing *Lactobacillus rhamnosus* GG versus placebo is also currently underway. The study is aimed at evaluating the effects of probiotic supplements on improvement in MELD score and gut mucosal integrity in patients with MELD score less than 21 and will collect valuable information that will potentially help to document the natural history of moderate AH (NCT01922895).

Targeting liver regeneration to counteract apoptosis and necrosis phenomena that take place in AH as a potentially new approach to treating the disease has also received considerable attention. In that regard, a phase 2a open-label single-arm clinical trial to test the safety and efficacy of F-652 has already been completed. F-652 is a recombinant fusion protein containing human interleukin-22 (IL-22) and human immunoglobulin G2 fragment crystallizable with antioxidant, antiapoptotic, antisteatotic,

Table 3
Ongoing clinical trials in patients with moderate alcoholic hepatitis

NCT Identifier	Treatment	Mechanism	Study Design	Definition of Moderate AH	Primary Endpoint
03157388	Combination of vancomycin, gentamycin, and meropenem in oral formulation	Microbiome modulation	Open-label, single-arm treatment	All spectrum of AH, potentially including patients with moderate disease. Not severity cutoff specified	Evaluate the effect of gut sterilization on macrophage activation (difference in serum levels of macrophage activation markers sCD163)
01922895	L rhamnosus GG vs placebo	Microbiome modulation	Double-blind, randomised controlled trial with parallel assignment	MELD < 20	Evolution of MELD score at 30 d
02655510	IL-22 (F-652)	Hepatocyte regeneration	Open-label, single-arm treatment, dose escalating study	All spectrum of AH Includes a subgroup of patients with MELD 11–20	Safety and tolerability
02039219	Obeticholic acid vs placebo	Amelioration of bile-acid injury	Double-blind, randomised controlled trial with parallel assignment	MELD > 11 and <20	Evolution of MELD score at 6 wk along with safety and tolerability
03432260	DUR-928	Small molecule. Epigenetic modulator regulating multiple biological pathways involved in metabolic homeostasis, inflammatory response, cell survival, and tissue regeneration	Open-label, single-arm treatment, dose escalating study	All spectrum of AH. MELD 11–30, inclusive	Safety and tolerability

antimicrobial, and proliferative effect. In this dose-escalating study, 9 patients with moderate AH defined as MELD score 11 to 20 were included and received the investigational drug at different doses. Preliminary results already published suggest that F-652 is safe in doses up to 45 μg/kg, and it is associated with a high rate of improvement as determined by Lille and MELD score, a reduction in markers of inflammation, and an increase in markers of hepatic regeneration.[61] A phase 2b trial is currently underway (NCT02655510).

Obeticholic acid (OCA) has been a drug that has received special interest from the liver research community in the past few years. It is a potent selective agonist of the farnesoid X receptor, a nuclear receptor that is thought to be a key regulator of bile acids and of the inflammatory, fibrotic, and metabolic pathways.[62] Because of its ameliorating effect on cholestasis in other liver diseases, such as primary biliary cholangitis and nonalcoholic steatohepatitis, OCA has been proposed as a new therapy for AH. A phase 2 double-blind, placebo-controlled trial of OCA in patients with moderate AH, defined as MELD score greater than 11 and less than 20, has already been completed. The study is primarily aimed at evaluating the impact on MELD score as well as its safety in this population, but the results have yet to be reported (NCT02039219).

Finally, a small molecule called DUR-928 is being tested in an open-label dose-escalation phase 2 multicentric trial in patients with AH, including less severe forms of the disease (MELD 11–30, inclusive). DUR-928 acts as an epigenetic modulator regulating multiple biological pathways involved in metabolic homeostasis, inflammatory response, cell survival, and tissue regeneration. The study is aimed at assessing the dose-related safety, pharmacokinetics, and pharmacodynamics of DUR 928 in patients with moderate and severe AH. The trial is currently under recruitment (NCT03432260).

The ongoing clinical trials evaluating new therapies in all the spectrum of patients with AH have been further reviewed elsewhere.[30] **Table 3** shows a summary of the clinical trials that are underway recruiting patients with moderate AH.

SUMMARY

Moderate AH is a frequent disease with a probable underestimated incidence compared with its severe form. Recent evidence supports that it is not a benign disease because it has a mortality in the short to medium term of up to 3% to 7% and as high as 13% to 20% at 1 year. Accordingly, a different nomenclature, such as "moderate alcoholic hepatitis," "alcoholic hepatitis of intermediate severity," or "moderately severe alcoholic hepatitis," has been proposed. A homogeneous definition of severity according to the different available prognostic scores is lacking as well. The use of a single score to determine the severity of the disease could help to better classify these patients and fully characterize this less severe form of the disease in terms of epidemiology and natural history. In addition, the systematic use of a single prognostic score could potentially identify new cutoffs to categorize these patients into 3 groups of risk, that is, nonsevere, moderate, and severe. In this regard, MELD score seems to be the most accurate prognostic score. Long-term abstinence is the main goal of the treatment because it is the main driver for disease progression and an independent predictor of long-term survival in these patients. Along with adequate nutritional support, the management of the underlying liver disease is critical, considering that up to 80% of patients will die during follow-up because of liver-related complications, including severe infections. New pathophysiologic-oriented therapies for the treatment of less severe forms of AH are being evaluated in several different ongoing clinical trials. Although the results of these investigations have yet to be reported, it is hoped they will provide new insights about the natural history of the disease as well as new effective treatments that improve the outcomes of these patients in terms of morbidity and mortality.

CLINICS CARE POINTS

- AH should be suspected in patients with history of sustained heavy alcohol use and acute onset of jaundice. Other signs and symptoms may be present (malaise, tender hepatomegaly, and liver-related complications such as ascites, encephalopathy, infections or variceal bleeding).
- Tipical laboratory findings are elevation of serum bilirubin (>3 mg/dL), AST >50 IU/mL and AST/ALT >1.5 (usually >2). AST and ALT do not typically exceed 400 IU/mL, and when that is the case, an alternative cause should be considered. Screening of other potential causes of jaundice should be part of the general differential diagnosis workup.
- A histologic confirmation is recommended when other confounding factors or concomitant diseases cannot be excluded by clinical criteria, laboratory findings, and imaging procedures.
- MELD score should be the elective prognostic score to stratify the severity of the disease. A cut-off of 21 discriminates severe ($\geq$21) from nonsevere or moderate (<21) forms of the disease.
- Cirrhosis is present in up to 70% of cases and 80% of patients will die during follow-up because of liver-related complications. Besides the treatment of acute liver-related complications, prophylactic therapies, to prevent new decompensations or the recurrence of current complications, should be initiated during admission when indicated. Enrollment in screening programs for the early detection of gastroesophageal varices or HCC should be considered as well.
- There are not specific therapies for moderate AH. Long-term abstinence is the main goal of the treatment since it is an independent predictor of long-term survival. It must be closely monitored after discharge and based on a multidisciplinary approach. Inpatient detoxification should be considered as well as pharmacologic treatment to prevent alcohol relapse, being acamprosate and baclofen the preferred drugs for their safety profile. The use of biomarkers to detect relapse episodes may be useful since alcohol consumption is often underreported.

DISCLOSURE

Ana Clemente-Sánchez is supported by an international scholarship sponsored by the Spanish Association of the Study of the Liver (AEEH).

Ramón Bataller is supported by NIAAA grants 1U01AA026978-01, 1U01AA026972-02, 5U01AA026264-02, NIH R01 (ENaC regulation by biliary factors), NIDDK 1R01DK117881-01, and NIEHS R35 (Xenobiotic Receptors in the Crossroad of Xenobiotic Metabolism and Endobiotic Metabolism).

REFERENCES

1. Asrani SK, Devarbhavi H, Eaton J, et al. Burden of liver diseases in the world. J Hepatol 2019;70(1):151–71.
2. Hammer JH, Parent MC, Spiker DA, World Health Organization. Global status report on alcohol and health65, 2018. p. 2018. https://doi.org/10.1037/cou0000248.

3. Rehm J, Samokhvalov AV, Shield KD. Global burden of alcoholic liver diseases. J Hepatol 2013;59(1):160–8.

4. Altamirano J, Bataller R. Alcoholic liver disease: pathogenesis and new targets for therapy. Nat Rev Gastroenterol Hepatol 2011;8(9):491–501.

5. Seitz HK, Bataller R, Cortez-Pinto H, et al. Alcoholic liver disease. Nat Rev Dis Prim 2018;4(1):16.

6. Maddrey WC, Boitnott JK, Bedine MS, et al. Corticosteroid therapy of alcoholic hepatitis. Gastroenterology 1978;75(2):193–9.

7. Carithers RL, Herlong F, Diehl AM, et al. Methylprednisolone therapy in patients with severe alcoholic hepatitis. A randomized multicenter trial. Ann Intern Med 1989. https://doi.org/10.7326/0003-4819-110-9-685.

8. Dunn W, Jamil LH, Brown LS, et al. MELD accurately predicts mortality in patients with alcoholic hepatitis. Hepatology 2005;41(2):353–8.

9. Forrest EH, Evans CDJ, Stewart S, et al. Analysis of factors predictive of mortality in alcoholic hepatitis and derivation and validation of the Glasgow Alcoholic Hepatitis Score. Gut 2005;54(8):1174–9.

10. Rincon D, Lo Iacono O, Ripoll C, et al. Prognostic value of hepatic venous pressure gradient for in-hospital mortality of patients with severe acute alcoholic hepatitis. Aliment Pharmacol Ther 2007;25(7):841–8.

11. Dominguez M, Rincón D, Abraldes JG, et al. A new scoring system for prognostic stratification of patients with alcoholic hepatitis. Am J Gastroenterol 2008;103(11): 2747–56.

12. Altamirano J, Miquel R, Katoonizadeh A, et al. A histologic scoring system for prognosis of patients with alcoholic hepatitis. Gastroenterology 2014; 146(5):e1–6.

13. Samala N, Gawrieh S, Tang Q, et al. Clinical characteristics and outcomes of mild to moderate alcoholic hepatitis. GastroHep 2019;1(4):161–5.

14. Bennett K, Enki DG, Thursz M, et al. Systematic review with meta-analysis: high mortality in patients with non-severe alcoholic hepatitis. Aliment Pharmacol Ther 2019;50(3):249–57.

15. Degre D, Stauber RE, Englebert G, et al. Long-term outcomes in patients with decompensated alcohol-related liver disease, steatohepatitis and Maddrey's discriminant function <32. J Hepatol 2020;72(4):636–42.

16. Thursz MR, Richardson P, Allison M, et al. Prednisolone or pentoxifylline for alcoholic hepatitis. N Engl J Med 2015;372(17):1619–28.

17. Parker R, Kim SJ, Im GY, et al. Obesity in acute alcoholic hepatitis increases morbidity and mortality. EBioMedicine 2019;45:511–8.

18. Louvet A, Naveau S, Abdelnour M, et al. The Lille model: a new tool for therapeutic strategy in patients with severe alcoholic hepatitis treated with steroids. Hepatology 2007;45(6):1348–54.

19. Crabb DW, Bataller R, Chalasani NP, et al. Standard definitions and common data elements for clinical trials in patients with alcoholic hepatitis: recommendation from the NIAAA Alcoholic Hepatitis Consortia. Gastroenterology 2016;150(4): 785–90.

20. Malinchoc M, Kamath PS, Gordon FD, et al. A model to predict poor survival in patients undergoing transjugular intrahepatic portosystemic shunts. Hepatology 2000;31(4):864–71.

21. Sandahl TD, Jepsen P, Ott P, et al. Validation of prognostic scores for clinical use in patients with alcoholic hepatitis. Scand J Gastroenterol 2011;46(9):1127–32.

22. Papastergiou V, Tsochatzis EA, Pieri G, et al. Nine scoring models for short-term mortality in alcoholic hepatitis: cross-validation in a biopsy-proven cohort. Aliment Pharmacol Ther 2014;39(7):721–32.

23. Palaniyappan N, Subramanian V, Ramappa V, et al. The utility of scoring systems in predicting early and late mortality in alcoholic hepatitis: whose score is it anyway? Int J Hepatol 2012;2012:624675.

24. Forrest EH, Atkinson SR, Richardson P, et al. Application of prognostic scores in the STOPAH trial: discriminant function is no longer the optimal scoring system in alcoholic hepatitis. J Hepatol 2018;68(3):511–8.

25. Altamirano J, López-Pelayo H, Michelena J, et al. Alcohol abstinençe in patients surviving an episode of alcoholic hepatitis: prediction and impact on long-term survival. Hepatology 2017;66(6):1842–53.

26. Infante-Rivard C, Esnaola S, Villeneuve J-P. Clinical and statistical validity of conventional prognostic factors in predicting short-term survival among cirrhotics. Hepatology 1987;7(4):660–4.

27. Hughes E, Hopkins LJ, Parker R. Survival from alcoholic hepatitis has not improved over time. PLoS One 2018;13(2):e0192393.

28. Theise ND. Histopathology of alcoholic liver disease. Clin Liver Dis 2013; 2(2):64–7.

29. Louvet A, Thursz MR, Kim DJ, et al. Corticosteroids reduce risk of death within 28 days for patients with severe alcoholic hepatitis, compared with pentoxifylline or placebo—a meta-analysis of individual data from controlled trials. Gastroenterology 2018;155(2):458–68.e8.

30. Sehrawat TS, Liu M, Shah VH. The knowns and unknowns of treatment for alcoholic hepatitis. Lancet Gastroenterol Hepatol 2020;5(5):494–506.

31. Louvet A, Labreuche J, Artru F, et al. Main drivers of outcome differ between short term and long term in severe alcoholic hepatitis: a prospective study. Hepatology 2017;66(5):1464–73.

32. Atkinson SR, Hamesch K, Spivak I, et al. Serum transferrin is an independent predictor of mortality in severe alcoholic hepatitis. Am J Gastroenterol 2020;115(3): 398–405.

33. Pessione F, Ramond MJ, Peters L, et al. Five-year survival predictive factors in patients with excessive alcohol intake and cirrhosis. Effect of alcoholic hepatitis, smoking and abstinence. Liver Int 2003;23(1):45–53.

34. Chedid A, Mendenhall CL, Gartside P, et al. Prognostic factors in alcoholic liver disease. VA Cooperative Study Group. Am J Gastroenterol 1991;86(2):210–6.

35. Lackner C, Spindelboeck W, Haybaeck J, et al. Histological parameters and alcohol abstinence determine long-term prognosis in patients with alcoholic liver disease. J Hepatol 2017;66(3):610–8.

36. Potts JR, Howard MR, Verma S. Recurrent severe alcoholic hepatitis: clinical characteristics and outcomes. Eur J Gastroenterol Hepatol 2013;25(6):659–64.

37. Potts JR, Goubet S, Heneghan MA, et al. Determinants of long-term outcome in severe alcoholic hepatitis. Aliment Pharmacol Ther 2013;38(6):584–95.

38. Deltenre P, Trépo E, Fujiwara N, et al. Gene signature-MELD score and alcohol relapse determine long-term prognosis of patients with severe alcoholic hepatitis. Liver Int 2020;40(3):565–70.

39. Khan A, Tansel A, White DL, et al. Efficacy of psychosocial interventions in inducing and maintaining alcohol abstinence in patients with chronic liver disease: a systematic review. Clin Gastroenterol Hepatol 2016;14(2):191–202.e1-4.

40. Simonetto DA, Shah VH, Kamath PS. Outpatient management of alcohol-related liver disease. Lancet Gastroenterol Hepatol 2020;5(5):485–93.

41. Peeraphatdit TB, Kamath PS, Karpyak VM, et al. Alcohol rehabilitation within 30 days of hospital discharge is associated with reduced readmission, relapse, and death in patients with alcoholic hepatitis. Clin Gastroenterol Hepatol 2020; 18(2):477–85.e5.

42. Mellinger JL, Winder GS. Alcohol use disorders in alcoholic liver disease. Clin Liver Dis 2019;23(1):55–69.

43. Addolorato G, Leggio L, Ferrulli A, et al. Effectiveness and safety of baclofen for maintenance of alcohol abstinence in alcohol-dependent patients with liver cirrhosis: randomised, double-blind controlled study. Lancet 2007;370(9603): 1915–22.

44. Yamini D, Lee SH, Avanesyan A, et al. Utilization of baclofen in maintenance of alcohol abstinence in patients with alcohol dependence and alcoholic hepatitis with or without cirrhosis. Alcohol Alcohol 2014;49(4):453–6.

45. Chaignot C, Zureik M, Rey G, et al. Risk of hospitalisation and death related to baclofen for alcohol use disorders: comparison with nalmefene, acamprosate, and naltrexone in a cohort study of 165 334 patients between 2009 and 2015 in France. Pharmacoepidemiol Drug Saf 2018;27(11):1239–48.

46. Cabezas J, Lucey MR, Bataller R. Biomarkers for monitoring alcohol use. Clin Liver Dis 2016;8(3):59–63.

47. European Association for the Study of the Liver. EASL Clinical Practice Guidelines on nutrition in chronic liver disease. J Hepatol 2019;70(1):172-93.

48. Trépo E, Ouziel R, Pradat P, et al. Marked 25-hydroxyvitamin D deficiency is associated with poor prognosis in patients with alcoholic liver disease. J Hepatol 2013;59(2):344–50.

49. Shen YC, Chang YH, Fang CJ, et al. Zinc supplementation in patients with cirrhosis and hepatic encephalopathy: a systematic review and meta-analysis. Nutr J 2019;18(1):34.

50. Moreno C, Deltenre P, Senterre C, et al. Intensive enteral nutrition is ineffective for patients with severe alcoholic hepatitis treated with corticosteroids. Gastroenterology 2016;150(4):903–10.e8.

51. Singal AK, Bataller R, Ahn J, et al. ACG clinical guideline: alcoholic liver disease. Am J Gastroenterol 2018;113(2):175–94.

52. Crabb DW, Im GY, Szabo G, et al. Diagnosis and treatment of alcohol-associated liver diseases: 2019 practice guidance from the American Association for the Study of Liver Diseases. Hepatology 2020;71(1):306–33.

53. European Association for the Study of the Liver. EASL Clinical Practice Guidelines: Management of alcohol-related liver disease. J Hepatol 2018;69(1):154-81.

54. European Association for the Study of the Liver EASL Clinical Practice Guidelines for the management of patients with decompensated cirrhosis. J Hepatol 2018;69(2):406-60.

55. Michelena J, Altamirano J, Abraldes JG, et al. Systemic inflammatory response and serum lipopolysaccharide levels predict multiple organ failure and death in alcoholic hepatitis. Hepatology 2015;62(3):762–72.

56. Vergis N, Atkinson SR, Knapp S, et al. In patients with severe alcoholic hepatitis, prednisolone increases susceptibility to infection and infection-related mortality, and is associated with high circulating levels of bacterial DNA. Gastroenterology 2017;152(5):1068–77.e4.

57. Garcia-Tsao G, Abraldes JG, Berzigotti A, et al. Portal hypertensive bleeding in cirrhosis: risk stratification, diagnosis, and management: 2016 practice guidance by the American Association for the Study of Liver Diseases. Hepatology 2017; 65(1):310–35.

58. Marrero JA, Kulik LM, Sirlin CB, et al. Diagnosis, staging, and management of hepatocellular carcinoma: 2018 practice guidance by the American Association for the Study of Liver Diseases. Hepatology 2018;68(2):723–50.
59. European Association for the Study of the Liver EASL clinical practice guidelines: management of hepatocellular carcinoma. J Hepatol 2018;69(1):182-236.
60. Mathurin P, Lucey MR. Liver transplantation in patients with alcohol-related liver disease: current status and future directions. Lancet Gastroenterol Hepatol 2020;5(5):507–14.
61. Arab JP, Sehrawat TS, Simonetto DA, et al. An open-label, dose-escalation study to assess the safety and efficacy of IL-22 agonist F-652 in patients with alcohol-associated hepatitis. Hepatology 2020;72(2):441–53.
62. Fiorucci S, Di Giorgio C, Distrutti E. Obeticholic Acid: An Update of Its Pharmacological Activities in Liver Disorders. Handbook of experimental pharmacology 2019;256:283–95.

Malnutrition and Alcohol-Associated Hepatitis

Craig J. McClain, MD[a,b,c,d,e,*], Cristian D. Rios, MD[a], Sally Condon, MD[a],
Luis S. Marsano, MD[a,c]

KEYWORDS

- Nutrition • Malnutrition • Alcohol-associated hepatitis (AH) • Micronutrients
- Standard drink

KEY POINTS

- Malnutrition is common in alcohol-associated hepatitis (AH).
- Malnutrition increases with severity of AH and is associated with worse outcomes.
- Nighttime snacks help prevent muscle loss.

INTRODUCTION

The role of alcohol in liver injury is complex and influenced by multiple factors, including dose of alcohol consumed, duration and pattern of drinking (eg, binge drinking), and, as reviewed in this article, potential interactions with nutrition. From a nutrition perspective, alcohol is an important source of calories, but these should be considered "empty" calories, that is, they contain little or no macronutrients, such as protein or fat, and basically no micronutrients, such as vitamins and minerals.[1] Regular alcohol intake can be a major source of unwanted calories; for example, beer has approximately 150 kcal per 12-ounce can, and a mixed drink has approximately 125 kcal per drink. The 2020 to 2025 Dietary Guidelines for Americans highlighted the concept of the standard drink (14 g alcohol) and the fact that if alcohol is consumed, it should be in moderation (ie, up to 1 drink per day for women and 2 drinks per day for men).[1] If subjects have underlying liver disease, no alcohol intake is safe or acceptable. Moreover, alcohol intake may have more adverse outcomes if subjects are overweight or obese. It is known that many patients with alcohol-associated

[a] Division of Gastroenterology, Hepatology and Nutrition, University of Louisville School of Medicine, 505 South Hancock Street, Louisville, KY 40202, USA; [b] UofL Alcohol Research Center, University of Louisville, Louisville, KY, USA; [c] Department of Medicine, University of Louisville, Louisville, KY, USA; [d] Hepatobiology and Toxicology Center, University of Louisville, Louisville, KY, USA; [e] Robely Rex Veterans Affairs Medical Center, Louisville, KY 40207, USA
* Corresponding author. Division of Gastroenterology, Hepatology and Nutrition, University of Louisville School of Medicine, 505 South Hancock Street, Louisville, KY 40202.
E-mail addresses: craig.mcclain@louisville.edu; cjmccl01@louisville.edu

Clin Liver Dis 25 (2021) 557–570
https://doi.org/10.1016/j.cld.2021.03.002
1089-3261/21/Published by Elsevier Inc.

liver.theclinics.com

hepatitis (AH) are drinking approximately 15 drinks per day, which amounts to about 2000 empty calories per day[1] (**Fig. 1**). Patients with AH often have inadequate protein intake and may have nutritionally imbalanced fat intake, with excess omega-6 and low omega-3 intake.[1] Diets are also often deficient in micronutrients, such as zinc.[1] Thus, alcohol and altered nutrition intersect at many levels to cause AH and its complications. This article reviews the following: (1) definition of malnutrition and diagnostic tests; (2) prevalence; (3) gut-liver axis and AH; (4) inpatient management, including impact on prognosis; (5) outpatient management; and (6) selected vitamins and trace metals in AH.

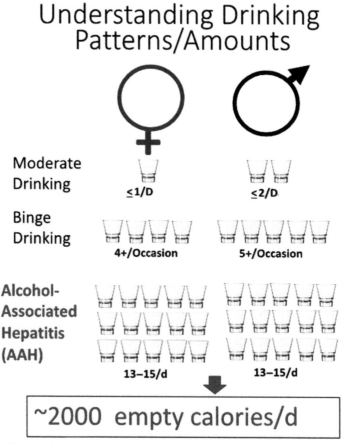

Fig. 1. Drinking levels and their consequences. In the United States, drinking levels are expressed in terms of standard drinks consumed, that is, the number of alcoholic beverages drank, each containing about 0.6 fluid ounce or 14 g of pure alcohol. The Dietary Guidelines for Americans 2015 to 2020 defined moderate drinking as consuming up to 2 drinks per day for men and up to 1 drink per day for women. The Substance Abuse and Mental Health Services Administration defines binge drinking as consuming 5 or more (for men) or 4 or more (for women) alcoholic drinks on the same occasion on at least 1 day in the past 30 days. Patients hospitalized for severe AH in the NIAAA-funded DASH study were drinking approximately 13 to 15 drinks per day. (Data from http://www.rethinkingdrinking.niaaa.nih.gov).

DISCUSSION
Definition of Malnutrition and Diagnostic Tests

Malnutrition is classically defined as a disorder of inadequate nutrition intake or uptake that leads to a decrease in body cell mass. Sarcopenia has generally been the clinical phenotype of malnutrition in AH. However, as obesity has increased in the United States, sarcopenia is often more difficult to discern clinically. Indeed, data from the National Institute on Alcohol Abuse and Alcoholism (NIAAA)-sponsored DASH consortium showed that the average body mass index (BMI) of patients with severe AH was about 30 (McClain, unpublished data, 2021). Patients may also be malnourished because of isolated micronutrient deficiency, such as zinc deficiency.

The most extensive studies of malnutrition in liver disease are in alcohol-associated liver disease (ALD), mainly in patients with AH. Patients with severe AH and cirrhosis have the most severe nutritional deficiencies, indicating that advanced disease is associated with more severe malnutrition.

There are several diagnostic tests that can be used to diagnose malnutrition in AH, although many of them have accuracy limitations in liver disease (**Box 1**). Anthropometry, which includes BMI, change in body weight, and triceps skin fold, is widely used to evaluate nutritional status. However, if patients have fluid retention with edema or ascites, this can overestimate BMI or underestimate weight loss. Biological parameters, such as visceral proteins, are commonly used to indicate prognosis and nutritional status. These visceral proteins most commonly include albumin, prealbumin, and retinol-binding protein. All these proteins are produced in the liver, which makes them inaccurate markers of malnutrition, and they correlate better with the severity of underlying liver disease than with malnutrition.

Various imaging modalities are being used to assess muscle mass and body composition. A single cross-sectional computed tomography (CT) slice has been validated as an accurate method to measure whole-body skeletal muscle and fat mass. Psoas thickness on CT has been used to predict muscle mass and has been shown to be predictive of mortality in cirrhotic patients.[2] Dual-energy x-ray absorption (DEXA) testing can assess whole-body and regional distribution of lean tissue and fat. DEXA is more often used in the outpatient setting.

Twenty-four-hour creatinine height index is another method of assessing muscle mass. It is the ratio of measured 24-hour urine creatinine excretion in a patient compared with expected excretion in a normal individual of the same sex and height.

Box 1
Selected methods for assessing malnutrition in alcohol-associated hepatitis

- Anthropometry (BMI, weight change, triceps skinfold)
- Biological parameters (visceral proteins)
- Dual-energy x-ray absorptiometry, computed tomography
- 24-hour urinary creatinine height index
- Assessment of muscle strength
- Subjective global assessment
- Bioelectrical impedance
- Energy balance
- Metabolomics

A study by Pirlich and coworkers[3] showed a strong correlation between muscle cell mass as assessed by creatinine and body cell mass as assessed by total body potassium count. Liver dysfunction did not alter urinary creatinine, but renal dysfunction did. Measurement of handgrip strength using a handgrip dynamometer is a quick and easy method to quantify muscle strength. It has been correlated with other markers of malnutrition in liver disease and is an indicator of functional status.

Subjective global assessment (SGA) is a regularly used, simple method, which includes patient history regarding weight loss, usual dietary intake, gastrointestinal symptoms, and evidence of malnutrition of physical examination, such as muscle wasting or presence of edema.[4] Bioelectrical impedance (BIA) is increasingly used for body composition analysis. The theory behind it is that each body tissue has a specific electrical conductivity that is directly related to the water and electrolyte content of that tissue. Pirlich and coworkers[3] showed a strong correlation between BIA and the gold standard of total body potassium for assessing malnutrition. Advances have made this method more accurate, even in patients with ascites, which was previously a limiting factor. This technology is simple to use and provides not only information on muscle mass but also extracellular water.

The assessment of energy intake/balance and nitrogen balance can be useful in determining if patients are meeting energy and protein targets. These targets come in the form of calorie counts in the inpatient setting, and food diaries in the outpatient setting. Air-displacement plethysmography calculates the density of the body using mass and body volume to assess body composition. Last, metabolomics is a quantitative analysis of all metabolites, which can be endogenous or from multiple outside sources, including food and the environment. Metabolomic assays provide an opportunity not only for identifying patients with malnutrition but also for identifying metabolic pathways that lead to malnutrition.

Prevalence

Studies have examined the prevalence of malnutrition in ALD, and although there were multiple methods of assessment, all consistently found high prevalence of malnutrition in patients along the whole spectrum of ALD. Prevalence in AH reaches 100%, which was shown by 2 large studies from the Veterans Administration (VA). The first study showed that in more than 280 patients, every patient had some evidence for malnutrition. Patients were divided in groups with mild, moderate, or severe alcohol-associated hepatitis based on clinical and biochemical markers. The mean alcohol consumption among these patients was 228 g per day, meaning approximately 50% of energy intake was from alcohol. The severity of malnutrition correlated closely with complications of liver disease, including encephalopathy, ascites, hepatorenal syndrome, and overall mortality.[5,6] Similar data were observed in a follow-up VA study.[5–9] Over time, these result trends have remained consistent. Singal and colleagues[10] found that among 261 patients with alcohol-associated cirrhosis undergoing transplant, 84% had malnutrition when assessed with the SGA.

Gut-Liver Axis

Bacteria, fungi, and other microorganisms make up the human gut microbiome, with the bacterial microbiome being the best studied. Intestinal bacterial dysbiosis is defined as an imbalance among the different microbial entities in the intestine with a disruption of symbiosis.[11] There are 3 major types of dysbiosis, including pathobiont expansion, reduced diversity, and loss of beneficial microbes, and they are not mutually exclusive. Early animal studies documented that the gut flora/bacterial dysbiosis and gut-derived toxins play a critical role in the development of both liver disease and its complications. Indeed, more than a half a century ago, it was shown that germ-free rodents or rodents treated with antibiotics to "sterilize the gut" were resistant to nutritional and toxin-induced liver injury. Elegant studies by Broitman and coworkers[12] showed that rats fed a choline-deficient diet developed cirrhosis, which could be prevented by oral neomycin.[12] However, when endotoxin was added to the water supply, neomycin could no longer prevent the development of liver injury and fibrosis. Most recent studies use some variation of the Lieber DeCarli liquid diet alcohol feeding mouse model. Using this alcohol feeding paradigm, the authors demonstrated a decline in the abundance of both *Bacteroidetes* and *Firmicutes* phyla, with a proportional increase in the gram-negative *Proteobacteria* and Gram-positive *Actinobacteria* phyla.[13] Bacterial genera analysis showed the greatest expansion in gram-negative alkaline-tolerant *Alcaligenes* and gram-positive *Corynebacterium*. These alterations were accompanied by an increase in colonic pH and liver steatosis and injury.[13] Treatment with the probiotic, *Lactobacillus rhamnosus* GG, attenuated dysbiosis, gut barrier dysfunction, and liver injury.[13–15] The authors also analyzed polar metabolites in the feces from mice fed with or without alcohol. Taurine, nicotinic acid, and several major short chain fatty acids (SCFAs) were significantly decreased in mice fed alcohol.[16] Thus, fecal metabolites are also a likely target for AH treatment. Indeed, studies from Schabl's laboratory demonstrated the importance of cytolysin, an exotoxin secreted by *Enterococcus faecalis*, in the pathogenesis of hepatocyte death in AH, and the potential for bacteriophage therapy.[17]

Alcohol abuse was reported to cause small intestinal bacterial overgrowth in humans more than 3 decades ago using culture techniques.[18] Development of sequencing techniques greatly advanced the gut bacterial studies. In a study of 244 patients with alcohol-associated cirrhosis, investigators found that intestinal dysbiosis was more severe in patients with decompensated cirrhosis compared with compensated cirrhosis.[19] Studies from the NIAAA-funded TREAT consortium documented that there are distinct changes in the fecal microbiome associated with the development, but not severity of AH. There also were clear changes in fecal metabolites, such as decreased SCFAs and altered tryptophan metabolites, similar to findings described above in alcohol-fed mice.[20]

Restoration of gut eubiosis is the major aim of gut microbiota–based therapies in AH. Several approaches, including diet modulation, probiotics/prebiotics/antibiotics intervention, fecal bacteria transplantation, bacteriophage therapy, and engineered bacteria therapy, have proven to be effective in alleviating experimental alcohol-induced liver injury through positively modifying gut microbiota, and pilot studies are ongoing in human AH.[11,13,17,21–24]

Inpatient Management

Patients with AH are frequently malnourished at baseline and are at risk of worsening malnutrition during hospitalization, especially when in the intensive care unit. Thus, hospitalized patients should be evaluated for nutritional status on a regular basis. Nutritional therapy in the inpatient with ALD is challenging. Most of these patients are admitted because of acute hepatic decompensation (hepatic encephalopathy, ascites, and so forth) or because of severe AH. The mechanisms for malnutrition are multiple and listed in **Box 2**. The barriers to nutritional therapy include preexisting nutritional deficiencies, high risk of refeeding syndrome, poor appetite, altered taste, nausea, early satiety, development of alcohol withdrawal syndrome, lack of understanding of the severity of the illness, and desire to keep some control during hospitalization, at least over one's own diet.

Box 2
Major causes of malnutrition

- Anorexia/altered taste/smell
- Nausea/vomiting/delayed gastric emptying
- Diarrhea/malabsorption/bacterial overgrowth
- Poor food availability/quality/unpalatable diets (Na, protein)
- Hormones/cytokine effects
- Complications of liver disease (hepatic encephalopathy, ascites)
- Fasting for procedures/interruption in feeding

It is important to gain early patient cooperation concerning the need for nutrition as a critical component of their treatment plan (**Box 3**). It is useful to educate the most severely ill patients about their mortality risk, and in severe AH this can be achieved by calculating their prognosis using the "Mayo Mortality Risk from Alcoholic Hepatitis Calculator" (https://www.mayoclinic.org/medical-professionals/transplant-medicine/calculators/meld-score-and-90-day-mortality-rate-for-alcoholic-hepatitis/itt-20434719), and sharing the information with them to increase their willingness to accept a feeding tube if they do not achieve their nutrition goals. The refeeding syndrome risk is also a potential problem because it forces an initial conservative approach in ramping-up caloric and protein intake.

It is imperative to rapidly diagnose metabolic disturbances, including electrolyte disorders, and to monitor food consumption and use oral nutritional supplements, including a nighttime snack, in patients to ensure optimal protein/energy requirements by the oral route. The use of a probiotic yogurt twice a day can help in maintaining stable intestinal flora and decreasing the risk of overt hepatic encephalopathy.[25] A 24-hour

---

Box 3
Nutrition support goals for hospitalized patients with alcohol-associated hepatitis

- Early nutrition assessment and evaluation of serum electrolytes
- Aggressive replacement of electrolytes to prevent refeeding syndrome
- Formulate water and electrolyte intake to individual needs, renal function, diuretic sensitivity
- Total energy intake goal: ~1.0 to 1.4 × resting energy expenditure or ~25 to 40 Kcal/kg body weight per day
- Protein: ~1.2 to 2.0 g/kg per day
- Fat: ~30 to 40% of nonprotein energy
- Replace vitamins and minerals as indicated and avoid excessive iron, copper, and vitamin A supplementation
- Supplement daily oral intake with enteral feedings (parenteral if enteral route otherwise contraindicated), if oral intake is insufficient
- Hypocaloric, high-protein diet for obese subjects
- Nutrition education with dietitian, including implementation of nighttime snacks

---

calorie count or estimate of caloric intake helps to rapidly identify the need for a feeding tube for enteral nutrition (EN). In patients with inadequate oral intake, early EN support is especially important because it has the potential to reduce complications and length of stay, and to positively impact patient outcomes. Two randomized clinical trials of EN therapy provide important insight into in-hospital nutrition support in AH. The first was a multicenter randomized study from Spain of EN versus corticosteroids in patients with AH. These patients had their enteral feeding supplements delivered by feeding tube. Results indicated a similar overall short-term mortality (1-month survival, primary endpoint).[26] Importantly, those receiving EN (rich in branched chain amino acids [BCAAs]) had a better long-term outcome. In the most recent multicenter trial, patients with biopsy-documented severe AH were treated with either intensive EN plus methyl-prednisolone or conventional nutrition plus methylprednisolone.[27] In the intensive EN group, EN was given via feeding tube for 14 days. Although the investigators concluded in the title that intensive EN was ineffective, the 6-month mortality (primary endpoint) was numerically lower in the EN group (44.4%) compared with the control group (52.1%). Importantly, patients from either group receiving less than 21.5 kcal/kg per day had significantly lower survival rates, as did those receiving less than 77.6 g of protein per day. There were frequent tube feeding adverse events, highlighting the importance of experience with this technology and use of oral supplements if possible.[27] Importantly, EN is favored over parenteral nutrition (PN) because of risk of infections, cost, and maintenance of the gut barrier function. If PN is used, the authors recommend returning to the enteral route as soon as the small bowel shows evidence of recovered function. It is important to remember that in patients taking lactulose, the radiologist will often diagnose "ileus" because of air-fluid levels seen in the bowel. If the patient has bowel movements, they do not have a true ileus, and enteral feeding should be given.

EN support should be initiated within 24 to 48 hours following hospitalization in patients unable to maintain oral nutritional intake, with the aim to provide greater than 80% of estimated or calculated goal energy and protein within 48 to 72 hours. Whole protein formulas are generally recommended. More concentrated formulas are preferable in patients with ascites to avoid positive fluid balance. BCAA-enriched formulas could be considered in patients with encephalopathy arising during EN and without any other explanation,[28] but this will be rare.

When using EN by feeding tube, it is useful to specify both the total volume of formula to be given in a day and the rate to be delivered. It is a good practice to calculate the feeding rate as a 20-hour course, allowing 4 hours for feeding interruption because of the multiple diagnostic and therapeutic interventions that the patient may need. The tube should be flushed forcefully with 30 mL of water each time the feeding is interrupted, to prevent "tube clogging."

Protein intake is usually recommended at 1.2 to 1.5 g/kg body weight per day (g/kg BW/d). A caloric target of 35 to 40 Kcal/kg body weight per day (cal/kg BW/d) is recommended in hospitalized nonobese patients.[28] Interrupting feeding for diagnostic tests or nurse procedures should be minimized. Obese patients with AH represent a nutrition challenge. Current guidelines recommend hypocaloric, high-protein nutrition therapy in an attempt to preserve lean body mass, to mobilize fat stores, and to minimize overfeeding complications in these at-risk obese patients with liver disease.[29] Energy targets are low in patients with BMI of 30 to 50, usually 65% to 70% of requirements as measured by indirect calorimetry or approximately 11 to 14 kcal/kg BW/d. However, protein requirements are high, usually projected at 2.0 to 2.5 g/kg of ideal body weight per day.[29]

It is important to assess for electrolyte disturbances on admission, not only for increased risk of refeeding syndrome related to chronic alcoholism but also because patients with AH usually have abnormalities with electrolytes. Guidelines recommend assessing the risk of refeeding syndrome on admission (**Box 4**), and screening should be repeated weekly (National Institute for Health and Clinical Excellence [NICE] 2006).[30] The correction of electrolytes abnormalities must occur before starting of feeding (table mineral and electrolyte replacement). For example, in a 70-kg person with normal renal function, the amount of oral minerals he or she will be receiving at the time of starting feeding (unless prefeeding levels were high) will be as follows:

- Mg oxide 400 mg: 1 tablet 3 times a day (will give 60 mEq a day)
- K-Phos original 500 mg: 2 tablets 4 times a day (will give 60 mEq of phosphate + 30 mEq of K)
- KCl 750 mg: 3 tablets 3 times a day or 4 times a day (will give 90 or 120 mEq of K as KCl plus 30 mEq from the K-Phos Original = 120 or 150 mEq per day, respectively)

In patients with high risk for refeeding syndrome, EN should be started slowly (percentage of estimated target energy and protein needs depends on severity of risk), and it should be built up to meet full needs over some period of time (2–7 days). Is also important to restore circulatory volume and monitoring fluid balance closely (see **Box 4**; NICE 2006).[30]

Outpatient Management

The cornerstones of treatment of malnutrition in patients with AH in the outpatient setting are nutritional intervention and alcohol cessation. Outpatient management of malnutrition, specifically in AH, is not well studied but can be extrapolated from data on malnutrition in patients with alcohol-associated cirrhosis. Studies show improved outcomes with nutritional support. In Hirsch and colleagues,[31] outpatients who supplemented their diet with an enteral product containing 1000 kcal (4.2 MJ/d) and 34 g protein had significantly improved protein intake and fewer hospitalizations, as well as improved immunity.[32] The early VA studies indicate that 85 g of

---

Box 4
Risk for refeeding syndrome

Risk of refeeding syndrome

Extremely high risk
- BMI less than 14kg/m^2
- Negligible intake greater than 15 days

High risk (NICE criteria for refeeding syndrome)
- One or more of the following:
  1. BMI less than 16 kg/m^2
  2. Unintentional weight loss greater than 15% over the last 6 months
  3. Little or no nutritional intake for greater than 10 days
  4. Low K, PO_4, or Mg before feeding.
- Two or more of the following:
  1. BMI less than 18.5 kg/m^2
  2. Unintentional weight loss greater than 10% over the last 6 months
  3. Little or no nutritional intake in greater than 5 days
  4. History of alcohol abuse, or use of the following drugs: insulin, chemotherapy, diuretics, or antiacids with Mg or Al

NICE, National Institute for Health and Clinical Excellence.[30]

protein per day or more is required to maintain nitrogen balance in AH, but both inpatients and outpatients were eating 20 g/d less than this.[7] A study in Japan evaluated more than 200 patients with cirrhosis, covering multiple causes, including alcohol, who received either standard-of-care or nutritional counseling from a dietician following a nutritional assessment. After 5 years, the patients in the nutritional counseling arm had improved survival. ESPEN Nutritional Guidelines recommend a calorie intake of 35 to 40 kcal/kg BW/d and a protein intake of 1.2 to 1.5 g/kg BW/d.[28] If patients are overweight, caloric goals should be reduced.

An important aspect in the dietary management of AH, as well as other forms of ALD, is to avoid long periods of time without food intake. During these periods, patients with advanced liver disease can enter a "starvation mode" with decreased glucose oxidation and increased protein and fat catabolism. A study by Owen and coworkers[33] outlined the reasoning behind an important intervention. Patients with cirrhosis (it can be inferred that patients with AH will react similarly) develop a "starvation" metabolic state overnight, whereas a healthy person takes 2 to 3 days of fasting to develop "starvation." A late evening snack can block the overnight catabolic state of patients with AH, as well as other forms of liver disease, and improve body protein stores/muscle mass. Optimally, these patients should have 3 meals, 3 snacks, and that bedtime snack. Breakfast early in the morning can improve cognitive function in subclinical hepatic encephalopathy.[34] Plank and colleagues[35] documented improvement in muscle mass with nighttime supplements by randomizing 103 cirrhotic patients to receive 2 cans of Ensure Plus (710 kcal with 26 g protein) or 2 cans of Diabetic Resource (500 kcal with 30 g protein), either during the day or at bedtime for 1 year. The addition of the nighttime snack was associated with a gain of muscle mass and improvement in quality of life over that year, which was not shown with the daytime snack.[35] This finding highlights the importance of supplementation with a high-nutrient bedtime snack in patients with AH.

A diet high in omega-6 unsaturated fat is a risk factor for the development and progression of experimental ALD and is correlated with severity. Alternatively, omega-3 unsaturated fat enrichment and dietary DHA and EPA (specific types of omega-3 fat) supplementation have been shown to alleviate alcohol-induced liver injury.[36,37] This result suggests that eating foods with omega-3s may be beneficial in patients with AH, but human studies are needed.[38] Data have increasingly suggested beneficial effects of prebiotics (nondigestible food substances to promote growth of beneficial bacteria) and probiotics (live microorganisms that are favorable to the host) in ALD. As discussed earlier, gut microbiota plays an etiologic role in AH, suggesting that prebiotics and probiotics may be effective therapy.[39]

In patients with AH, meeting caloric needs is frequently difficult with ongoing alcohol intake. Abstinent patients have a higher caloric intake compared with those with ongoing alcohol use. Abstinence may increase the beneficial effects of nutritional support on cell-mediated immunity.[32] Developing more effective treatment options for alcohol cessation would have important effects on malnutrition in AH.

Vitamins and Trace Metals

Vitamin A

In ALD, vitamin A storage and release are impaired. The liver is the major storage site for vitamin A (retinol) mostly found in stellate cells. Venu and colleagues[40] found most patients evaluated for liver transplantation in a single center had vitamin A and D deficiency without documentation of night blindness. Abbott-Johnson and colleagues[41] found impaired dark adaptation in almost 50% of patients with liver diseases and also showed patients with ALD had the greatest impairment of dark adaptation. Most patients with impairment were asymptomatic. It is important to monitor levels of vitamin A when a patient with AH is undergoing vitamin A supplementation because of the risk of vitamin A–induced liver toxicity.

Vitamin D

The primary function of vitamin D is regulation of intestinal calcium absorption. Vitamin D undergoes 25-hydroxylation in the liver, yielding the 25-hydroxyvitamin D peptide before it undergoes hydroxylation in the kidneys. Patients with liver diseases frequently suffer from vitamin D deficiency and are at high risk for osteoporosis. The prevalence of osteopenia in ALD is between 34% and 48%, and the prevalence of osteoporosis is between 11% and 36%.[42] Vitamin D also plays an important role in immune function and may help maintain gut barrier function in ALD.

Vitamin B12/Folate

The liver plays an important role in the storage and transport of vitamin B12. Elevated serum levels of B12 are often found in patients with AH, cirrhosis, and hepatocellular carcinoma. This elevated level is due to the release of stored cobalamin through hepatocyte degradation.[43] Folate participates in DNA methylation and replication. It is stored in the liver. Chronic alcoholics are often folate deficient because of reduced dietary intake, intestinal malabsorption, reduced liver uptake and storage, and increased urinary excretion.[44]

Vitamin E

Vitamin E is a potent lipid-soluble antioxidant that prevents the propagation of free radicals.[45] Multiple studies in experimental ALD documented a clear link between oxidative stress and liver damage, and antioxidants, including vitamin E, have been protective in experimental ALD. Vitamin E has been shown to reduce hepatic fat and inflammation in human nonalcoholic steatohepatitis. However, Mezey and colleagues[46] tested the effects of vitamin E (1000 IU) on laboratory parameters of liver function in patients with mild to moderate AH and found no beneficial effect.

Zinc

Zinc deficiency is found in approximately 83% of patients with cirrhosis, correlating with disease severity and with decrease transplant-free survival.[47] Zinc deficiency may present in multiple diverse fashions, including skin lesions, impaired wound healing, altered mental status, or altered immune function.[48] The underlying mechanisms are multiple and include increased urinary zinc excretion, decreased absorption in the intestine, and decreased dietary intake owing to alcohol "empty calories." Zinc deficiency plays a major role in gut barrier dysfunction and dysbiosis in experimental ALD.[49] The dose of zinc used for treatment of AH is usually 50 mg of elemental zinc per day.

Magnesium

Magnesium is an intracellular cation essential for multiple enzymatic reactions. Hypomagnesemia frequently occurs in alcoholics because of vomiting, diarrhea, excessive urinary loss, and an inadequate diet. Prior studies showed that magnesium treatment may decrease levels of AST/ALT and could potentially increase handgrip muscle strength.[50,51] Magnesium deficiency is often associated with muscle cramps, a frequent complaint in patients with AH. Muscle cramps may be treated with 400 mg of magnesium oxide.

SUMMARY

Malnutrition is a common complication of AH, and it correlates directly with degree of liver disease and mortality. Studies have shown that virtually 100% of patients with AH have some degree of malnutrition. Malnutrition is generally defined by a state of inadequate protein and/or calorie intake that results in sarcopenia. The contributing factors to this are numerous and include anorexia/nausea, high intake of empty calories, complications of severe liver disease, and unpalatable or incorrectly recommended diets. Adequate nutrition can be argued as the most critical form of treatment for AH other than abstinence. A prompt evaluation of nutrition risk should be performed in the inpatient setting and in clinic. EN is always preferable, and tube feedings should be considered when oral intake is inadequate. In both the inpatient and outpatient setting, the bedtime snack helps to prevent overnight starvation and muscle breakdown. Patients with AH are at increased risk to develop deficiency of multiple vitamins and minerals. Identification and replacement of these can be critical. Importantly, new observations concerning the gut-liver axis and dysbiosis should lead to exciting potential therapies in the form of prebiotics/probiotics, among others. Overall, nutritional support improves nutritional status and may improve liver function and decrease the risk for liver-related complications and mortality.

FUNDING

C.J. McClain has received funding grants (NIH 1P50AA024337-01, 1P20GM113226-01, 1U01AA026980-01, 1U01AA026934-01, 1U01AA026926-01, 1U01AA026934-01; VA [1I01BX002996-01A2])

CLINICS CARE POINTS

- Alcohol is a major source of empty calories.
- Patients with AH often consume a diet inadequate in protein, and loss of muscle mass is common in AH.
- Nighttime snacks should be prescribed to help prevent muscle loss.
- Deficiencies in micronutrients such as zinc are common in AH, and deficiencies should be replaced with supplementation.

REFERENCES

1. Barve S, Chen SY, Kirpich I, et al. Development, prevention, and treatment of alcohol-induced organ injury: the role of nutrition. Alcohol Res 2017;38(2): 289–302.

2. Durand F, Buyse S, Francoz C, et al. Prognostic value of muscle atrophy in cirrhosis using psoas muscle thickness on computed tomography. J Hepatol 2014;60(6):1151–7.

3. Pirlich M, Schütz T, Spachos T, et al. Bioelectrical impedance analysis is a useful bedside technique to assess malnutrition in cirrhotic patients with and without ascites. Hepatology 2000;32(6):1208–15.

4. Makhija S, Baker J. The Subjective Global Assessment: a review of its use in clinical practice. Nutr Clin Pract 2008;23(4):405–9.

5. Mendenhall CL, Anderson S, Weesner RE, et al. Protein-calorie malnutrition associated with alcoholic hepatitis. Veterans Administration cooperative study group on alcoholic hepatitis. Am J Med 1984;76(2):211–22.

6. Mendenhall CL, Tosch T, Weesner RE, et al. VA Cooperative Study on alcoholic hepatitis. II: prognostic significance of protein-calorie malnutrition. Am J Clin Nutr 1986;43(2):213–8.

7. Mendenhall CL, Moritz TE, Roselle GA, et al. A study of oral nutritional support with oxandrolone in malnourished patients with alcoholic hepatitis: results of a Department of Veterans Affairs cooperative study. Hepatology 1993;17(4): 564–76.

8. Mendenhall CL, Moritz TE, Roselle GA, et al. Protein energy malnutrition in severe alcoholic hepatitis: diagnosis and response to treatment. The VA Cooperative Study Group #275. JPEN J Parenter Enteral Nutr 1995;19(4):258–65.

9. Mendenhall C, Roselle GA, Gartside P, et al. Relationship of protein calorie malnutrition to alcoholic liver disease: a reexamination of data from two Veterans Administration Cooperative Studies. Alcohol Clin Exp Res 1995;19(3):635–41.

10. Singal AK, Kamath PS, Francisco Ziller N, et al. Nutritional status of patients with alcoholic cirrhosis undergoing liver transplantation: time trends and impact on survival. Transpl Int 2013;26(8):788–94.

11. Li F, McClain CJ, Feng W. Microbiome dysbiosis and alcoholic liver disease. Liver Res 2019;3(3):218–26.

12. Broitman SA, Gottlieb LS, Zamcheck N. Influence of neomycin and ingested endotoxin in the pathogenesis of choline deficiency cirrhosis in the adult rat. J Exp Med 1964;119:633–42.

13. Bull-Otterson L, Feng WK, Kirpich I, et al. Metagenomic analyses of alcohol induced pathogenic alterations in the intestinal microbiome and the effect of Lactobacillus rhamnosus GG treatment. PLoS One 2013;8(1):e53028.

14. Wang Y, Kirpich I, Liu Y, et al. Lactobacillus rhamnosus GG treatment potentiates intestinal hypoxia-inducible factor, promotes intestinal integrity and ameliorates alcohol-induced liver injury. Am J Pathol 2011;179(6):2866–75.

15. Shao T, Zhao C, Li F, et al. Intestinal HIF-1alpha deletion exacerbates alcoholic liver disease by inducing intestinal dysbiosis and barrier dysfunction. J Hepatol 2018;69(4):886–95.

16. He L, Li F, Yin X, et al. Profiling of polar metabolites in mouse feces using four analytical platforms to study the effects of cathelicidin-related antimicrobial peptide in alcoholic liver disease. J Proteome Res 2019;18(7):2875–84.

17. Duan Y, Llorente C, Lang S, et al. Bacteriophage targeting of gut bacterium attenuates alcoholic liver disease. Nature 2019;575(7783):505–11.

18. Bode JC, Bode C, Heidelbach R, et al. Jejunal microflora in patients with chronic alcohol abuse. Hepato-Gastroenterol. 1984;31(1):30–4.

19. Bajaj JS, Hylemon P, Heuman DM, et al. The cirrhosis dysbiosis ratio provides insight into gut microbiome changes across the spectrum of cirrhosis: a prospective study of 250 patients. Hepatology 2013;58:274a.

20. Smirnova E, Puri P, Muthiah MD, et al. Fecal microbiome distinguishes alcohol consumption from alcoholic hepatitis but does not discriminate disease severity. Hepatology 2020;72(1):271–86.

21. Adachi Y, Moore LE, Bradford BU, et al. Antibiotics prevent liver injury in rats following long-term exposure to ethanol. Gastroenterology 1995;108(1):218–24.

22. Keshavarzian A, Choudhary S, Holmes EW, et al. Preventing gut leakiness by oats supplementation ameliorates alcohol-induced liver damage in rats. J Pharmacol Exp Ther 2001;299(2):442–8.

23. Nanji AA, Khettry U, Sadrzadeh SM. Lactobacillus feeding reduces endotoxemia and severity of experimental alcoholic liver (disease). Proc Soc Exp Biol Med 1994;205(3):243–7.

24. Sehrawat TS, Liu M, Shah VH. The knowns and unknowns of treatment for alcoholic hepatitis. Lancet Gastroenterol Hepatol 2020;5(5):494–506.

25. Bajaj JS, Saeian K, Christensen KM, et al. Probiotic yogurt for the treatment of minimal hepatic encephalopathy. Am J Gastroenterol 2008;103(7):1707–15.

26. Cabre E, Rodriguez-Iglesias P, Caballeria J, et al. Short- and long-term outcome of severe alcohol-induced hepatitis treated with steroids or enteral nutrition: a multicenter randomized trial. Hepatology 2000;32(1):36–42.

27. Moreno C, Deltenre P, Senterre C, et al. Intensive enteral nutrition is ineffective for patients with severe alcoholic hepatitis treated with corticosteroids. Gastroenterology 2016;150(4):903–910 e908.

28. Plauth M, Cabre E, Riggio O, et al. ESPEN guidelines on enteral nutrition: liver disease. Clin Nutr 2006;25(2):285–94.

29. McClave SA, Taylor BE, Martindale RG, et al. Guidelines for the provision and assessment of nutrition support therapy in the adult critically ill patient: Society of Critical Care Medicine (SCCM) and American Society for Parenteral and Enteral Nutrition (A.S.P.E.N.). JPEN J Parenter Enteral Nutr 2016;40(2): 159–211.

30. Excellence NIfHaC. Nutrition support in adults Clinical guideline CG32. 2006 2006. Available at: www.nice.org.uk/page.aspx?o=cg032. Accessed November 23, 2020.

31. Hirsch S, Bunout D, de la Maza P, et al. Controlled trial on nutrition supplementation in outpatients with symptomatic alcoholic cirrhosis. JPEN J Parenter Enteral Nutr 1993;17(2):119–24.

32. Hirsch S, de la Maza MP, Gattas V, et al. Nutritional support in alcoholic cirrhotic patients improves host defenses. J Am Coll Nutr 1999;18(5):434–41.

33. Owen OE, Trapp VE, Reichard GA Jr, et al. Nature and quantity of fuels consumed in patients with alcoholic cirrhosis. J Clin Invest 1983;72(5): 1821–32.

34. Vaisman N, Katzman H, Carmiel-Haggai M, et al. Breakfast improves cognitive function in cirrhotic patients with cognitive impairment. Am J Clin Nutr 2010; 92(1):137–40.

35. Plank LD, Gane EJ, Peng S, et al. Nocturnal nutritional supplementation improves total body protein status of patients with liver cirrhosis: a randomized 12-month trial. Hepatology 2008;48(2):557–66.

36. Wang M, Zhang X, Ma LJ, et al. Omega-3 polyunsaturated fatty acids ameliorate ethanol-induced adipose hyperlipolysis: a mechanism for hepatoprotective effect against alcoholic liver disease. Biochim Biophys Acta Mol Basis Dis 2017; 1863(12):3190–201.

37. Huang W, Wang B, Li X, et al. Endogenously elevated n-3 polyunsaturated fatty acids alleviate acute ethanol-induced liver steatosis. Biofactors 2015;41(6): 453–62.

38. Kirpich IA, Miller ME, Cave MC, et al. Alcoholic liver disease: update on the role of dietary fat. Biomolecules 2016;6(1):1.

39. Llopis M, Cassard AM, Wrzosek L, et al. Intestinal microbiota contributes to individual susceptibility to alcoholic liver disease. Gut 2016;65(5):830–9.

40. Venu M, Martin E, Saeian K, et al. High prevalence of vitamin A deficiency and vitamin D deficiency in patients evaluated for liver transplantation. Liver Transpl 2013;19(6):627–33.

41. Abbott-Johnson WJ, Kerlin P, Abiad G, et al. Dark adaptation in vitamin A-deficient adults awaiting liver transplantation: improvement with intramuscular vitamin A treatment. Br J Ophthalmol 2011;95:544–8.

42. Kizilgul M, Ozcelik O, Delibasi T. Bone health and vitamin D status in alcoholic liver disease. Indian J Gastroenterol 2016;35(4):253–9.

43. Ermens AA, Vlasveld LT, Lindemans J. Significance of elevated cobalamin (vitamin B12) levels in blood. Clin Biochem 2003;36(8):585–90.

44. Medici V, Halsted CH. Folate, alcohol, and liver disease. Mol Nutr Food Res 2013; 57(4):596–606.

45. Beier JI, Arteel GE, McClain CJ. Advances in alcoholic liver disease. Curr Gastroenterol Rep 2011;13(1):56–64.

46. Mezey E, Potter JJ, Rennie-Tankersley L, et al. A randomized placebo controlled trial of vitamin E for alcoholic hepatitis. J Hepatol 2004;40(1):40–6.

47. Sengupta S, Wroblewski K, Aronsohn A, et al. Screening for zinc deficiency in patients with cirrhosis: when should we start? Dig Dis Sci 2015;60(10):3130–5.

48. Mohammad MK, Zhou Z, Cave M, et al. Zinc and liver disease. Nutr Clin Pract 2012;27(1):8–20.

49. Zhong W, Wei X, Hao L, et al. Paneth cell dysfunction mediates alcohol-related steatohepatitis through promoting bacterial translocation in mice: role of zinc deficiency. Hepatology 2020;71(5):1575–91.

50. Poikolainen K, Alho H. Magnesium treatment in alcoholics: a randomized clinical trial. Subst Abuse Treat Prev Policy 2008;3:1.

51. Gullestad L, Dolva LO, Soyland E, et al. Oral magnesium supplementation improves metabolic variables and muscle strength in alcoholics. Alcohol Clin Exp Res 1992;16(5):986–90.

Diagnosis of Alcohol-Associated Hepatitis
When Is Liver Biopsy Required?

Juan Pablo Arab, MD[a,b], Marco Arrese, MD[a,b],
Ashwani K. Singal, MD, MS[c],*

KEYWORDS

- Histology • Alcohol-associated liver disease • Alcohol-associated hepatitis
- Acute on chronic liver failure

KEY POINTS

- Liver biopsy is recommended to determine the diagnosis of alcohol-associated hepatitis (AH) in asymptomatic patients with either transaminitis and/or with steatosis.
- Among patients with alcohol-associated liver disease presenting with jaundice, liver biopsy is recommended to establish the diagnosis of AH if the clinical diagnosis is uncertain.
- When needed, transjugular route is recommended to biopsy in symptomatic patients suspected to have AH.
- Clinical evaluation and scoring systems are used to gauge the prognosis and disease severity of patients with AH, and liver biopsy currently is not recommended for this purpose.

INTRODUCTION

Alcohol-associated liver disease (ALD) is caused by heavy alcohol consumption defined as three or more drinks in males and two or more drinks in females within the last at least 12 months.[1,2] The histologic spectrum of ALD includes steatosis, steatohepatitis, fibrosis, and cirrhosis.[3] Alcohol-associated hepatitis (AH) is a unique

Grant support: J.P. Arab and M. Arrese are supported by the Chilean government through the Fondo Nacional de Desarrollo Científico y Tecnológico (FONDECYT 1200227 and 1191145) and the Commission Nacional de Investigación Científica y Tecnológica (CONICYT, AFB170005, and CARE Chile UC).
Conflict of Interest: The authors declare no conflict of interest.
[a] Department of Gastroenterology and Hepatology, Escuela de Medicina, Pontificia Universidad Católica de Chile, Av Libertador Bernardo O'Higgins 340, Santiago, Región Metropolitana, Chile; [b] Departamento de Biología Celular y Molecular, Centro de Envejecimiento y Regeneración (CARE), Facultad de Ciencias Biológicas, Pontificia Universidad Católica de Chile, Santiago, Chile; [c] University of South Dakota Sanford School of Medicine, McKennan University Hospital Transplant Institute, Cliff Ave., Sioux Falls, SD 57105, USA
* Corresponding author.
E-mail address: ashwanisingal.com@gmail.com
Twitter: @singal_ashwani (A.K.S.)

inflammatory clinical entity in patients with excessive and prolonged alcohol consumption. Among asymptomatic patients, the diagnosis of AH is determined on liver biopsy. Symptomatic AH is characterized by rapid onset of jaundice, often associated with features of systemic inflammatory response syndrome, leading to severe liver injury, with a mortality of up to 40% in those with acute on chronic liver failure (ACLF).[3–6] Over the past decade, consensus on clinical criteria for the diagnosis of AH,[7] and emerging data on the noninvasive biomarkers for the diagnosis and prognosis assessment of patients with ALD, has led to a decrease in the use of liver biopsy.[8–10] In this review, we summarize these data and provide clinical guidance on when to perform liver biopsy in patients with AH.

DIAGNOSIS OF ASYMPTOMATIC ALCOHOL-ASSOCIATED HEPATITIS

Steatosis is the initial histologic feature of ALD with accumulation of fat globules in the liver (macrovesicular steatosis), which may be associated with asymptomatic elevation of alanine aminotransferase and/or aspartate aminotransferase (AST). Over a period of 5 to 10 years, about 25% to 30% develop AH and 10% to 15% progress to cirrhosis.[11–13] Diagnosis of asymptomatic AH can only be made on liver biopsy, which is characterized by steatosis, hepatocyte ballooning with Mallory-Denk bodies, predominantly neutrophilic lobular inflammation, and variable degrees of pericellular fibrosis (**Fig. 1**).[3,4,14]

Although, the histopathologic features of AH may resemble those observed in nonalcoholic steatohepatitis (NASH), there are subtle differences. Mallory-Denk

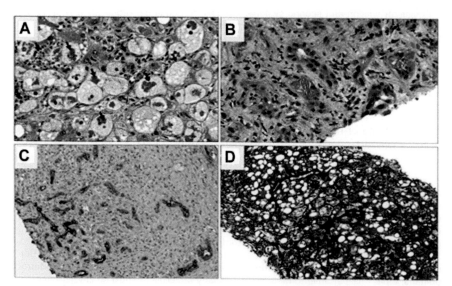

Fig. 1. Histologic findings in alcohol-associated hepatitis. Macrovesicular steatosis is the earliest and most commonly seen histologic feature. Hepatocellular injury is characterized by lobular infiltration of neutrophils (*A, blue arrows*) with ballooned hepatocytes that often contain amorphous eosinophilic inclusions called Mallory-Denk bodies (*A, black arrows*), bilirubin stasis (*B*), ductular reaction (*C*), and liver fibrosis, which is typically described as pericellular and sinusoidal ("chicken wire" appearance) (*D*). (*Adapted from*: Arab JP, Roblero JP, Altamirano J, et al. Alcohol-related liver disease: Clinical practice guidelines by the Latin American Association for the Study of the Liver (ALEH). Ann Hepatol. 2019;18(3):518-535. https://doi.org/10.1016/j.aohep.2019.04.005.)

bodies, neutrophilic infiltrate, and cholestasis are more often found in AH than in NASH.[15] ASH-NASH index based on gender, mean corpuscular volume, and liver enzymes may differentiate AH from NASH.[16] Furthermore, the natural history of AH is worse than other liver diseases including NASH, with higher risk of progression to cirrhosis and its complications.[17–20] Patients with ALD also present more often at an advanced stage of cirrhosis or complications compared with other liver diseases.[18,20,21] For these reasons and nonfeasibility of performing liver biopsy in everyone at risk of ALD including those with steatosis or liver enzyme abnormalities, the true health care burden of asymptomatic AH in the general population remains unknown.

Noninvasive Assessment of Fibrosis

Fibrosis is the most important determinant of long-term outcome in patients with ALD, as in other liver disease.[13,22] Several commercially available patented serum biomarkers, such as enhanced liver fibrosis (ELF), FibroTest, and Hepascore, are useful to assess risk of advanced fibrosis among patients with ALD.[8,9,23] ELF and FibroTest are about 90% accurate in excluding advanced fibrosis in patients with ALD at respective cutoff value less than 10.5 and 0.58.[23] However, patented biomarkers require obtaining special laboratory tests and are also not widely available. For example, ELF requires testing for serum tissue inhibitor of metalloproteinase, amino-terminal procollagen III propeptide, and hyaluronic acid; and FibroTest requires testing for α_2-macroglobulin, haptoglobin, and apolipoprotein. When these patented serum biomarkers are not available, nonpatented serum markers, such as the AST to platelet ratio index, Forn index, and Fibrosis-4 score, are used. A Fibrosis-4 score less than 3.25 is used to exclude advanced fibrosis (**Fig. 2**).[23] Although, nonpatented scores can be calculated using the standard of care laboratory values, their accuracy is lower than patented serum biomarkers.[23]

Liver stiffness measurement (LSM) by transient elastography (TE) or FibroScan is an important tool for the assessment of fibrosis.[8,13,24,25] The advantages of TE are its

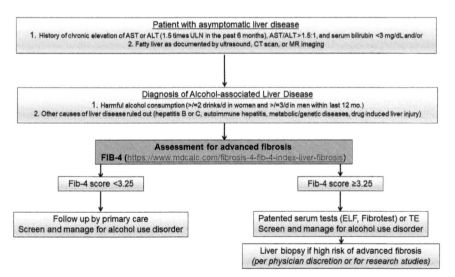

Fig. 2. Proposed algorithm in the assessment of fibrosis in patients with early asymptomatic alcohol-associated liver disease. ALT, alanine aminotransferase; CT, computed tomography; Fib-4, Fibrosis-4 score; TE, transient elastography; ULN, upper limit of normal.

availability, ability to be used as a point-of-care test, simple technique to learn by nurses and advanced providers, lower cost compared with other radiologic-based liver stiffness assessments, and standardization across different machines. The cutoff value of LSM to define advanced fibrosis and cirrhosis is higher in patients with ALD at 12.5 to 15.0 kPa, with sensitivity and specificity of 86% and 94%, respectively, for diagnosis of advanced fibrosis or cirrhosis.[23] Elevated AST and/or bilirubin levels and recent alcohol intake should be accounted for while interpreting the TE results, because these factors may be associated with falsely higher LSM values. If needed, elastography may be repeated after abstaining alcohol for 2 weeks.[9] Serum biomarkers and ultrasound-based LSM assessment are accurate in identifying patients with ALD at low to intermediate risk of advanced fibrosis. Magnetic resonance elastography has better accuracy compared with TE to diagnose advanced fibrosis in patients with ALD.[26] With ability to obtain two- or three-dimensional view, magnetic resonance elastography provides the LSM of the entire liver, and is performed in patients with morbid obesity and those with ascites. However, this technique is more expensive and is available only at specialized centers. Unlike chronic viral hepatitis and nonalcoholic fatty liver disease, combination approach of using serum and radiologic evaluation does not increase the accuracy of fibrosis assessment.[9,23] A sequential approach with TE in those at high risk of advanced fibrosis based on serum biomarkers is a cost-effective strategy, and significantly reduces the need for liver biopsy (see **Fig. 2**).

DIAGNOSIS OF SYMPTOMATIC ALCOHOL-ASSOCIATED HEPATITIS
When to Consider Specific Diagnosis of Alcohol-Associated Hepatitis in Decompensated Patients with Alcohol-Associated Liver Disease

Because most patients with AH have underlying advanced fibrosis or cirrhosis,[14,27] it may be important to differentiate whether the decompensation and precipitation of acute worsening is because of AH or secondary to non-AH-related precipitants, such as sepsis or infections, drug-induced liver injury, ischemic hepatitis or portal vein thrombosis, trauma, or development of hepatocellular carcinoma.[6,28-30] Alcohol including AH is also an underreported precipitant of ACLF in patients with chronic liver disease and cirrhosis.[31] Biliary obstruction and cholangitis can mimic clinical presentation of AH, and should be ruled out with appropriate imaging.[14,32]

Corticosteroids are the only available and recommended treatment of patients with severe AH (modified discriminant function score >32 or Model for End-Stage Liver Disease [MELD] score >20).[1,33,34] However, this treatment has several limitations: (1) contraindications in 30% to 40% patients because of ongoing infection/sepsis, gastrointestinal bleeding, and hepatorenal syndrome; (2) unpredictable response rate of around 40% to 60%, evaluable at Day 4 or 7 of treatment using the Lille score; (3) risk of bacterial and/or fungal infections especially among nonresponders to treatment; and (4) survival benefit among responders lasting for a limited period of only 1 month.[35-41] Hence, corticosteroids use is heterogeneous worldwide, and may also vary based on center-specific protocol or provider discretion.[42] Among patients eligible for corticosteroid therapy, it is recommended to have clinical and/or histologic diagnosis of AH.[1,34] Given limited treatment options for AH, several ongoing clinical trials are ongoing to develop effective and safe therapies targeting gut-liver axis, inflammatory signaling, apoptosis, oxidative stress, and hepatic regeneration.[43] Because patients with moderate AH (MELD score <21) may have 1-year mortality risk of 10% to 20%,[44] these trials are also enrolling patients with moderate AH.[43,45] A clinical and/or histologic diagnosis of AH should be determined to decide eligibility of corticosteroids and/or recruitment into clinical trials. Among patients ineligible for steroids and for the clinical trials including those considered for early liver transplantation via exception pathway (not requiring minimum 6 months of abstinence), the treating physician may be at discretion on the need to determine specific diagnosis of AH.

Approach to Diagnosis of Symptomatic Alcohol-Associated Hepatitis

Although liver biopsy is the definitive tool for confirming the diagnosis of AH, it may not be safely feasible in symptomatic patients, especially those with ascites and/or coagulopathy.[7,46] Furthermore, the histologic findings should be correlated with clinical data. For example, in one study 13 of 68 patients with histologic findings of AH did not have clinical syndrome of AH.[28] Histologic findings of AH has also been reported on 22% to 53% of explants from patients undergoing liver transplantation for ALD cirrhosis and greater than or equal to 6 months of abstinence.[47,48]

The National Institute on Alcohol Abuse and Alcoholism (NIAAA) funded consortia in the United States has proposed a set of clinical criteria for the diagnosis of AH (**Box 1**).[7] Obtaining self-reported alcohol consumption including quantity and last alcohol drink may be challenging because of underreporting, the social stigmatization associated with alcohol use disorder, and altered mental status caused by alcohol withdrawal and/or hepatic encephalopathy.[49,50] Hence, this information should be corroborated with family members, close friends, and other providers.[1,51] Biomarkers with objective measurement of alcohol consumption may be more accurate compared with self-reported data.[52] Indirect markers of alcohol consumption, such as serum γ-glutamyltransferase, AST, mean corpuscular volume, and carbohydrate-deficient transferrin, have low specificity.[34,52,53] Emerging biomarkers of alcohol metabolism, such as ethyl glucuronide, ethyl sulfate, and phosphatidylethanol, have better specificity. Ethyl glucuronide and ethyl sulfate, nonvolatile water-soluble metabolites, estimation in urine samples has a sensitivity of 62% to 89% and a specificity of 93% to 99% to identify alcohol use in the last 4 days.[1,34,52–54] Phosphatidylethanol, a phospholipid metabolite of alcohol in red blood cells, can detect alcohol consumption over the last 28 days with a sensitivity of 90% to 99% and specificity of 100%.[34,52,54] It is also important to rule out other causes of liver disease, which may concomitantly be present in patients with ALD or those with heavy alcohol consumption.[55] For example, hepatitis C virus infection has been reported as a cofactor in up to 25% of cases with liver disease.[56–59] Moreover, it is possible that alcohol

---

Box 1
Clinical criteria proposed by the National Institute of Alcoholism and Alcohol Abuse for the diagnosis of alcoholic hepatitis

- Active ongoing alcohol consumption of >2 drinks in women and >3 drinks in men for >6 months.
- Last alcohol drink within previous 60 days before the onset of jaundice.
- Elevated serum levels of AST and ALT greater than 50 IU/L but less than 400 IU/L, with AST/ALT ratio greater than 1.5.
- Sudden onset or worsening of jaundice (serum bilirubin level >3 mg/dL).
- Excluding causes of liver disease other than caused by alcohol consumption.

Abbreviation: ALT, alanine aminotransferase.

constitutes an underreported cause of ACLF, especially in those patients categorized as ACLF of unknown origin.[31] The presence of obesity, type 2 diabetes mellitus, metabolic syndrome, hepatitis B or C infection, and other preexistent chronic liver disease can contribute to the development of severe AH, lowering the threshold of alcohol amount required to cause liver injury.[60] Because the clinical diagnosis of AH may be inaccurate in 4% to 46% cases,[28,61,62] liver biopsy is recommended in those who do not meet one or more of the NIAAA criteria.[7] It may be noted that liver biopsy may also be performed based on practice pattern of individual physicians and centers or as an inclusion criterion for enrollment to a specific clinical trial (**Fig. 3**).

Liver Biopsy in Diagnosis of Symptomatic Alcohol-Associated Hepatitis

Histologically, AH is characterized by the presence of ballooned hepatocytes and polymorphonuclear neutrophils infiltration, detection of Mallory-Denk bodies, and bilirubin stasis and a pericellular/perisinusoidal ("chicken wire") pattern of fibrosis (see **Fig. 1**).[4,14,17,63] In a review of 11 randomized controlled trials on 1668 patients with biopsy-proven AH, clinical diagnosis was accurate in 84.5% patients, and this accuracy increased to 96% in patients with total serum bilirubin greater than 80 μmol/L or greater than 4.7 mg/dL.[61] In another study, 70% of patients with severe AH meeting clinical criteria of AH had histologic confirmation on liver biopsy.[64] However, both these studies are abstract publications. In a recent peer reviewed report on post hoc analysis of a subgroup of 161 patients from the STOPAH study with biopsy-conformed AH, authors made similar observations. In this study, the accuracy of clinical diagnosis using the cutoff bilirubin level of 4.7 mg/dL was 100% in patients with MELD score greater than or equal to 25 and liver biopsy performed before the administration of corticosteroids.[65,66] However, the accuracy was only about 80% in patients with MELD 21 to 24 or after administration of corticosteroids.[65]

LIVER BIOPSY IN PREDICTING PROGNOSIS OF ALCOHOL-ASSOCIATED HEPATITIS

Clinical evaluation and several scoring systems in predicting disease severity and prognosis of patients with AH are available, and these are discussed in detail elsewhere in

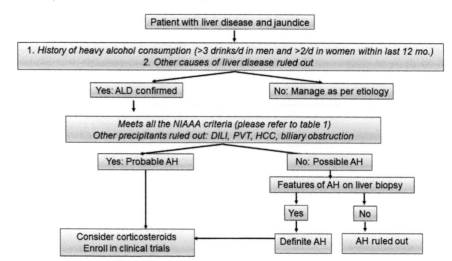

Fig. 3. Proposed algorithm with emphasis on the role of liver biopsy for the diagnosis of severe AH. DILI, Drug Induced Liver Injury; HCC, hepatocellular carcinoma; PVT, Portal Vein Thrombosis.

this issue.[1,33,34,67] Liver biopsy may also predict the disease severity and prognosis based on bilirubin stasis, fibrosis, neutrophilic infiltration, and presence of megamitochondria. The Alcoholic Hepatitis Histologic Score (AHHS) is a semiquantitative tool that was created as a prediction model from a multicentric and international cohort to assess prognosis in AH.[68] Bilirubin stasis and fibrosis were associated with the severity of the disease, whereas neutrophilic infiltration and megamitochondria protected from developing severe disease.[68,69] The observation of the neutrophilic infiltration might be counterintuitive because increased serum white blood cell count confers higher risk of mortality and acute kidney injury in patients with AH.[27,70,71] In another study, AHHS risk stratified patients for 90-day mortality: low-risk group (AHHS 0–3) with mortality rate at 3%, the intermediate-risk group (AHHS 4–5) at 19%, and the high-risk group (AHHS 6–9) at 51%.[68] Similar findings have been reported in other studies.[65,72] One of these studies also examined the role of the Laennec staging system.[72] After controlling for patient age and MELD score, the AHHS and Laennec stage were not associated with short-term survival.[72,73] Note that the AHHS was comparable with the validated modified discriminant function and MELD scores, but did not increase the accuracy of these clinical noninvasive scores in predicting short-term mortality in patients with severe AH.[65,68] However, the AHHS was useful in stratifying patients with moderate AH for 90-day survival at 72% among patients with AHHS greater than 5 and 94% survival among those with AHHS less than or equal to 5.[68]

Histologic findings in severe AH of ballooning degeneration and Mallory-Denk bodies may also help identify patients likely to respond to corticosteroids.[69] However, the AHHS in another study was similar between responders and nonresponders to corticosteroids.[68] Specifically, none of the individual histologic features of the AHHS were associated with the treatment response. Cholestasis ductular or canalicular cholestasis has been shown to be associated with occurrence of bacterial infections in patients with AH.[68]

The agreement between pathologists on reporting cholestasis is excellent with kappa statistics of 0.86 (95% confidence interval [CI], 0.75–0.97). However, the agreement is modest for neutrophilic infiltration in the lobules and poor for presence of megamitochondria, with respective kappa statistics of 0.6 (95% CI, 0.42–0.78) and 0.46 (95% CI, 0.27–0.65), respectively.[68] The kappa statistics on interpretation of liver biopsy by pathologists on histologic findings of AH in another study was 0.89 (95% CI, 0.85–0.92) for steatosis grade, 0.60 (95% CI, 0.49–0.69) for portal fibrosis, 0.65 (95% CI, 0.55–0.73) for lobular inflammation, 0.68 (95% CI, 0.59–0.76) for Mallory-Denk bodies, and 0.40 (95% CI, 0.27–0.52) for hepatocyte ballooning.[74] For accurate interpretation and diagnosis of AH on the liver biopsy, the liver tissue should be adequate with at least five portal triads, and the histology be interpreted by a pathologist with expertise in hepatopathology. Often such an expertise may need to be obtained by sending the frozen sections or stained slides to the specialized centers. Fortunately, the histopathologic features of AH may persist for several months after alcohol cessation, thus providing a wide diagnostic window.[47,48,61,62] However, as mentioned these histologic features may change quickly after treatment with corticosteroids,[65] and this factor must be taken into consideration while interpreting the histologic features.

NONINVASIVE BIOMARKERS IN DIAGNOSIS AND PROGNOSIS OF ALCOHOL-ASSOCIATED HEPATITIS

When needed, liver biopsy is performed via transjugular access, which is technically more feasible in these patients, especially those with ascites and/or coagulopathy.[1,4,14,46,63] The success rate in obtaining adequate biopsy for interpretation is 96% to 98% with a median of 2.7 passes, with an excellent safety pro-file.[75–77] In a systematic review, analysis of more than 7500 transjugular liver biopsy pro-cedures, rates of minor complications, major bleeding, and mortality were encountered in 6.5%, 0.6%, and 0.09%, respectively, which were similar to percutaneous proced-ure.[77] Furthermore, transjugular approach allows measurement of portal pressure that is also helpful to estimate short-term prognosis, because the degree of portal hyperten-sion and hyperdynamic circulation relates to AH severity.[67,78] However, transjugular ac-cess may not be widely available because this requires the expertise of an interventional radiologist, which may only be available in specialized tertiary centers.

Recognizing the need for noninvasive accurate prognostication of patients with AH, several biomarkers have emerged in the last few years for the diagnosis of AH and to assess their prognosis.[10] In a study on 58 patients with suspected AH (43 confirmed on liver biopsy), a white cell count greater than 10.8 and platelet count of greater than 148 in 19 patients had 100% positive predictive value to diagnosis AH. A white cell count less than 6 and platelet count less than 86 in six patients had 83% negative predictive value in excluding the diagnosis of AH. Importantly, the white cell and platelet count were not helpful in 33 patients, where AH diagnosis needed liver biopsy assessment.[79] In another retrospective study, elevated white cell count combined with a nodular liver surface on imaging identified patients with AH with a specificity of 86%, a sensitivity of 59%, and an area under the receiver operating characteristic curve of 0.72. The spec-ificity for diagnosis of AH was 100% with white cell count cutoff at 10 in patients with nodular liver on imaging and 14 in those without nodularity of liver surface.[74]

MicroRNA or noncoding RNA (especially microRNA-30a, 122, and 192) associated with exosomes/extracellular vesicles isolated from sera samples is associated with a diagnosis of AH in decompensated patients with ALD.[80] In another study, quantifying plasma exosomes/extracellular vesicles and sphingolipid cargo signature was useful in differentiating AH from heavy drinkers, decompensated alcoholic cirrhosis, and other etiologies of liver cirrhosis, and in predicting the 90-day survival.[81] Dynamic quantification of exosomes/extracellular vesicles on follow-up has also been shown to be associated with response to therapy in a clinical trial investigating the safety and efficacy of interleukin-22 in patients with AH.[82]

Several other biomarkers, such as serum malondialdehyde (a by-product of lipid per-oxidation),[83] cytokeratin-18 (a marker of hepatocyte apoptosis),[84] osteopontin (protein that mediates diverse biologic functions),[85] serum levels of CCL-20 (a proinflammatory cytokine that mediates lipopolysaccharide-induced liver injury),[10,86] serum interleukin-6 levels,[87] macrophages subtypes with MI:M2 ratio,[88] and changes in the gut microbiota[89] have been examined for the diagnosis and prognosis of AH. Breath levels of volatile com-pounds (eg, trimethylamine, pentane, 2-propranolol, acetone, acetaldehyde, and ethanol) have also been assessed as noninvasive biomarkers for diagnosis of AH; how-ever, these have not shown to be useful in predicting the disease severity.[90] Mitochondrial function and oxygen consumption rate in the purified circulating monocytes has been shown to be useful in diagnosis of AH in decompensated patients with ALD.[10,91] Genetic polymorphisms especially of the patatin-like phospholipase domain protein 3 (*PNPLA3*) with an isoleucine-to-methionine substitution at position 148 (rs738409 C>G), TM6SF2, MBOAT7, and HSD17B13 have been shown to be associated with propensity to devel-opment of AH and are discussed in detail elsewhere in this issue.[92–95]

SUMMARY

Among patients with decompensated ALD, there should be low threshold for suspect-ing AH. Advances have been made to diagnose AH using the clinical criteria proposed by the NIAAA. However, liver biopsy may be required when the clinical diagnosis is uncertain, especially in patients with moderate AH. When needed, a transjugular route is preferred in these sick patients with ascites and/or coagulopathy. Over the last decade or so, conflicting data have emerged on the role of liver biopsy in estimating disease severity and outcomes. Data are also emerging on several noninvasive biomarkers for diagnosis and prognostication of patients with AH. However, the use of these biomarkers in clinical practice is limited because of lack of validation in large patient cohorts, difficult technique, availability only for research studies, and high cost.[10,95] Multicentric prospective studies are needed to examine combination of clinical and histologic assessment versus either alone and validated simple noninvasive biomarkers in predicting the prognosis of AH. In this regard, the data obtained from ongoing clinical trials requiring liver biopsy for patient recruitment will be useful to further substantiate the role of liver biopsy in patients with AH.

CLINICS CARE POINTS

- Among patients with decompensated alcohol-associated liver disease, liver biopsy is recommended to diagnose when the clinical diagnosis of alcoholic hepatitis as a precipitant of decompensation is uncertain.
- Liver biopsy is not recommended for estimating the prognosis of alcoholic hepatitis.
- There is a clinical unmet need for non-invasive simple accurate biomarkers for diagnosis and predicting prognosis of alcoholic hepatitis among patients with decompensated alcohol-associated liver disease.

REFERENCES

1. Singal AK, Bataller R, Ahn J, et al. ACG clinical guideline: alcoholic liver disease. Am J Gastroenterol 2018;113(2):175–94.
2. Global status report on alcohol and health. World Health Organization; 2018.
3. Gao B, Bataller R. Alcoholic liver disease: pathogenesis and new therapeutic targets. Gastroenterology 2011;141(5):1572–85.
4. Lucey MR, Mathurin P, Morgan TR. Alcoholic hepatitis. N Engl J Med 2009; 360(26):2758–69.
5. Thursz MR, Richardson P, Allison M, et al. Prednisolone or pentoxifylline for alcoholic hepatitis. N Engl J Med 2015;372(17):1619–28.
6. Singal AK, Arora S, Wong RJ, et al. Increasing burden of acute-on-chronic liver failure among alcohol-associated liver disease in the young population in the United States. Am J Gastroenterol 2020;115(1):88–95.
7. Crabb DW, Bataller R, Chalasani NP, et al. Standard definitions and common data elements for clinical trials in patients with alcoholic hepatitis: recommendation from the NIAAA alcoholic hepatitis consortia. Gastroenterology 2016;150(4): 785–90.
8. Altamirano J, Qi Q, Choudhry S, et al. Non-invasive diagnosis: non-alcoholic fatty liver disease and alcoholic liver disease. Transl Gastroenterol Hepatol 2020;5:31.
9. Moreno C, Mueller S, Szabo G. Non-invasive diagnosis and biomarkers in alcohol-related liver disease. J Hepatol 2019;70(2):273–83.
10. Singal AK, Bailey SM. Cellular abnormalities and emerging biomarkers in alcohol-associated liver disease. Gene Expr 2018;19(1):49–60.
11. Teli MR, Day CP, Burt AD, et al. Determinants of progression to cirrhosis or fibrosis in pure alcoholic fatty liver. Lancet 1995;346(8981):987–90.

12. Deleuran T, Gronbaek H, Vilstrup H, et al. Cirrhosis and mortality risks of biopsy-verified alcoholic pure steatosis and steatohepatitis: a nationwide registry-based study. Aliment Pharmacol Ther 2012;35(11):1336–42.

13. Parker R, Aithal GP, Becker U, et al. Natural history of histologically proven alcohol-related liver disease: a systematic review. J Hepatol 2019;71:586–93.

14. Singal AK, Louvet A, Shah VH, et al. Grand rounds: alcoholic hepatitis. J Hepatol 2018;69(2):534–43.

15. Tannapfel A, Denk H, Dienes HP, et al. Histopathological diagnosis of non-alcoholic and alcoholic fatty liver disease. Virchows Arch 2011;458(5):511–23.

16. Dunn W, Angulo P, Sanderson S, et al. Utility of a new model to diagnose an alcohol basis for steatohepatitis. Gastroenterology 2006;131(4):1057–63.

17. Arab JP, Roblero JP, Altamirano J, et al. Alcohol-related liver disease: clinical practice guidelines by the Latin American Association for the Study of the Liver (ALEH). Ann Hepatol 2019;18(3):518–35.

18. Shoreibah M, Raff E, Bloomer J, et al. Alcoholic liver disease presents at advanced stage and progresses faster compared to non-alcoholic fatty liver disease. Ann Hepatol 2016;15(2):183–9.

19. Dam-Larsen S, Franzmann M, Andersen IB, et al. Long term prognosis of fatty liver: risk of chronic liver disease and death. Gut 2004;53(5):750–5.

20. Shah ND, Ventura-Cots M, Abraldes JG, et al. Alcohol-related liver disease is rarely detected at early stages compared with liver diseases of other etiologies worldwide. Clin Gastroenterol Hepatol 2019;17(11):2320–9.e2312.

21. Askgaard G, Leon DA, Kjaer MS, et al. Risk for alcoholic liver cirrhosis after an initial hospital contact with alcohol problems: a nationwide prospective cohort study. Hepatology 2017;65(3):929–37.

22. Lackner C, Spindelboeck W, Haybaeck J, et al. Histological parameters and alcohol abstinence determine long-term prognosis in patients with alcoholic liver disease. J Hepatol 2017;66(3):610–8.

23. Thiele M, Madsen BS, Hansen JF, et al. Accuracy of the enhanced liver fibrosis test vs FibroTest, elastography, and indirect markers in detection of advanced fibrosis in patients with alcoholic liver disease. Gastroenterology 2018;154(5):1369–79.

24. Nguyen-Khac E, Thiele M, Voican C, et al. Non-invasive diagnosis of liver fibrosis in patients with alcohol-related liver disease by transient elastography: an individual patient data meta-analysis. Lancet Gastroenterol Hepatol 2018;3(9):614–25.

25. Thiele M, Detlefsen S, Sevelsted Moller L, et al. Transient and 2-dimensional shear-wave elastography provide comparable assessment of alcoholic liver fibrosis and cirrhosis. Gastroenterology 2016;150(1):123–33.

26. Bensamoun SF, Leclerc GE, Debernard L, et al. Cutoff values for alcoholic liver fibrosis using magnetic resonance elastography technique. Alcohol Clin Exp Res 2013;37(5):811–7.

27. Sujan R, Cruz-Lemini M, Altamirano J, et al. A validated score predicts acute kidney injury and survival in patients with alcoholic hepatitis. Liver Transpl 2018;24(12):1655–64.

28. Mookerjee RP, Lackner C, Stauber R, et al. The role of liver biopsy in the diagnosis and prognosis of patients with acute deterioration of alcoholic cirrhosis. J Hepatol 2011;55(5):1103–11.

29. Gustot T, Jalan R. Acute-on-chronic liver failure in patients with alcohol-related liver disease. J Hepatol 2019;70(2):319–27.

30. Singal AK, Kamath PS. Acute on chronic liver failure in non-alcoholic fatty liver and alcohol associated liver disease. Transl Gastroenterol Hepatol 2019;4:74.

31. Moreau R, Jalan R, Gines P, et al. Acute-on-chronic liver failure is a distinct syndrome that develops in patients with acute decompensation of cirrhosis. Gastroenterology 2013;144(7):1426–37, 1437 e1421-1429.
32. Singal AK, Shah VH. Therapeutic strategies for the treatment of alcoholic hepatitis. Semin Liver Dis 2016;36(1):56–68.
33. Crabb DW, Im GY, Szabo G, et al. Diagnosis and treatment of alcohol-related liver diseases: 2019 practice guidance from the American Association for the Study of Liver Diseases. Hepatology 2019;71:306–33.
34. EASL Clinical Practice Guidelines on nutrition in chronic liver disease. J Hepatol 2019;70(1):172–93.
35. Singh S, Murad MH, Chandar AK, et al. Comparative effectiveness of pharmacological interventions for severe alcoholic hepatitis: a systematic review and network meta-analysis. Gastroenterology 2015;149(4):958–70.e912.
36. Thursz M, Morgan TR. Treatment of severe alcoholic hepatitis. Gastroenterology 2016;150(8):1823–34.
37. Louvet A, Thursz MR, Kim DJ, et al. Corticosteroids reduce risk of death within 28 days for patients with severe alcoholic hepatitis, compared with pentoxifylline or placebo-a meta-analysis of individual data from controlled trials. Gastroenterology 2018;155(2):458–68.e458.
38. Louvet A, Naveau S, Abdelnour M, et al. The Lille model: a new tool for therapeutic strategy in patients with severe alcoholic hepatitis treated with steroids. Hepatology 2007;45(6):1348–54.
39. Louvet A, Wartel F, Castel H, et al. Infection in patients with severe alcoholic hepatitis treated with steroids: early response to therapy is the key factor. Gastroenterology 2009;137(2):541–8.
40. Hmoud BS, Patel K, Bataller R, et al. Corticosteroids and occurrence of and mortality from infections in severe alcoholic hepatitis: a meta-analysis of randomized trials. Liver Int 2016;36(5):721–8.
41. Vergis N, Atkinson SR, Knapp S, et al. In patients with severe alcoholic hepatitis, prednisolone increases susceptibility to infection and infection-related mortality, and is associated with high circulating levels of bacterial DNA. Gastroenterology 2017;152(5):1068–77.e1064.
42. Singal AK, Salameh H, Singal A, et al. Management practices of hepatitis C virus infected alcoholic hepatitis patients: a survey of physicians. World J Gastrointest Pharmacol Ther 2013;4(2):16–22.
43. Singal AK, Shah VH. Current trials and novel therapeutic targets for alcoholic hepatitis. J Hepatol 2019;70(2):305–13.
44. Degre D, Stauber RE, Englebert G, et al. Long-term outcomes in patients with decompensated alcohol-related liver disease, steatohepatitis and Maddrey's discriminant function <32. J Hepatol 2020;72:636–42.
45. Thursz M, Kamath PS, Mathurin P, et al. Alcohol-related liver disease: areas of consensus, unmet needs and opportunities for further study. J Hepatol 2019; 70(3):521–30.
46. Rockey DC, Caldwell SH, Goodman ZD, et al. Liver biopsy. Hepatology 2009; 49(3):1017–44.
47. Wells JT, Said A, Agni R, et al. The impact of acute alcoholic hepatitis in the explanted recipient liver on outcome after liver transplantation. Liver Transpl 2007; 13(12):1728–35.
48. Tome S, Martinez-Rey C, Gonzalez-Quintela A, et al. Influence of superimposed alcoholic hepatitis on the outcome of liver transplantation for end-stage alcoholic liver disease. J Hepatol 2002;36(6):793–8.

49. Kranzler HR, Soyka M. Diagnosis and pharmacotherapy of alcohol use disorder: a review. JAMA 2018;320(8):815–24.

50. O'Connor EA, Perdue LA, Senger CA, et al. Screening and behavioral counseling interventions to reduce unhealthy alcohol use in adolescents and adults: updated evidence report and systematic review for the US preventive services task force. JAMA 2018;320(18):1910–28.

51. Mathurin P, Lucey MR. Liver transplantation in patients with alcohol-related liver disease: current status and future directions. Lancet Gastroenterol Hepatol 2020;5(5):507–14.

52. Wozniak MK, Wiergowski M, Namiesnik J, et al. Biomarkers of alcohol consumption in body fluids: possibilities and limitations of application in toxicological analysis. Curr Med Chem 2019;26(1):177–96.

53. Staufer K, Andresen H, Vettorazzi E, et al. Urinary ethyl glucuronide as a novel screening tool in patients pre- and post-liver transplantation improves detection of alcohol consumption. Hepatology 2011;54(5):1640–9.

54. Fleming MF, Smith MJ, Oslakovic E, et al. Phosphatidylethanol detects moderate-to-heavy alcohol use in liver transplant recipients. Alcohol Clin Exp Res 2017; 41(4):857–62.

55. Russ KB, Chen NW, Kamath PS, et al. Alcohol use after liver transplantation is independent of liver disease etiology. Alcohol Phosphatidyl ethanol 2016;51(6):698–701.

56. Jamal MM, Saadi Z, Morgan TR. Alcohol and hepatitis C. Dig Dis 2005;23(3–4):285–96.

57. Singal AK, Anand BS. Mechanisms of synergy between alcohol and hepatitis C virus. J Clin Gastroenterol 2007;41(8):761–72.

58. Shoreibah M, Anand BS, Singal AK. Alcoholic hepatitis and concomitant hepatitis C virus infection. World J Gastroenterol 2014;20(34):11929–34.

59. Singal AK, Kuo YF, Anand BS. Hepatitis C virus infection in alcoholic hepatitis: prevalence patterns and impact on in-hospital mortality. Eur J Gastroenterol Hepatol 2012;24(10):1178–84.

60. Altamirano J, Michelena J. Alcohol consumption as a cofactor for other liver diseases. Clin Liver Dis (Hoboken) 2013;2(2):72–5.

61. Hamid RF. Is histology required for the diagnosis of alcoholic hepatitis? A review of published randomized controlled trials. Gut 2011;60:A233.

62. Elphick DA, Dube AK, McFarlane E, et al. Spectrum of liver histology in presumed decompensated alcoholic liver disease. Am J Gastroenterol 2007;102(4):780–8.

63. Axley P, Russ K, Singal AK. Severe alcoholic hepatitis: atypical presentation with markedly elevated alkaline phosphatase. J Clin Transl Hepatol 2017;5(4):414–5.

64. Dhanda AD, Collins PL, McCune CA. Is liver biopsy necessary in the management of alcoholic hepatitis? World J Gastroenterol 2013;19(44):7825–9.

65. Forrest EP, Austin A, Lloyd K, et al. The diagnostic and prognostic significance of liver histology in alcoholic hepatitis. Aliment Pharmacol Ther 2021;53(3):426–31.

66. Haiar JS. Liver biopsy in alcoholic hepatitis: more clarity on when to do it. Aliment Pharmacol Ther 2021;53(5):630–1.

67. Singal AK, Shah VH. Alcoholic hepatitis: prognostic models and treatment. Gastroenterol Clin North Am 2011;40(3):611–39.

68. Altamirano J, Miquel R, Katoonizadeh A, et al. A histologic scoring system for prognosis of patients with alcoholic hepatitis. Gastroenterology 2014;146(5):1231–9, e1231-1236.

69. Shasthry SM, Rastogi A, Bihari C, et al. Histological activity score on baseline liver biopsy can predict non-response to steroids in patients with severe alcoholic hepatitis. Virchows Arch 2018;472(4):667–75.
70. Michelena J, Altamirano J, Abraldes JG, et al. Systemic inflammatory response and serum lipopolysaccharide levels predict multiple organ failure and death in alcoholic hepatitis. Hepatology 2015;62(3):762–72.
71. Forrest EH, Evans CD, Stewart S, et al. Analysis of factors predictive of mortality in alcoholic hepatitis and derivation and validation of the Glasgow Alcoholic Hepatitis Score. Gut 2005;54(8):1174–9.
72. Dubois M, Sciarra A, Trépo E, et al. Histologic parameter score does not predict short-term survival in severe alcoholic hepatitis. United Eur Gastroenterol J 2020. 2050640620949737.
73. Palmer G, Singal AK. Refining criteria for liver biopsy in severe alcoholic hepatitis: moving the field forward. United Eur Gastroenterol J 2020. 2050640620957140.
74. Roth NC, Saberi B, Macklin J, et al. Prediction of histologic alcoholic hepatitis based on clinical presentation limits the need for liver biopsy. Hepatol Commun 2017;1(10):1070–84.
75. Esposito AA, Nicolini A, Meregaglia D, et al. Role of transjugular liver biopsy in the diagnostic and therapeutic management of patients with severe liver disease. Radiol Med 2008;113(7):1008–17.
76. Soyer P, Fargeaudou Y, Boudiaf M, et al. Transjugular liver biopsy using ultrasonographic guidance for jugular vein puncture and an automated device for hepatic tissue sampling: a retrospective analysis of 200 consecutive cases. Abdom Imaging 2008;33(6):627–32.
77. Kalambokis G, Manousou P, Vibhakorn S, et al. Transjugular liver biopsy–indications, adequacy, quality of specimens, and complications: a systematic review. J Hepatol 2007;47(2):284–94.
78. Rincon D, Lo Iacono O, Ripoll C, et al. Prognostic value of hepatic venous pressure gradient for in-hospital mortality of patients with severe acute alcoholic hepatitis. Aliment Pharmacol Ther 2007;25(7):841–8.
79. Hardy T, Wells C, Kendrick S, et al. White cell count and platelet count associate with histological alcoholic hepatitis in jaundiced harmful drinkers. BMC Gastroenterol 2013;13(1):55.
80. Momen-Heravi F, Saha B, Kodys K, et al. Increased number of circulating exosomes and their microRNA cargos are potential novel biomarkers in alcoholic hepatitis. J Transl Med 2015;13:261.
81. Sehrawat TS, Arab JP, Liu M, et al. Circulating extracellular vesicles carrying sphingolipid cargo for the diagnosis and dynamic risk profiling of alcoholic hepatitis. Hepatology 2021;73(2):571–85.
82. Arab JP, Sehrawat TS, Simonetto DA, et al. An open label, dose escalation study to assess the safety and efficacy of IL-22 agonist F-652 in patients with alcoholic hepatitis. Hepatology 2020;74:441–53.
83. Perez-Hernandez O, Gonzalez-Reimers E, Quintero-Platt G, et al. Malondialdehyde as a prognostic factor in alcoholic hepatitis. Alcohol Simonetta 2017; 52(3):305–10.
84. Woolbright BL, Bridges BW, Dunn W, et al. Cell death and prognosis of mortality in alcoholic hepatitis patients using plasma keratin-18. Gene Expr 2017;17(4): 301–12.
85. Morales-Ibanez O, Dominguez M, Ki SH, et al. Human and experimental evidence supporting a role for osteopontin in alcoholic hepatitis. Hepatology 2013;58(5):1742–56.

86. Affo S, Morales-Ibanez O, Rodrigo-Torres D, et al. CCL20 mediates lipopolysaccharide induced liver injury and is a potential driver of inflammation and fibrosis in alcoholic hepatitis. Gut 2014;63(11):1782–92.

87. Rachakonda V, Gabbert C, Raina A, et al. Stratification of risk of death in severe acute alcoholic hepatitis using a panel of adipokines and cytokines. Alcohol Clin Exp Res 2014;38(11):2712–21.

88. Wan J, Benkdane M, Alons E, et al. M2 Kupffer cells promote hepatocyte senescence: an IL-6-dependent protective mechanism against alcoholic liver disease. Am J Pathol 2014;184(6):1763–72.

89. Puri P, Liangpunsakul S, Christensen JE, et al. The circulating microbiome signature and inferred functional metagenomics in alcoholic hepatitis. Hepatology 2018;67(4):1284–302.

90. Hanouneh IA, Zein NN, Cikach F, et al. The breathprints in patients with liver disease identify novel breath biomarkers in alcoholic hepatitis. Clin Gastroenterol Hepatol 2014;12(3):516–23.

91. Chacko BK, Kramer PA, Ravi S, et al. The Bioenergetic Health Index: a new concept in mitochondrial translational research. Clin Sci (Lond) 2014;127(6):367–73.

92. Salameh H, Raff E, Erwin A, et al. PNPLA3 gene polymorphism is associated with predisposition to and severity of alcoholic liver disease. Am J Gastroenterol 2015;110(6):846–56.

93. Liangpunsakul S, Beaudoin JJ, Shah VH, et al. Interaction between the patatin-like phospholipase domain-containing protein 3 genotype and coffee drinking and the risk for acute alcoholic hepatitis. Hepatol Commun 2018;2(1):29–34.

94. Atkinson SR, Way MJ, McQuillin A, et al. Homozygosity for rs738409:G in PNPLA3 is associated with increased mortality following an episode of severe alcoholic hepatitis. J Hepatol 2017;67(1):120–7.

95. Kirpich IA, Warner DR, Feng W, et al. Mechanisms, biomarkers and targets for therapy in alcohol-associated liver injury: from genetics to nutrition: summary of the ISBRA 2018 symposium. Alcohol 2020;83:105–14.

Assessing the Severity and Prognosis of Alcoholic Hepatitis

Arnab Mitra, MD, MS*, Lauren Myers, MMSc, PA-C,
Joseph Ahn, MD, MS, MBA

KEYWORDS

• Alcoholic hepatitis • Severity • Prognosis

KEY POINTS

- Alcoholic hepatitis can be associated with increased short-term mortality especially with associated risk of acute kidney injury and infection.
- Multiple models and scoring systems, including Maddrey's discriminant function and the MELD score, have been validated to predict mortality and determine whether corticosteroid therapy should be considered.
- Multiple other biomarkers are being investigated as possible alternatives that might better inform severity and prognosis compared with current tools available.

INTRODUCTION

Acute alcoholic hepatitis (AAH) is a clinical entity of increasing importance. It is defined as an acute inflammatory syndrome with associated jaundice and liver injury in the context of significant alcohol consumption.[1] The clinical impact of AAH is readily apparent, as it accounts for approximately 4 out of every 100,000 US hospital admissions and approximately 10% of deaths secondary to alcohol-related liver disease.[2,3] There are varying degrees of severity leading to varying clinical outcomes.

Several scoring systems and criteria have been used to inform the severity and prognosis of AAH, including the Model for End-Stage Liver Disease (MELD) Score and Maddrey's discriminant function (MDF). These 2 scores are the most commonly used by practitioners, with other scoring systems, such as the ABIC (age, serum bilirubin, international normalized ratio [INR], and serum creatinine) score, Glasgow Alcoholic Hepatitis Score (GAHS), and MELD-Lille, also demonstrated to be helpful tools. This review discusses the aforementioned validated models to inform severity and prognosis and bring to light other biomarkers that are currently being studied.

Division of Gastroenterology and Hepatology, Department of Medicine, Oregon Health and Science University, 3181 Southwest Sam Jackson Park Road, L461, Portland, OR 97239-3098, USA
* Corresponding author.
E-mail address: mitraa@ohsu.edu

Clin Liver Dis 25 (2021) 585–593
https://doi.org/10.1016/j.cld.2021.03.004
1089-3261/21/© 2021 Elsevier Inc. All rights reserved.
liver.theclinics.com

NATURAL HISTORY

AAH has a wide spectrum of severity. Mild to moderate disease often improves with alcohol cessation and nutritional support but is still associated with a short-term mortality that is not insignificant, reported to be 10% to 15%.[4] Severe AAH however can certainly be more problematic, as it is associated with acute kidney injury and increased risk of infection. Mortality associated with severe AAH in earlier studies has been reported to be 30% to 50% at 28 days, and potentially up to 70% at 6 months in the presence of persistent hepatic impairment/nonresponse to medical therapy.[5–7] More recent studies suggest short-term mortality could be closer to 14% to 18%.[8–12] Corticosteroid therapy is often considered in the setting of severe AAH, because it can lead to significant improvement in liver tests and overall clinical course, potentially with a short-term mortality benefit. The use of steroids can be associated with harm given an increased reported rate of infections, reported up to 50%.[13,14] For those who do not respond to corticosteroid therapy, liver transplant is being increasingly considered as an option, with similar 1- and 3-year survival compared with those transplanted for other indications.[15]

ESTABLISHED MODELS/SCORING SYSTEMS
Maddrey's Discriminant Function

MDF is used heavily in determining the severity of AAH. This model was originally derived from an early clinical trial for patients with alcoholic hepatitis, demonstrating a 28-day mortality reaching 30% to 50% above a score of 32 in addition to a mortality benefit for those receiving corticosteroid therapy.[5] Short-term mortality benefit for prednisolone therapy in severe AAH has been in question and previously shown in other studies, with 6% mortality at 28 days compared with 35% in the placebo group.[16] In the largest to-date placebo-controlled trial for corticosteroid therapy in alcoholic hepatitis, the STOPAH trial initially on cross-sectional analysis did not demonstrate mortality benefit. However, on post hoc analysis, it reported an approximate 40% mortality improvement at 28 days, although no mortality benefit was seen at 90 days or 1 year.[13] MDF scores less than 32 are associated with lower risk of short-term mortality although are still associated with an increased mortality approaching 50% at 5 years.[17] Although short-term mortality can be assessed using the MDF calculation, it is not a reliable estimator of long-term mortality. Limitations in using MDF include lower specificity, especially compared with MELD (60 vs 84%).[18] In addition, it is a static score and also requires identification of prothrombin time (PT), which is not commonly reported in the United States.

Lille Score

The Lille score is often used in conjunction with the MDF and comes with a unique aspect in that it incorporates bilirubin measurements at 2 different time points. The score is based off data suggesting that early bilirubin improvement after initiation of corticosteroid therapy is associated with improved prognosis.[19] Furthermore, it is also helpful in predicting those with severe AAH who are unlikely to benefit from further corticosteroid therapy after 7 days. A Lille score calculated to be greater than 0.45 after 7 days of therapy indicates a lack of response to steroids, and associated mortality of 75%.[7] There are newer data to suggest a calculated Lille score at day 4 of corticosteroid therapy has similar accuracy to the calculated score at day 7, potentially reducing unnecessary corticosteroid therapy.[20] A calculated Lille score less than 0.45 indicates a good response to merit continuation of corticosteroid therapy, and furthermore, a score less than 0.25 indicates an improved mortality to 25% at 6 months.[1] The dynamic nature of the Lille score with comparison of bilirubin at days 0 and 7 provides a unique understanding of the trajectory of this illness and generally becomes a very important part of the assessment.

Model for End-Stage Liver Disease Score

The MELD score has also been shown to be a useful tool in assessing prognosis and severity in AAH. MELD has had similar performance to MDF in predicting mortality at 30 days with 86% sensitivity and specificity.[21,22] Furthermore, a score ≥21 predicts a 90-day mortality of 20% with sensitivity and specificity of 75%.[23] Generally, a calculation of MELD and/or MELD-Na on presentation is mostly helpful in determining prognosis. Drawbacks of using MELD include variability in laboratory measurements between institutions,[24] and potential overestimation of mortality if renal function is impaired while liver function improves. Furthermore, there are other factors that can affect the creatinine value, including gender, nutritional status, and age, which can lead to misrepresentations of the MELD score as well.

Glasgow Alcoholic Hepatitis Score

GAHS incorporates variables, including total bilirubin, blood urea nitrogen (BUN), age, PT, and white blood cell count (WBC). The initial study describing this score demonstrated that with a GAHS ≥9, 28-day survival for untreated patients was 52% and 78% in those on corticosteroids.[25] The latter shows that GAHS does provide some insight into short-term mortality and guidance into the threshold of when to initiate corticosteroid therapy. Compared with MDF, an initial study demonstrated that GAHS ≥9 had a lower sensitivity in predicting short-term mortality but a higher specificity (61 vs 27%).[26] This model has only been validated in studies from the United Kingdom, but may be considered to potentially help narrow the pool of patients who steroid therapy may be beneficial in.

Age, Serum Bilirubin, International Normalized Ratio, Serum Creatinine Model

The ABIC model is a predictive score that can help assess short- and longer-term mortality. In the initial study, the ABIC score helped to determine mortality risk at 90 days in those on corticosteroids. Furthermore, these patients were stratified into 3 groups, including low risk (100% survival), medium risk (70% survival) and high risk (25% survival). In addition, patients were able to be further classified according to risk of death at 1 year.[27] This model was validated in a cohort of patients with biopsy-proven alcoholic hepatitis.[28] Given this was studied in a patient population already on corticosteroids, it may be helpful in assessing prognosis while on therapy but not necessarily in the decision-making process in whether therapy should be started.

Model for End-Stage Liver Disease Score–Lille

Studies have also demonstrated the combination of static (MELD) and dynamic (Lille) models as important tools in predicting survival. The MELD-Lille model was shown to be superior to other combinations, including MDF/Lille and ABIC/Lille, with the highest area under the receiver operating characteristic (AUROC) of 0.77 in predicting survival at 2 and 6 months.[29] Patients with MELD 21/Lille 0.45 had almost 2 times the risk of death compared with those patients with MELD 21/Lille 0.16. The advantage of this model is it uniquely provides a continuum for mortality assessment, which is helpful and quite different than other validated prognostic models.

Alcoholic Hepatitis Histologic Score

In addition to laboratory-based markers, histology has also been incorporated as a potential tool to predict prognosis. The development of the Alcoholic Hepatitis Histologic Score incorporated histologic findings, such as degree of fibrosis, neutrophilic infiltration, type of bilirubinostasis, and presence of megamitochondria, that correlated with outcome and prediction of 90-day mortality. Scores of 0 to 3 were associated with 3% mortality, 4 to 5 with 19% mortality, and 6 to 9 with 51% mortality.[30] Although certainly this can be used in prognostication, this does subject the patient to in an invasive procedure that may otherwise not be needed in making the diagnosis of alcoholic hepatitis and furthermore does not provide guidance on potential initiation of therapy, including corticosteroids. **Table 1** summarizes the described scoring systems, including timing of use and associated clinical implications.

OTHER RELATED CLINICAL FACTORS

Infection-related biomarkers, such as serum lipopolysaccharide, bacterial DNA, high-sensitivity C-reactive protein, and procalcitonin, are also associated with increased risk of infection and 90-day mortality.[8] In addition, the presence of SIRS criteria on admission can potentially predict multiorgan failure, including acute kidney injury and death in the setting of severe alcoholic hepatitis.[8] Although these are not tests specific to AAH nor developed to guide decision making around steroids, it is important to be aware of these markers and other associated clinical conditions that would indicate a greater severity of AAH, and a greater potential need for therapeutic intervention.

OTHER PROGNOSTIC AND POTENTIALLY MORE NOVEL TOOLS

Although the aforementioned models and scoring systems have been validated and used readily in clinical settings, there are limitations as well that have been described. The latter underlies the importance of identifying other biomarkers that might be useful in characterizing the severity of condition and the threshold to consider medical therapy.

One biomarker of importance is keratin-18, which is found in epithelial cells and released from hepatocytes upon cell death. Keratin-18 is thought to better reflect the degree of hepatocyte death and severity of liver disease compared with traditional laboratory tests, such as liver enzymes. In AAH, the keratin 18/ALT ratio was found to be elevated compared with control healthy patients. Given its specificity for alcohol-related hepatitis, it may also be used as a marker to differentiate nonalcoholic steatohepatitis, in addition to potentially identifying patients with severe AAH at increased risk of death.[31] In a more recent study, K18 fragments were markedly elevated in severe AAH and were identified to be strong predictors of finding steatohepatitis on liver biopsy. Furthermore, keratin-18 had a strong association with 90-day mortality independent of age and MELD score in untreated patients, and above a threshold of 5 kIU/L, the K18-M30 biomarker predicted ~60% improvement from prednisone.[32]

MicroRNAs are newly emerging biomarkers in alcohol-related liver disease. Increased levels of miR-122, which is a microRNA found primarily in hepatocytes, have been seen in mouse models and humans with alcohol-related liver disease. However, it is hard to differentiate the underlying liver-related cause for elevation, given that it is a nonspecific marker for hepatocyte injury and damage.[33] Furthermore, other microRNAs, such as miR192 and miR-30a, are increased in patients with alcoholic hepatitis.[34] Beyond the above, other identified microRNAs have also been shown to be biomarkers in alcoholic cirrhosis.[35]

Table 1
Scores used in assessing severity and clinical decision making in acute alcoholic hepatitis

Score	Components	When to Use in Clinical Course	Interpretation	Limitations
MDF	• PT (measured and control) • Bilirubin (total)	Initial presentation	Score >32: • High short-term mortality • Consider steroids	Static, unable to estimate long-term mortality, and low specificity
MELD	• INR • Bilirubin (total) • Creatinine • Sodium	Initial presentation	MELD or MELD-Na $\geq$21: • High short-term mortality • Consider steroids	Overestimation of mortality because of incorporation of renal function, and other external factors that can influence creatinine
Lille	• Age • Bilirubin (initial and day 4 or 7) • Albumin • Creatinine • PT	Day 4 and/or day 7 of steroid therapy	Score <0.45: • Good response, continue steroids for 28-d course Score >0.45: • Stop steroids	
MELD-Lille model	Components as above for both scores	Initial presentation	• Provides continuum of mortality risk, potentially more precise • Best combination model at assessing 2 and 6 mo mortality risk	
GAHS	• Age • WBC • BUN • Bilirubin • PT (measured and control)	Initial presentation	Score $\geq$9: • Worse survival at 28 d • Consider steroids • Helpful as adjunct to MDF	Validated only in United Kingdom, less sensitive than MDF and/or MELD for predicting short-term mortality
ABIC	• Age • Bilirubin • INR • Creatinine	Early in clinical course if on steroids	Score >9: • Highest mortality risk Score 6.71–9: • Intermediate mortality risk Score <6.71: • Lowest mortality risk	Only studied in those patients already on corticosteroids, helpful only for prognosis
Alcoholic Hepatitis Histologic Score	Histologic findings	48 h after initial presentation	Scoring system predicts 90 d mortality	Requires invasive test

Cytokine levels have also been identified as potential biomarkers in alcoholic hepatitis, especially in the setting of significant inflammation seen with this condition. Particular cytokines studied include interleukin-8 (IL-8), tumor necrosis factor, and IL-1β, all of which have been shown to be elevated in severe alcoholic hepatitis.[36,37] Furthermore, a model incorporating IL-6, IL-13, and age was shown to be a better predictor of 90-day mortality with superior AUROC compared with the MELD score.[38] Elevated IL-6 in particular at increased levels has also been shown to be associated with increased mortality with MDF greater than 32.[39]

Other biomarkers related to inflammation and macrophage activation are also being studied as predictors of mortality. A recently published study demonstrated an elevation of indicators of gut microbial translocation (endotoxin, bacterial 16S rDNA) and host response indicators (CD14, lipopolysaccharide binding protein [LBP]) in patients with alcoholic hepatitis, with MELD and GAHS found to have a strong correlation with endotoxin levels. Other significant markers found to be elevated in patients with alcoholic hepatitis include High Mobility Group Protein 1 (HMGB1) and osteopontin (OPN), a multifunctional protein involved in neutrophil activation. In addition, a positive correlation of OPN was observed with MELD, GAHS, and LBP levels. Other markers of macrophage activation, such as sCD163 and sCD206, were also observed to have a positive correlation with OPN, HMGB1, LBP, MELD, and GAHS scores. A few biomarkers related to macrophage activation and OPN were significantly higher in nonsurvivors, with sCD14, sCD163, and OPN identified as predictors of organ failure, 90-day mortality, and infection.[40–43] This new research is promising and suggests the discovery of newer more specific biomarkers that have positive correlations with validated scoring systems as previously described.

SUMMARY

AAH is a clinical entity of significant importance. In its severe form, it can be associated with significantly increased short-term mortality. The ability to predict prognosis at time of presentation is crucial, as early intervention with potential corticosteroid therapy may be beneficial in reducing short-term mortality and potential need for liver transplant. MDF and MELD are validated and important models that help predict short-term mortality and guide clinical decision making regarding the use of steroids. Some limitations around MDF include its specificity and calculation of score, and limitations with MELD include incorporation of renal function assessment, which may be affected by other clinical factors and can lead to mischaracterization of mortality risk. The Lille score is an important tool in assessing response to corticosteroid therapy, with newer data suggesting score calculation at day 4 is accurate and can prevent unnecessary steroid use. GAHS can be used to determine if steroid therapy should be considered but has only been validated in the United Kingdom. ABIC can be used to determine level of response and mortality risk for those on corticosteroids. A combined MELD-Lille model was found to be superior to other combination models and offers a continuum to estimate mortality as opposed to other scoring systems. The Alcoholic Hepatitis Histologic Score can estimate the severity of disease and prognosis based off biopsy findings but involves an invasive test that may otherwise not be indicated in determining diagnosis. Other associated conditions with severe AAH, including infection, SIRS, and cytokines, have also been shown to predict mortality.

Overall, there are validated and important models that can help inform severity and prognosis in severe AAH, albeit with some limitations. Novel biomarkers, such as keratin-18, microRNAs, and cytokines, are being studied to identify potentially better and more specific ways to better assess mortality and indicate for corticosteroid therapy in severe AAH.

CLINICS CARE POINTS

- Alcoholic hepatitis is a clinical entity, which in its most severe form, may lead to increased mortality, acute kidney injury, and death.
- A Maddrey discriminant function (MDF) score greater than 32 or MELD-Na $\geq$ 21 predicts increased short-term mortality, and raises consideration for corticosteroid therapy.
- Other models can help to predict response to and associated mortality risk with corticosteroid therapy, estimate severity of disease based off histologic findings, and provide a continuum in estimating overall mortality.
- Other novel biomarkers are being studied to identify potential more specific ways to predict mortality and potential need for corticosteroid therapy.

DISCLOSURE

The authors have nothing to disclose.

REFERENCES

1. Im GY. Acute alcoholic hepatitis. Clin Liver Dis 2019;23(1):81–98.
2. Yang AL, Vadhavkar S, Singh G, et al. Epidemiology of alcohol-related liver and pancreatic disease in the United States. Arch Intern Med 2008;168:649–56.
3. Paula H, Asrani SK, Boetticher NC, et al. Alcoholic liver disease-related mortality in the United States: 1980-2003. Am J Gastroenterol 2010;105:1782–7.
4. Kulkarni K, Tran T, Medrano M, et al. The role of the discriminant factor in the assessment and treatment of alcoholic hepatitis. J Clin Gastroenterol 2004; 38(5):453–9.
5. Maddrey WC, Boitnott JK, Bedine MS, et al. Corticosteroid therapy for alcoholic hepatitis. Gastroenterology 1978;75:193–9.
6. Lucey MR, Mathurin P, Morgan TR. Alcoholic hepatitis. N Engl J Med 2009;360: 2758–69.
7. Louvet A, Naveau S, Abdelnour M, et al. The Lille model: a new tool for therapeutic strategy in patients with severe alcoholic hepatitis treated with steroids. Hepatology 2007;45:1348–54.
8. Michelena J, Altamirano J, Abraldes JG, et al. Systemic inflammatory response and serum lipopolysaccharide levels predict multiple organ failure and death in alcoholic hepatitis. Hepatology 2015;62:762–72.
9. Rambaldi A, Saconato HH, Christensen E, et al. Systematic review: glucocorticosteroids for alcoholic hepatitis—a Cochrane Hepato-Biliary Group systematic review with meta-analyses and trial sequential analyses of randomized clinical trials. Aliment Pharmacol Ther 2008;27:1167–78.
10. Christensen E, Gluud C. Glucocorticoids are ineffective in alcoholic hepatitis: a meta-analysis adjusting for confounding variables. Gut 1995;37:113–8.
11. Pavlov CS, Varganova DL, Casazza G, et al. Glucocorticosteroids for people with alcoholic hepatitis. Cochrane Database Syst Rev 2017;11:CD001511.
12. Mathurin P, Mendenhall CL, Carithers RL Jr, et al. Corticosteroids improve short-term survival in patients with severe alcoholic hepatitis (AH): individual data analysis of

the last three randomized placebo controlled double blind trials of corticosteroids in severe AH. J Hepatol 2002;36:480–7.

13. Thursz MR, Richardson P, Allison M, et al. Prednisolone or pentoxifylline for alcoholic hepatitis. N Engl J Med 2015;372:1619–28.

14. Louvet A, Wartel F, Castel H, et al. Infection in patients with severe alcoholic hepatitis treated with steroids: early response to therapy is the key factor. Gastroenterology 2009;137(2):541–8.

15. Lee BP, Mehta N, Platt L, et al. Outcomes of early liver transplantation for patients with severe alcoholic hepatitis. Gastroenterology 2018;155:422–30.

16. Carithers RL, Herlong HF, Diehl AM, et al. Methylprednisolone therapy in patients with severe alcoholic hepatitis. A randomized multicenter trial. Ann Intern Med 1989;110(9):685–90.

17. Degre D, Stauber RE, Englebert G, et al. Long-term outcomes in patients with decompensated alcohol-related liver disease, steatohepatitis, and Maddrey's discriminant function < 32. J Hepatol 2020;72(4):636–42.

18. Srikureja W, Kyulo NL, Runyon BA, et al. MELD score is a better prognostic model than Child-Turcotte-Pugh score or discriminant function score in patients with alcoholic hepatitis. J Hepatol 2005;42:700–6.

19. Mathurin P, Abdelnour M, Ramond M-J, et al. Early change in bilirubin levels is an important prognostic factor in severe alcoholic hepatitis treated with prednisolone. Hepatology 2003;38(6):1363–9.

20. Garcia-Saenz-de-Secilia M, Duvoor C, Altamirano J, et al. A day-4 Lille model predicts response to corticosteroids and mortality in severe alcoholic hepatitis. Am J Gastroenterol 2017;112:306–15.

21. Sheth M, Riggs M, Patel T. Utility of the Mayo End-Stage Liver Disease (MELD) score in assessing prognosis of patients with alcoholic hepatitis. BMC Gastroenterol 2002;2:2.

22. Mathurin P, O'Grady J, Carithers RL, et al. Corticosteroids improve short-term survival in patients with severe alcoholic hepatitis: meta-analysis of individual patient data. Gut 2011;60(2):255–60.

23. Dunn W, Jamil LH, Brown LS, et al. MELD accurately predicts mortality in patients with alcoholic hepatitis. Hepatology 2005;41:353–8.

24. Lisman T, van Leeuwen Y, Adelmeijer J, et al. Interlaboratory availability in assessment of the model of end-stage liver disease score. Liver Int 2008;28:1344–51.

25. Forrest EH, Morris AJ, Stewart S, et al. The Glasgow Alcoholic Hepatitis Score identifies patients who may benefit from corticosteroids. Gut 2007;56(2):1743–6.

26. Forrest EH, Evans CDJ, Stewart S, et al. Analysis of factors predictive of mortality in alcoholic hepatitis and derivation and validation of the Glasgow Alcoholic Hepatitis Score. Gut 2005;54(8):1174.

27. Dominguez M, Rincón D, Abraldes JG, et al. A new scoring system for prognostic stratification of patients with alcoholic hepatitis. Am J Gastroenterol 2008;103(11):2747–56.

28. Papastergiou V, Tsochatzis EA, Pieri G, et al. Nine scoring models for short-term mortality in alcoholic hepatitis: cross-validation in a biopsy-proven cohort. Aliment Pharmacol Ther 2014;39(7):721–32.

29. Louvet A, Labreuche J, Artru F, et al. Combining data from liver disease scoring systems better predicts outcomes of patients with alcoholic hepatitis. Gastroenterology 2015;149(2):398–406.e8.

30. Altamirano J, Miquel R, Katoonizadeh A, et al. A histologic scoring system for prognosis of patients with alcoholic hepatitis. Gastroenterology 2014;146(5): 1231–9.
31. Vatsalya V, Cave MC, Kong M, et al. Keratin 18 is a diagnostic and prognostic factor for acute alcoholic hepatitis. Clin Gastroenterol Hepatol 2020;18(9): 2046–54.
32. Atkinson SR, Grove JI, Liebig S, et al. In severe alcoholic hepatitis, serum keratin-18 fragments are diagnostic, prognostic, and theragnostic biomarkers. Am J Gastroenterol 2020. https://doi.org/10.14309/ajg.0000000000000912.
33. Bala S, Szabo G. MicroRNA signature in alcoholic liver disease. Int J Hepatol 2012;2012:498232.
34. Momen-Heravi F, Saha B, Kodys K, et al. Increased number of circulating exosomes and their microRNA cargos are potential novel biomarkers in alcoholic hepatitis. J Transl Med 2015;13:261.
35. Moreno C, Mueller S, Szabo G. Non-invasive diagnosis and biomarkers in alcohol-related liver disease. J Hepatol 2019;70(2):273–83.
36. Achur RN, Freeman WM, Vrana KE. Circulating cytokines as biomarkers of alcohol abuse and alcoholism. J Neuroimmune Pharmacol 2010;5:83–91.
37. McClain CJ, Song Z, Barve SS, et al. Recent advances in alcoholic liver disease. IV. Dysregulated cytokine metabolism in alcoholic liver disease. Am J Physiol Gastrointest Liver Physiol 2004;287(3):G497–502.
38. Tornai D, Mitchell MC, McClain CJ, et al. A novel composite score of biomarkers and age predicts mortality in severe alcoholic hepatitis patients. Hepatology 2019;70:835A–6A.
39. Rachakonda V, Gabbert C, Raina A, et al. Stratification of risk of death in severe acute alcoholic hepatitis using a panel of adipokines and cytokines. Alcohol Clin Exp Res 2014;38(11):2712–21.
40. Saha B, Tornai D, Kodys K, et al. Biomarkers of macrophage activation and immune danger signals predict clinical outcomes in alcoholic hepatitis. Hepatology 2019;70(4):1134–49.
41. Forrest E, Storey N, Sinha R, et al. Baseline neutrophil-to-lymphocyte ratio predicts response to corticosteroids and is associated with infection and renal dysfunction in alcoholic hepatitis. Journal of Hepatology 2019;70(1):e47.
42. Tyson LD, Atkinson S, Pechlivanis A, et al. Serum bile acid profiles distinguish severe alcoholic hepatitis from decompensated alcohol-related cirrhosis. Journal of Hepatology 2019;70(15):e108.
43. Perez-Hernandez O, González-Reimers E, Quintero-Platt G, et al. Malondialdehyde as a prognostic factor in alcoholic hepatitis. Alcohol 2017;52:305–10.

Current Therapies for Alcohol-Associated Hepatitis

Haripriya Maddur, MD

KEYWORDS

- Alcohol-associated hepatitis • Corticosteroids • NAC • G-CSF • Pentoxifylline

KEY POINTS

- Treatment options for alcohol-associated hepatitis remain limited at the current time.
- The mainstay of treatment remains corticosteroid therapy.
- Granulocyte colony-stimulating factor has shown promise but warrants study in a more heterogenous population before more widespread use.

INTRODUCTION

Alcohol-associated hepatitis (AAH) remains a difficult-to-treat malady, particularly among those individuals with severe disease. Current treatment options remain limited despite extensive study. Many previously studied therapeutic options have been limited in scope due to minimal efficacy or association with worsening outcomes, that is, increased risk of infection. The following article discusses currently available treatment options for severe AAH in addition to therapies that have been used or studied in the recent past (the treatment of moderate disease is discussed elsewhere in this book).

CORTICOSTEROID THERAPY

The mainstay of treatment of severe AAH remains corticosteroid therapy. The mechanism of action includes inhibition of transcription factors associated with the inflammatory process, such as nuclear factor kappa B, thus leading to decreased levels of circulatory proinflammatory cytokines, specifically, interleukin-8 and tumor necrosis factor alpha (TNF-alpha).[1,2] In addition, corticosteroids have been linked to reductions in intracellular adhesion molecules within hepatic venous blood and hepatocyte membranes.[3]

Initial studies using corticosteroid therapy for treatment of AAH yielded conflicting results.[4–6] Variable results can be attributed to early studies with lack of cohesive treatment targets, that is, use of hepatic encephalopathy as an assessment of treatment response and inclusion of those with mild disease. The preferred corticosteroid

Department of Gastroenterology and Hepatology, Northwestern University Feinberg School of Medicine, 676 North Street Clair, Suite 1900, Chicago, IL 60611, USA
E-mail address: Hmaddur@nm.org

Clin Liver Dis 25 (2021) 595–602
https://doi.org/10.1016/j.cld.2021.03.005
1089-3261/21/© 2021 Elsevier Inc. All rights reserved.

agent was also variable, with some studies including methylprednisolone, whereas others using prednisolone.[4,5] In addition, many early studies included a small number of patients and thus were not powered to a significant degree, hence not supporting widespread use. Meta-analyses performed early on also yielded different conclusions, and thus use of corticosteroid therapy was not a universal practice.[7,8]

However, with the incorporation of the Maddrey discriminant function and tailoring therapy to those with severe disease (ie, discriminant function >32), improved response rates have been reported. A more recent analysis of 3 randomized placebo-controlled clinical trials yielded positive results, with 1-month survival of 84.6% versus 65.1% in the placebo arm.[9] Accordingly, corticosteroid use is currently recommended by both the American Association for the Study of Liver Diseases and European Association of the Study of Liver Diseases for patients with severe AAH without infection.[10,11] It should be noted, however, that controversy remains regarding the use of corticosteroids, with the STOPAH trial (pentoxifylline vs prednisolone) showing favorable treatment effects with corticosteroid therapy, although a subsequent Cochrane review deemed corticosteroids to be ineffective.[12,13] Nonetheless, corticosteroids remain the standard of care for treatment of severe AAH.

Because of the risk of infection, however, a protracted course of therapy is not feasible. The current standard treatment duration is prednisolone for 28 days (with or without taper over a 3-week period).[14] Studies have shown that the risk of infection following a standard course of therapy is highest at 30 to 90 days following therapy.[15] Given the high risk of infection, judicious use of corticosteroids is imperative, thus serving as the impetus for models determining treatment response.

The Lille model was first described in 2007 by Louvet and colleagues, to determine steroid response following 7 days of therapy. By means of logistic regression analysis, this model can determine which patients are nonresponders to therapy at day 7 (approximately 40% of patients). In addition, this model can determine 6-month survival (25% in those with a Lille score of >45 at day 7 vs 85% in those with a Lille score <45 at day 7).[16] More recent literature has suggested that the Lille score calculated at day 4 is equally efficacious at determining 28- and 90-day mortality.[17] The latter is helpful in determining patient disposition in those who are admitted with a diagnosis of AAH in which follow-up is unclear, such that the risk of infection with protracted therapy can be mitigated.

In addition to infection, studies examining corticosteroid therapy have excluded patients with renal failure and gastrointestinal bleeding. Unfortunately, many patients with severe AAH are excluded from therapy based on such criteria, and thus alternate therapies have been explored, among them being pentoxifylline (PTX). In regard to gastrointestinal bleeding, however, there has been one study that demonstrated that once gastrointestinal bleeding has been adequately treated, the use of corticosteroids was safe, with no worsening of survival at 1, 3, and 6 months.[18] It should also be noted that the avoidance of corticosteroid therapy in patient with renal dysfunction is not based on the potential for worsening renal function with treatment, but rather, the lack of appreciable benefit with the use of corticosteroids in the setting of renal dysfunction.[19] Indeed, in the STOPAH trial patients with renal failure were excluded only if creatinine was greater than 5.7 mg/dL.

ANTITUMOR NECROSIS FACTOR TARGETS
Pentoxifylline

Initial interest in the use of pentoxifylline stemmed from its anti-TNF properties, with fewer side effects as compared with corticosteroid therapy. In the recent past, PTX was often used in those patients who had significant contraindications to corticosteroids, although data reported from the STOPAH trial (prednisolone or pentoxifylline for alcoholic hepatitis) has made its use less favorable.[13] That being said, there has been renewed interest in PTX in current clinical trials, and thus it may reemerge as a potential adjunctive agent in the future.

In addition to its anti-TNF properties, studies have demonstrated that PTX enhances blood flow by allowing for deformability of red blood cell membranes, thus contributing to enhanced renal perfusion.[20] Interestingly, despite widespread use in the past, the use of PTX has been based on the results of a single randomized controlled. In this trial, 101 patients were randomized to PTX, 400 mg, three times daily or placebo, with short-term survival better in the treatment arm (75.5%) versus 53.9% in the placebo arm. In addition, those patients randomized to the PTX treatment arm exhibited a decreased incidence of hepatorenal syndrome. Of note, there were no measurable decreases in TNF levels.[21]

Interestingly, when the use of PTX and corticosteroid therapy was reported in the STOPAH trial, PTX was not found to be efficacious.[13] In this trial, a 2 x 2 factorial design was used to examine the efficacy of treatment with corticosteroids and pentoxifylline. A total of 1103 patients with severe AAH were randomized to PTX- and prednisolone-matched placebo, versus prednisolone with a PTX-matched placebo, versus PTX with a prednisolone-matched placebo, versus PTX with prednisolone. There was no mortality reduction with use of PTX. Based on the results of this ground-breaking trial, the use of PTX is not currently recommended. In regard to corticosteroid therapy, although mortality reduction was noted with corticosteroid use at 28 days, it was not statistically significant and was not appreciated at 90 days or at 1 year.

Biological Inhibition of Tumor Necrosis Factor

Other agents that have been explored based on TNF inhibition include etanercept and infliximab. Etanercept, which is a fusion protein that binds to TNF receptors, and infliximab, which is a mono-clonal antibody against TNF, were initially thought to be promising based on pilot data.[22,23] Unfortunately, a subsequent randomized controlled trial with infliximab in conjunction with corticosteroid therapy was halted due to an increased incidence of infection within the treatment arm.[24] It was posited that high-dose infliximab therapy (10 mg/kg) in conjunction with steroid therapy contributed to the increased rate of infection and that more favorable outcomes may have been appreciated with lower dose therapy or the exclusion of adjunctive steroids. Nonetheless, further study with the use of infliximab has not been conducted. In regard to etanercept, randomized controlled trial data not only was associated with increased infection rate but also increased 6-month mortality as compared with placebo.[25] Based on unfavorable randomized controlled data, anti-TNF therapy is not currently recommended as a therapeutic option.

N-ACETYLCYSTEINE

N-acetylcysteine(NAC) is used in the treatment and prevention of acetaminophen (APAP)-induced liver injury based on its ability to restore glutathione and enhance hepatic perfusion.[26] Additional study in the treatment of patients with non–APAP-induced acute liver failure has yielded favorable outcomes.[27] Theorized to enhance recovery based on its antioxidant properties, NAC was trialed in conjunction with glucocorticoid therapy and compared with glucocorticoids alone. Although mortality benefit was appreciated at 1 month (8% in the combination arm vs 24% in the steroid arm alone), this was not sustained long term (no statistically significant reduction in mortality was appreciated at 3 and 6 months posttreatment). Interestingly, fewer deaths related to hepatorenal syndrome were appreciated in the NAC-glucocorticoid arm, in addition to a decreased rate of infection. Although NAC is not currently used as an approved therapy for AAH, there have been recent trials using NAC as adjunctive therapy, including as an adjunct to granulocyte colony-stimulating factor (G-CSF).[28] The latter did not reveal added benefit with the use of NAC, although there may be potential for reexploration as a suitable therapy based on its potential for improving renal function.

GRANULOCYTE COLONY-STIMULATING FACTOR

More recently, there has been significant interest in the role of G-CSF for the treatment of AAH. The basis for the use of G-CSF is recruitment of bone-marrow derived stem cells, thus allowing for hepatocyte cell regeneration by differentiation of bone marrow precursor cells into hepatocytes. Outcomes with the use of G-CSF were initially reported in 2008 in patients with alcohol-associated steatohepatitis.[29] In this study, increases in CD34+ cells (markers of hematopoietic stem cells) were noted in addition to an increase in hepatocyte progenitor cells on histologic sample evaluation. Interestingly, there were no significant improvements in liver function, although this was theorized to be due to lack of power with recommendation for further study to be undertaken.

Subsequent studies using G-CSF have had varying results. In a study evaluating patients with acute-on-chronic liver failure, the use of G-CSF yielded positive results.[30] Additional studies undertaken in Europe using G-CSF for the treatment of acute-on-chronic liver failure and cirrhosis (including a cohort with AAH) have had less favorable results and, in fact, were associated with adverse outcomes, including variceal bleed, adverse cardiovascular events and decompensation of liver disease, and an overall worsening of mortality.[31,32]

Nonetheless, ongoing interest in the use of G-CSF has been seen, and, in 2018, investigators in India published a randomized controlled pilot study evaluating the effect of G-CSF administration versus standard of care (including steroids and/or PTX). The results of this study were positive, with survival of 78.3% in the treatment arm as compared with 30.4% in the standard treatment arm. Significant improvements in Model for End-Stage Lives Disease (MELD) score, discriminant function, and Child-Turcotte-Pugh scores were also seen. Moreover, similar to the initial randomized controlled trial published in 2008, increases in CD34+ cells were seen. Interestingly, exclusionary criteria were similar to that used with corticosteroid therapy (patients with sepsis, gastrointestinal bleeding, and renal failure were excluded).[33]

In a subsequent study evaluating the role of adjunctive NAC to G-CSF that was previously mentioned, although GCSF was superior to standard medical therapy, there was no added benefit of GCSF in regard to a reduction in discriminant function.[28] That being said, additional support for the use of G-CSF in the treatment of AAH was reported in 2019 by the same investigators who reported favorable pilot data in 2018. In this study, patients with histologically proven AAH were administered G-CSF versus placebo for 28 days. Improvements in MELD and discriminant function were appreciated at 90 days in addition to reduction in mortality (35.7%) versus 71.4% within the placebo arm. Moreover, the incidence of infection was less in the G-CSF group (28%) versus 71% in the control group.[34]

Interestingly, there have been 2 recent meta-analyses with differing conclusions. One such recent meta-analysis substantiated the findings that G-CSF improved 90-day mortality with improvements in indices measuring severity (MELD, Child Pugh score, and discriminant function); however, this only included one European study, with the remaining 3 studies from Asia.[35] Another meta-analysis that included patients treated with G-CSF for ACLF and cirrhosis (selecting only those with AAH) showed dissimilar results, with improvements in mortality only seen in patients from Asia and not seen in patients from Europe. In addition, although infection risk was decreased in patients from Asia, this again was not seen in patients included from the European cohort.[36] Although G-CSF seems to be extremely promising, further research in a more heterogenous population is needed before further widespread use can be considered, as favorable results cannot currently be extrapolated to those within the Western hemisphere.

Additional Therapies

Although pharmacologic therapy is often used as first-line therapy, the role of alcohol abstinence is often overlooked. By removing the offending agent, this may allow for prevention of further, ongoing hepatic insult. Alcohol abstinence is often difficult to accomplish in patients with alcohol use disorder, and thus efforts should be made to provide assistance with engaging in alcohol abstinence. Although pharmacotherapy is often considered first, the role of psychotherapy is often overlooked and should be offered.[37] In regard to pharmacologic agents, many are associated with worsening of hepatic function, that is, naltrexone, primarily in those with decompensated disease. Nonetheless, there are agents that have been found to be safe and effective in patients with end-stage liver disease, that is, baclofen, initiated at a starting dose of 5 mg three times daily and accelerated upward as tolerated to reduce alcohol craving.[38] In addition, nutritional support is also often forgotten despite the fact that optimal nutrition is key to improving outcomes. In fact, recent study has indicated that adherence to optimal nutrition management in patients with AAH is quite low (a more in-depth discussion on the role of nutrition in the management of patients with AAH is provided elsewhere in this book).[39,40]

Approach to Treatment

Although extensive study has been undertaken, current treatment options remain limited for patients with AAH. In those patients with severe AAH (ie, discriminant function >32 or MELD >21) alcohol abstinence should be recommended in addition to optimization of nutritional status. If no contraindications to steroid therapy are noted, that is, infection, gastrointestinal bleeding, or renal dysfunction, then consideration for corticosteroid therapy with prednisolone, 40 mg, po daily should be initiated. The Lille score should be calculated at either day 4 or 7, and, if favorable (<0.45), therapy should be continued for a total of 28 days.

In patients who have contraindications to corticosteroid therapy or have an unfavorable Lille score, alternate approaches should be considered. Among these therapies include referral for early liver transplantation, particularly in those individuals with first presentation of AAH, as recently reported outcomes have been quite favorable (a more extensive discussion is noted elsewhere in this book).[41] If the patient is not deemed to be a transplant candidate and continues to show evidence of decompensation, then enrollment in clinical trials should be considered.

SUMMARY

Severe AAH remains a difficult-to-treat condition. Advancements with therapy have been plagued by increased rates of infection and lack of clinical efficacy. Treatment with steroids should be offered as first-line therapy if no contraindications are evident.

Evidence for alternate therapies such as pentoxifylline, NAC, and G-CSF do not have significant supporting evidence and are not currently recommended. Nonetheless, ongoing studies seem promising, and the landscape of treatment options may continue to evolve.

CLINICS CARE POINTS

- Patients presenting with severe alcohol associated hepatitis should be placed on steroid therapy if no contraindications to treatment.
- If gastrointestinal bleeding is amongst the contraindications for steroid therapy, steroids can be initiated once the bleed has been adequately controlled.
- Patients with severe disease with no response or contraindication to steroid therapy should be considered for liver transplant referral.

DISCLOSURE

None.

REFERENCES

1. Barnes PJ, Karin M. Nuclear factor-kappaB: a pivotal transcription factor in chronic inflammatory diseases. N Engl J Med 1997;336(15):1066–71.
2. Taïeb J, Mathurin P, Elbim C, et al. Blood neutrophil functions and cytokine release in severe alcoholic hepatitis: effect of corticosteroids. J Hepatol 2000; 32(4):579–86.
3. Spahr L, Rubbia-Brandt L, Pugin J, et al. Rapid changes in alcoholic hepatitis histology under steroids: correlation with soluble intercellular adhesion molecule-1 in hepatic venous blood. J Hepatol 2001;35(5):582–9.
4. Carithers RL, Herlong HF, Diehl AM, et al. Methylprednisolone therapy in patients with severe alcoholic hepatitis. A randomized multicenter trial. Ann Intern Med 1989;110(9):685–90.
5. Depew W, Boyer T, Omata M, et al. Double-blind controlled trial of prednisolone therapy in patients with severe acute alcoholic hepatitis and spontaneous encephalopathy. Gastroenterology 1980;78(3):524–9.
6. Lesesnse HR, Bozymski EM, Fallon HJ. Treatment of alcoholic hepatitis with hepatic encephalopathy. Comparison of prednisolone with caloric supplements. Gastroenterology 1978;74(2):169–73.
7. Christensen E, Gluud C. Glucocorticoids are ineffective in alcoholic hepatitis: a meta-analysis adjusting for confounding variables. Gut 1995;37(1):113–8.
8. Imperiale TF, McCullough AJ. Do corticosteroids reduce mortality from alcoholic hepatitis? A meta-analysis of the randomized trials. Ann Intern Med 1990;113(4): 299–307.
9. Mathurin P, O'Grady J, Carithers RL, et al. Corticosteroids improve short-term survival in patients with severe alcoholic hepatitis: meta-analysis of individual patient data. Gut 2011;60(2):255–60.
10. Crabb DW, Im GY, Szabo G, et al. Diagnosis and treatment of alcohol-associated liver diseases: 2019 practice guidance from the American Association for the Study of Liver Diseases. Hepatology 2020;71(1):306–33.
11. European Association for the Study of Liver. EASL clinical practical guidelines: management of alcoholic liver disease. J Hepatol 2012;57(2):399–420.
12. Pavlov CS, Varganova DL, Casazza G, et al. Glucocorticosteroids for people with alcoholic hepatitis. Cochrane Database Syst Rev 2017;11:CD001511.

13. Thursz MR, Richardson P, Allison M, et al. Prednisolone or pentoxifylline for alcoholic hepatitis. N Engl J Med 2015;372(17):1619–28.

14. Mathurin P, Abdelnour M, Ramond MJ, et al. Early change in bilirubin levels is an important prognostic factor in severe alcoholic hepatitis treated with prednisolone. Hepatology 2003;38(6):1363–9.

15. Cabré E, Rodríguez-Iglesias P, Caballería J, et al. Short- and long-term outcome of severe alcohol-induced hepatitis treated with steroids or enteral nutrition: a multicenter randomized trial. Hepatology 2000;32(1):36–42.

16. Louvet A, Naveau S, Abdelnour M, et al. The Lille model: a new tool for therapeutic strategy in patients with severe alcoholic hepatitis treated with steroids. Hepatology 2007;45(6):1348–54.

17. Garcia-Saenz-de-Sicilia M, Duvoor C, Altamirano J, et al. A day-4 lille model predicts response to corticosteroids and mortality in severe alcoholic hepatitis. Am J Gastroenterol 2017;112(2):306–15.

18. Rudler M, Mouri S, Charlotte F, et al. Prognosis of treated severe alcoholic hepatitis in patients with gastrointestinal bleeding. J Hepatol 2015;62(4):816–21.

19. Maher JJ. Treatment of alcoholic hepatitis. J Gastroenterol Hepatol 2002;17(4):448–55.

20. Ehrly AM. The effect of pentoxifylline on the deformability of erythrocytes and on the muscular oxygen pressure in patients with chronic arterial disease. J Med 1979;10(5):331–8.

21. Akriviadis E, Botla R, Briggs W, et al. Pentoxifylline improves short-term survival in severe acute alcoholic hepatitis: a double-blind, placebo-controlled trial. Gastroenterology 2000;119(6):1637–48.

22. Menon KV, Stadheim L, Kamath PS, et al. A pilot study of the safety and tolerability of etanercept in patients with alcoholic hepatitis. Am J Gastroenterol 2004;99(2):255–60.

23. Tilg H, Jalan R, Kaser A, et al. Anti-tumor necrosis factor-alpha monoclonal antibody therapy in severe alcoholic hepatitis. J Hepatol 2003;38(4):419–25.

24. Naveau S, Chollet-Martin S, Dharancy S, et al. A double-blind randomized controlled trial of infliximab associated with prednisolone in acute alcoholic hepatitis. Hepatology 2004;39(5):1390–7.

25. Boetticher NC, Peine CJ, Kwo P, et al. A randomized, double-blinded, placebo-controlled multicenter trial of etanercept in the treatment of alcoholic hepatitis. Gastroenterology 2008;135(6):1953–60.

26. Prescott LF, Illingworth RN, Critchley JA, et al. Intravenous N-acetylcystine: the treatment of choice for paracetamol poisoning. Br Med J 1979;2(6198):1097–100.

27. Ben-Ari Z, Vaknin H, Tur-Kaspa R. N-acetylcysteine in acute hepatic failure (non-paracetamol-induced). Hepatogastroenterology 2000;47(33):786–9.

28. Singh V, Keisham A, Bhalla A, et al. Efficacy of granulocyte colony-stimulating factor and N-acetylcysteine therapies in patients with severe alcoholic hepatitis. Clin Gastroenterol Hepatol 2018;16(10):1650–6.e2.

29. Spahr L, Lambert JF, Rubbia-Brandt L, et al. Granulocyte-colony stimulating factor induces proliferation of hepatic progenitors in alcoholic steatohepatitis: a randomized trial. Hepatology 2008;48(1):221–9.

30. Garg V, Garg H, Khan A, et al. Granulocyte colony-stimulating factor mobilizes CD34(+) cells and improves survival of patients with acute-on-chronic liver failure. Gastroenterology 2012;142(3):505–12.e1.

31. Newsome PN, Fox R, King AL, et al. Granulocyte colony-stimulating factor and autologous CD133-positive stem-cell therapy in liver cirrhosis (REALISTIC): an

open-label, randomised, controlled phase 2 trial. Lancet Gastroenterol Hepatol 2018;3(1):25–36.

32. Philips CA, Augustine P, Rajesh S, et al. Granulocyte colony-stimulating factor use in decompensated cirrhosis: lack of survival benefit. J Clin Exp Hepatol 2020;10(2):124–34.

33. Singh V, Sharma AK, Narasimhan RL, et al. Granulocyte colony-stimulating factor in severe alcoholic hepatitis: a randomized pilot study. Am J Gastroenterol 2014; 109(9):1417–23.

34. Shasthry SM, Sharma MK, Shasthry V, et al. Efficacy of granulocyte colony-stimulating factor in the management of steroid-nonresponsive severe alcoholic hepatitis: a double-blind randomized controlled trial. Hepatology 2019;70(3): 802–11.

35. Baig M, Walayat S, Dhillon S, et al. Efficacy of granulocyte colony stimulating factor in severe alcoholic hepatitis: a systematic review and meta-analysis. Cureus 2020;12(9):e10474.

36. Marot A, Singal AK, Moreno C, et al. Granulocyte colony-stimulating factor for alcoholic hepatitis: a systematic review and meta-analysis of randomised controlled trials. JHEP Rep 2020;2(5):100139.

37. Caputo F, Domenicali M, Bernardi M. Diagnosis and treatment of alcohol use disorder in patients with end-stage alcoholic liver disease. Hepatology 2019;70(1): 410–7.

38. Addolorato G, Leggio L, Ferrulli A, et al. Effectiveness and safety of baclofen for maintenance of alcohol abstinence in alcohol-dependent patients with liver cirrhosis: randomised, double-blind controlled study. Lancet 2007;370(9603): 1915–22.

39. Trieu JA, Bilal M, Lewis B, et al. Adherence to adequate nutrition in alcoholic hepatitis is low. Ann Hepatol 2018;17(5):752–5.

40. Uetrecht J. Idiosyncratic drug reactions: current understanding. Annu Rev Pharmacol Toxicol 2007;47:513–39.

41. Lee BP, Mehta N, Platt L, et al. Outcomes of early liver transplantation for patients with severe alcoholic hepatitis. Gastroenterology 2018;155(2):422–30.e1.

Emerging Therapies for Alcoholic Hepatitis

Ma Ai Thanda Han, MD[a], Nikolaos Pyrsopoulos, MD, PhD, MBA, FRCP (Edin)[b],*

KEYWORDS

- Alcoholic hepatitis • Therapeutic • Gut-liver axis • Antioxidant • Anti-inflammatory
- Anti-regenerative agents

KEY POINTS

- Novel therapies are emerging, owing to the high mortality of alcoholic hepatitis and limited available treatment options.
- Therapeutic agents focusing on different pathways targeting the pathogenesis of alcoholic hepatitis have been explored and studied.
- Combination therapies may provide a synergetic effect in improving efficacy and survival.

INTRODUCTION

Alcoholic liver disease remains a public health issue given the rising prevalence of alcohol use disorder.[1,2] Severe alcoholic hepatitis (sAH) is a high-mortality clinical syndrome presented with liver failure. A definitive diagnosis of alcoholic hepatitis (AH) is established by histologic confirmation in addition to a compatible clinical scenario, which includes an abrupt increase of the bilirubin greater than 3 mg/dL, high liver enzymes with an aspartate aminotransferase–to–alanine aminotransferase ratio of greater than 1.5:1 and a lack of individual liver enzymes above 500 IU/L, in the context of chronic heavy alcohol use for longer than 6 months with ongoing active use until at least 8 weeks prior to the presentation and the exclusion of other possible etiologies of liver disease. The histologic features for AH include neutrophilic infiltration, ballooning, and Mallory-Denk bodies, suggesting hepatic injury, cholestasis, and pericellular and sinusoidal hepatic fibrosis. Probable AH can be diagnosed without a liver biopsy if a patient meets the clinical criteria without any confounding factors indicating other potential liver diseases.[3,4] There are different scoring systems available to stratify the severity of AH, knowledge of which is essential for appropriate choice of pharmacologic agent, overall management, and prognosis.[5] Of those, the model for end-

[a] Division of Gastroenterology and Hepatology, Rutgers New Jersey Medical School, 185 South Orange Avenue, H-526, Newark, NJ 07103, USA; [b] Division of Gastroenterology and Hepatology, Rutgers New Jersey Medical School, 185 South Orange Avenue, H-536, Newark, NJ 07103, USA
* Corresponding author.
E-mail address: pyrsopni@njms.rutgers.edu

Clin Liver Dis 25 (2021) 603–624
https://doi.org/10.1016/j.cld.2021.03.006
1089-3261/21/© 2021 Elsevier Inc. All rights reserved.

stage disease (MELD) and modified Maddrey discriminant function (MDF) scores are the scores used most commonly in clinical practice. sAH is diagnosed if the MELD score is greater than or equal to 20, MDF score is greater than or equal to 32, or at the presence of hepatic encephalopathy. A high 90-day mortality rate (>50%) was found in patients with MDF score greater than or equal to 32 without intervention.[4,6,7] An early alteration of MELD score greater than or equal to 2 within the first week of hospitalization predicts in-patient outcomes.[8,9]

Management of AH includes mainly abstinence from alcohol, treatment of alcohol withdrawal symptoms, nutritional support, and potential pharmacologic options.[2] The current available treatment of sAH is corticosteroids. The randomized controlled Steroids or Pentoxifylline for Alcoholic Hepatitis (STOPAH) trial of 1103 clinically diagnosed sAH demonstrated a 28-day survival benefit of corticosteroids compared with placebo, with an odds ratio of 0.72, and a lack of clinical benefits of pentoxifylline. Corticosteroids have major limitations, however, due to unpredictable response, risk of complications (especially infection), and lack of a long-term (6-mo) survival benefit.[10–12] Lille score is used to predict treatment response to corticosteroids in sAH patients beyond 7 days. The cutoff of 0.45 predicts 75% of mortality at 6 months in patients treated with corticosteroids for 28 days.[10] Even though early liver transplantation showed a survival benefit in corticosteroid nonresponders, only a small percentage of patients with sAH are eligible to early liver transplantation.[13–16] Due to the limited benefit of pharmacologic agents[10] and the low accessibility of early liver transplantation,[13,14] novel therapies are emerging to salvage patients with AH. This review article discusses mainly emerging novel therapies for AH.

Alcohol induces liver damage through 4 main pathways (**Fig. 1**): (1) direct injury of hepatocytes, leading to the production of oxidative stress and apoptosis through acetaldehyde; (2) affecting the gut-liver axis by altering the intestinal flora and permeability of intestinal mucosa, resulting in bacterial and or bacterial products translocation; (3) activation of an inflammatory cascade through the activation of cytokines and inflammatory signaling pathways; and (4) hepatic regeneration through the stimulation of stellate cells and the alteration of nitric oxide in the hepatic circulation, causing

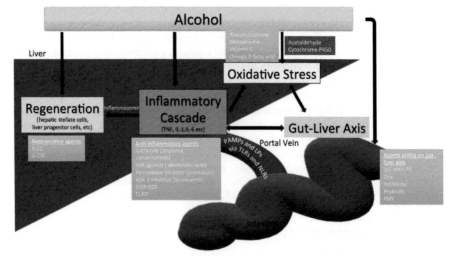

Fig. 1. Mechanistic pathways of AH with current and ongoing novel therapeutics in clinical trials. GCSF, granulocyte colony-stimulating factor; Ig, immunoglobulin.

hepatic fibrosis and portal hypertension.[17–21] Therapies targeting those pathways to control AH are emerging and can be delineated into 4 categories: agents that modulate the gut-liver axis, agents with anti-inflammatory activity, antioxidant activity, and anti-regenerative activity. Lists of completed and ongoing clinical trials for novel therapeutic agents are summarized in **Tables 1** and **2**, respectively.

AGENTS MODULATING THE GUT-LIVER AXIS

There is a constant interaction between the gut microbiota and the liver through the activation of the immune system, initiating liver injury.[22] Alcohol alters gut microbiota in the small and large intestines and disrupts the intestinal tight junctions, triggering an increase in intestinal permeability and inflammation. Excessive alcohol consumption promotes gut dysbiosis with the promotion of proinflammatory Enterobacteriaceae and the depletion of *Lactobacillus* and multiple types of Bacteroidetes.[22,23] Alcohol also alters the gut metabolome by reduction of saturated long-chain fatty acids and short-chain fatty acids, which is associated with an interruption of the intestinal barrier and increase of intestinal permeability, leading to bacterial translocation.[23,24] Antigens, mainly pathogen-associated molecular patterns (PAMPs) and lipopolysaccharides (LPSs) from the translocated bacteria, activate an inflammatory cascade by stimulating the nuclear factor κB via toll-like receptors (TLRs) and node-like receptors (NLRs). The release of inflammatory cytokines and chemokines triggers an inflammatory storm and leukocyte infiltration. Moreover, PAMPs promote and progress hepatic fibrosis through the activation of hepatic stellate cells.[25] Alcohol also alters bile acid concentration that results in activation of farnesoid X receptor (FXR), modulating inflammatory response, and glucose and lipid metabolism.[23] Hence, clinical trials have been conducting to identify therapies that modulate gut microbiota to ameliorate liver injury in AH.

1. Bovine colostrum (IMM-124E)
    Purified hyperimmune bovine colostrum (IMM-124E) includes immunoglobulin G (IgG) antibodies against LPSs, which are involved in the endotoxemia and activation of inflammatory cascades through the TLR4.[26] An open-label proof-of-concept trial of bovine colostrum and corticosteroids in 20 sAH patients with MDF score greater than or equal to 54 was performed in India (NCT02265328). It demonstrated a significant decrease in MDF score after 8 weeks of bovine colostrum treatment. The survival rates after 1 month and 3 months were 90% and 70%, respectively.[27] Recently, a phase 2a, proof-of-concept, randomized placebo-controlled trial (NCT01968382) completed enrollment of 57 patients with sAH (MELD score 20–28) to determine if there is a significant reduction in plasma LPSs after 6 months of receiving IMM-124E compared with placebo. Two different doses of IMM-124E, 2400 mg per day and 4800 mg per day, were given to patients with sAH. There were no significant differences in circulating LPS levels at day 28 or in 180-day mortality and change in MELD score at 180 days between patients receiving IMM-124E and those receiving placebo.[28] A phase 3, randomized, double-blind, placebo-controlled trial (NCT 02473341) has been recruiting patients with sAH defined as MDF score greater than or equal to 32 and MELD score greater than or equal to 21 to compare the primary endpoint of survival at 3 months between bovine colostrum and placebo. TLR4 antagonist would be another potential target in the future, because TLR4 activated by LPSs is an important step in the initiation of the inflammatory cascades.[17,21]
2. Zinc as an additional compound in patients receiving anakinra

Table 1
Summary of completed clinical trials of therapeutic agents in treatment of alcoholic hepatitis

Agent	Mechanism of Action	Study Design and Numbers of Patients (n)	Major Inclusion Criteria	Primary Outcomes
Bovine colostrum (IMM-124E)[27]	IgG against LPSs and bacterial translocation	Placebo-controlled RCT of bovine colostrum with CS (n = 20)	MDF ≥52	Significant decrease in MDF at 8 wk
		Placebo-controlled RCT of IMM-124E (n = 57)	MELD ≥20 but ≤28	Safe but no significant different in LPSs after 28 d and no 180-d mortality benefit
Rifaximin[38]	Antibiotic	Open label Rifampin + CS vs historical controls CS (n = 19)	MDF >32 or MELD >21	Reduction of infection rate (21% vs 32%) not statistically significant
Lactobacillus subtilis/ Streptococcus faecium[41]	Alteration in intestinal microbiota	Placebo-controlled RCT (n = 117)	AH	Liver enzymes reduced in both groups at d 7
FMT[43,44]	Alteration in intestinal microbiota	Open label FMT vs CS vs nutritional support vs pentoxifylline (n = 51)	Severe AH	Improved survival of FMT at 3 mo (75% vs 38% vs 29% vs 30%, respectively; $P = .036$)
		Open label FMT vs matched controls (standard-of-care) (n = 13)	Severe AH	Improved survival of FMT at 1 mo and 3 mo (100% vs 60%, respectively; $P = .016$, and 53.8% vs 25%, respectively; $P = .14$)
Anakinra[32]	Antagonist to IL-1 receptor	RCT IL-1R antagonist + zinc + pentoxyfylline vs CS (n = 103)	MDF >32 or MELD >20	180-d survival between combination group vs CS (69.7% vs 55.8%, respectively; HR = 0.69; $P = .28$)
Emricasan	Pan-caspase inhibitor	Placebo-controlled RCT (n = 5)	MELD = 21–34 or 35–40 if SOFA score <10	Phase II, terminated due to high drug level in sick patients
Selonsertib [GS-4997][68]	ASK-1 inhibitor	RCT selonsertib + CS vs CS (n = 99)	MDF = 32–60	No effect on survival (70.3% vs 81.7%, respectively; $P = .18$) at wk 24

	Mechanism	Study design	MELD/criteria	Outcome
DUR-928[71]	Endogenous sulfated oxysterol molecule that modulates lipid homeostasis, inflammation, and cell survival	Open label IV infusion with different doses 30 mg, 90 mg, or 150 mg at day 1 and day 4 (n = 19)	MELD = 11–30	Safe and well tolerated (at all doses) at d 28
ELAD[74]	Liver cellular support therapy	RCT ELAD vs standard-of-care (n = 203)	MDF ≥32, bilirubin ≥, MELD ≤35	No difference in adverse effect and survival (51.1% vs 49.5%, respectively; P = .9) at d 91
		RCT ELAD vs standard-of-care (n = 151)	MDF ≥32 (age 18–49, MELD <30, creatinine <1.3, and INR <2.5)	Phase III terminated due to failed primary endpoint Comparable overall survival rate (70.5% vs 69.9%, respectively; P = .76)
NAC[91]	Antioxidant	RCT NAC + CS vs CS (n = 174)	MDF ≥32	Not significant in 6-mo mortality (27% vs 38%, respectively; P = .07)
Metadoxine[96]	Antioxidant	RCT metadoxine vs CS vs pentoxifylline (n = 135)	MDF ≥32	Significantly better 3-mo and 6-mo survival in either metadoxine + CS or metadoxine + pentoxifylline
IL-22 infusion (F-652)[110]	Hepatic regeneration, anti-inflammatory, antioxidant	Open label, dose escalating (10 μg/kg, 30 μg/kg, or 45 μg/kg) (n = 18)	MELD = 21–28	Safe without significant adverse events at day 42
G-CSF (filgrastim)[92,115]	Hemopoietic stem cell mobilization and hepatic progenitor cells proliferation	Open label (ICU patients) G-CSF vs G-CSF + NAC vs standard therapy with pentoxiphylline (n = 57)	MDF ≥32	90-d survival benefit in both G-CSF and G-CSF + NAC vs standard therapy
		RCT G-CSF vs placebo (n = 28)	MDF ≥32 with steroid nonresponder	Comparable 28-d mortality rate (21.4% vs 28.6%, respectively; P = .69)

Abbreviations: CS, corticosteroids; RCT, randomized controlled trial.

Table 2
Summary of ongoing clinical trials of therapeutic agents in treatment of alcoholic hepatitis

Agent	Mechanism of Action	Study Design	Major Inclusion Criteria	Primary Endpoint	Status
Bovine colostrum (IMM-124E)	IgG against LPSs and bacterial translocation	Placebo-controlled RCT	MDF ≥32 and MELD ≥21	Survival at 3 mo	Phase III, recruiting
Augmentin	Antibiotic	RCT Augmentin vs CS	MELD >20	Survival at 2 mo	Phase III, active and recruiting
Lactobacillus	Alteration in intestinal microbiota	Placebo-controlled RCT	MELD <21	Change in MELD at 30 d	Phase III, active and recruiting
		Placebo-control RCT	AH	Change in liver enzymes at 7 d	Phase IV, active
FMT	Alteration in intestinal microbiota	RCT FMT vs CS	Severe AH, eligible for steroid	Overall survival at 3 mo	Active, finished recruiting
		Open label, non-RCT FMT vs standard-of-care	MDF >32 or grade I or grade II HE	Survival at 3 mo	Active, recruiting
Anakinra	Antagonist to IL-1 receptor	RCT IL-1R antagonist + zinc vs CS	MELD = 20–35	Survival at 90 d	Phase II, not recruiting yet
Canakinumab	Monoclonal antibody against IL-1β	Placebo-controlled RCT	MDF ≥32 and MELD <27	Histologic improvement after 28 d of therapy	Phase II, recruiting
OCA	FXR antagonist	Placebo-controlled RCT	MELD = 12–19	Change in MELD at 6 wk	Phase II, completed[a]
NAC	Antioxidant	RCT NAC + CS vs CS	MDF ≥32	Improvement in monocyte oxidative burst at 24 h and d 5	Phase III, recruiting
Vitamin C	Antioxidant and anti-inflammatory	RCT vitamin C vs placebo	AH with sepsis	Change in MELD at 96 h after infusion	Active, recruiting

Omega-5 fatty acid	Antioxidant and anti-inflammatory	RCT omega-5 fatty acid + CS vs CS	MDF >30	30-d survival	Active, recruiting
G-CSF (filgrastim)	Hemopoietic stem cell mobilization and hepatic progenitor cells proliferation	RCT G-CSF vs standard medical therapy	MDF ≥32	3-mo survival	Phase IV, recruiting
		RCT G-CSF + CS vs CS vs G-CSF	MDF ≥32	3-mo survival	Phase IV, recruiting
		RCT G-CSF + CS vs CS vs G-CSF	MDF ≥32 in either CS null responder or CS partial responder	2-mo survival in CS null responder, 6-mo survival in CS partial responder	Phase IV, recruiting

Abbreviations: CS, corticosteroids; HE, hepatic encephalopathy; RCT, randomized controlled trial.
[a] Completed study but the result has not yet been published.

Zinc is an important micronutrient for the stabilization of the intestinal barrier. Zinc deficiency is common in alcoholic patients, including AH. Zinc deficiency disrupts intestinal permeability, leading to endotoxemia, and facilitates caspase-3–mediated apoptosis and oxidative stress.[29–31] A multicenter, randomized, double-blind, placebo-controlled trial (NCT01809132) enrolled 103 sAH patients (MDF score >32 or MELD score >20). The study compared the efficacy of a zinc sulfate, 220-mg dose, administered daily for 180 days in addition to pentoxifylline administered for 28 days and an interleukin (IL)-1 receptor antagonist (anakinra) injection administered for 14 days to methyl prednisolone administered for 28 days. The 30-day mortality rate was comparable between the 2 groups (83.4% vs 81.2%, respectively; hazard ratio [HR] 0.91; $P = .85$). Even though the 180-day survival rate was not significantly different between the 2 groups (69.7% vs 55.8%, respectively; HR 0.69; $P = .28$), the study found a potential long-term mortality benefit of the combination group, with a separation of the survival curve noticed at day 90. The study also demonstrated an independent association of the baseline MELD score and 180-day survival for patients with a baseline MELD score below 25, regardless of therapies.[32] Zinc may have additional benefit on sAH if it is given adjunct to anakinra.

3. Antibiotics

The human intestine is colonized by multiple diverse microbiomes. Alcohol induces small bowel bacterial overgrowth from intestinal dysmotility and suppression of gastric acid. Moreover, alcohol causes dysbiosis of intestinal microbiota with an increasing prevalence of detrimental bacteria, including Actinobacteria and Firmicutes. In the setting of the leaky intestinal barrier due to alcohol, this intestinal dysbiosis stimulates immune dysregulation and a vicious cascade of hepatic injury in AH.[24,33] This mechanism provides potential therapeutic targets, including antibiotics, probiotics, and fecal microbiota transplantation (FMT).

Because infection is a major complication of sAH, either due to the immunocompromised state induced by sAH or due to the adverse effect of corticosteroids, antibiotic therapy is of interest for the management of sAH.[34,35] A multicenter, double-blind, randomized, placebo-controlled trial (NTC 02281929) of Augmentin (amoxicillin/clavulanic acid) and prednisolone for 30 days will recruit 280 patients with sAH (MDF score >32 or MELD score >20). Its primary endpoint is survival at 2 months. Another antibiotic, rifaximin, showed a significant benefit on portal hypertension and survival in decompensated alcoholic cirrhosis patients.[36,37] A small open-label pilot study of rifaximin plus standard therapy with corticosteroids compared with a historical cohort with corticosteroids in patients with sAH (MDF score >32 or MELD score >21) revealed a reduction of infection rates (21% vs 32%, respectively) and 90-day mortality rate (16% vs 47%, respectively) in a rifaximin group compared with historical controls, without statistically significant differences, due to a small sample size of 19 patients.[38]

4. Probiotics

Restoration to a healthy microbiota is a target of therapeutic intervention in AH. Preclinical data suggest a beneficial effect of Lactobacillus rhamnosus GG on the liver injury with a reduction in intestinal leakiness and oxidative stress.[39,40] A multicenter, randomized, placebo-controlled trial of probiotics (cultured Lactobacillus subtilis/Streptococcus faecium) given for 7 days to 117 AH patients suggested an improvement in LPSs and tumor necrosis factor (TNF)-α with potential repopulation of healthy intestinal microbiota at the end of therapy. The number of colony-forming units of *Escherichia coli* was reduced significantly in the probiotic group compared with the placebo group.[41] These data showed an efficacy of short-term therapy, but a majority of patients had a mild form of AH. Currently, there are 2 ongoing randomized clinical trials investigating probiotics in AH patients, summarized in **Table 2**.

5. Fecal microbiota transplant

A fairly new method of repopulation with healthy intestinal microbiota is FMT. A pilot, proof-of-concept study included 8 male patients with sAH (mean MELD–sodium score 33.6 ± 4.3) who were ineligible to receive corticosteroids but underwent FMT via nasoduodenal tube daily for 7 days. The study provided promising safety and efficacy data when compared with historical matched controls. Ascites and hepatic encephalopathy were resolved with an improvement in MELD–sodium scores and a survival benefit at 1 year (88% vs 33%, respectively; $P = .018$). Healthy microbiota from donors was found to concur with microbiota of the recipients. Reductions of Proteobacteria species with change in relative abundance of certain pathogenic species, such as *Klebsiella pneumonia*, were noted at 1-year post-FMT.[42] The same research group conducted another study of 51 male patients with sAH, comparing the efficacy of FMT to corticosteroids, nutritional support, and pentoxifylline. There was a statistically significant improvement in 3-month survival rates among patients receiving FMT compared with those receiving corticosteroids, nutritional support, and pentoxifylline (75% vs 38%, respectively, vs 29% vs 30%, respectively; $P = .036$). Stool analysis was performed in 16 patients who received FMT, indicating healthy microbiota diversity, and their metabolism up to 90 days post-FMT. There was a substantial decreased in Proteobacteria and Actinobacteria, with an increase in Firmicutes, which was persistent 30 days to 90 days post-FMT. In addition, reduction in pathogenic bacteria, such as *Enterobacter* and *Klebsiella*, and predominance of less pathogenic bacteria, such as *Bacteroides, Parabacteroides, Porphyromonas, Roseburia*, and *Micrococcus*, were found post-FMT. Modulations of amino acid metabolism and degradation pathway were noticed in post-FMT.[43] Another pilot study compared 13 patients with sAH treated with FMT via nasojejunal tube to 20 matched controls receiving standard-of-care. The 1-month and 3-month survival rates were better in the FMT group compared with the standard-of-care group (100% vs 60%, respectively; $P = .016$, and 53.8% vs 25%, respectively; $P = .14$). The FMT group showed resolution of hepatic encephalopathy and ascites.[44] There is an upcoming a randomized controlled trial (NCT03091010) of FMT compared with corticosteroids for sAH patients who are eligible to corticosteroids. The primary endpoint of the study is an overall 3-month survival. Another nonrandomized trial (NCT03827772) of FMT compared with standard-of-care has been recruiting 40 patients with sAH defined by MDF score greater than 32 or grade 1 or grade 2 hepatic encephalopathy. The primary endpoint is survival at 3 months.

AGENTS WITH ANTI-INFLAMMATORY ACTIVITY

One of the proposed mechanisms of alcohol-induced hepatic inflammation is activation of the immune system from bacterial translocation. PAMPs and LPSs bind TLRs (mainly TLR4) and NLRs activates of inflammatory cytokines, such as TNF, IL-1, and IL-6, as described previously.[25] During the activation of these inflammatory signaling pathways, chemokines, such as IL-8 and C-C chemokine ligand (CCL) type 2 (CCL2), recruit leukocytes in the liver, which amplifies the inflammatory cascades.[45,46] These inflammatory changes also enhance hepatic steatosis, apoptosis or hepatic necrosis.[47] Moreover, a triggering of adaptive immunity by stimulating splenic T cells and hepatic natural killer T cells advances cytotoxic response against hepatocytes through the Fas and TNF receptor 1 signaling pathway in AH.[48,49] Stellate cells also are involved in releasing inflammatory cytokines, such as CCL2, IL-8, TNF, and IL-1.[49,50] All these changes result in dysfunction of mitochondria and oxidative stress, which is part of the pathogenesis of AH.[50] Scientists have been exploring novel therapies targeting multiple steps in the mechanism of inflammatory cascades.

1. Inhibition of interleukin 1 signaling

IL-1β and IL-1 receptors have been found to induce inflammation via up-regulation of TLR4-dependent inflammatory signaling in macrophages and inflammatory chemokine in hepatocytes in animal studies. Inhibition of IL-1 signaling was found to attenuate inflammasome-dependent liver inflammation along with improved hepatocyte regeneration, resulting in rapid recovery in AH mice.[51,52]

Anakinra is a recombinant IL-1 receptor antagonist and its efficacy was studied in a recent multicenter randomized controlled trial in combination with zinc sulfate and pentoxifylline. The combination therapy in patients with sAH (MDF score >32 or MELD score >20) provided a potential 90-day survival benefit but a comparable short-term survival benefit compared with corticosteroid therapy, described previously.[32] There is an upcoming multicenter randomized controlled trial (NCT04072822) of anakinra plus zinc compared with prednisone for sAH patients (MELD score 20–35) to evaluate the 90-day survival rates as a primary endpoint.

Canakinumab is a monoclonal antibody against IL-1β that is involved in the inflammatory cascade. The drug has been used to treat autoinflammatory conditions, such as juvenile idiopathic arthritis and adult-onset Still disease.[53,54] A multicenter randomized placebo-controlled trial (NCT03775109) has been recruiting patients with sAH (MDF score ≥32 and MELD score <27) to evaluate histologic improvement after 28 days of treatment.

2. Farnesoid X receptor agonist

FXRs are found in the liver and intestine. They bind to bile acid, producing fibroblast growth factor 19, which plays a role in negative feedback controlling of bile acid synthesis, decreasing fatty acid synthesis, and promoting fatty acid oxidation in the liver. Moreover, FXR agonist showed anti-inflammatory activity, antioxidant activity, and hepatic hemodynamic benefits, with an improvement in portal hypertension in animal studies.[55–57] Obeticholic acid (OCA) is an FXR agonist and a semisynthetic derivative of the chenodeoxycholic acid; it was studied in patients with primary biliary cholangitis and nonalcoholic steatohepatitis (NASH), showing promising efficacy.[58,59] A recent randomized, placebo-controlled clinical trial (NCT02039219) using OCA (10 mg daily) for 6 weeks in moderately severe AH patients (MELD score = 12–19) was completed to evaluate the efficacy and safety of the medication. The results are not yet published.

3. Pan-caspase inhibitor (emricasan)

Caspases, cysteine proteases, participate in hepatic inflammation, apoptosis, and fibrosis. Inhibition of caspases was shown to attenuate hepatic inflammation, fibrosis, and portal hypertension in animal studies.[60,61] Emricasan is a pan-caspase inhibitor shown to improve liver enzymes in patients with chronic hepatitis C and NASH.[62,63] A multicenter, randomized, placebo-controlled study of emricasan administered for 3 months to 86 patients with cirrhosis (MELD score 11–18) demonstrated an improvement in liver function indicated by the MELD and Child-Pugh scores, international normalized ratio (INR), and bilirubin at 3 months of therapy. The study included only 38% of patients, however, with alcohol-associated cirrhosis, and most of the patients had low MELD score. The subgroup analysis for alcohol-associated liver disease showed a minimal but not statistically significant improvement in MELD score.[64] Moreover, it was difficult to identify a safe optimal dose of emricasan in sick patients with sAH. This was demonstrated in a phase 2, randomized, placebo-controlled trial (NCT01912404) of emricasan in patients with sAH (MELD score 21–34 or 35–40 if sequential organ failure assessment [SOFA] <10). The study was terminated prematurely after recruitment of 5 patients due to a poor pharmacokinetic profile with a markedly elevated level of drug compounds in those patients.[17]

4. Apoptosis signal-regulating kinase-1 inhibitor (selonsertib [GS-4997])

Apoptosis signal-regulating kinase-1 (ASK-1) is involved in hepatic apoptosis, cytokine-mediated inflammation, and fibrosis via hepatic stellate cells activation. Inhibition of ASK1 resulted in a reduction of inflammation, cell death, and fibrosis via the inflammasome activation pathway in preclinical studies.[65–67] The efficacy and safety of selonsertib, an ASK-1 inhibitor, in combination with prednisolone, 40 mg, administered daily, were studied in a phase 2, multi-center, randomized controlled trial of 102 patients with sAH (MDF score ≥32) compared with prednisolone alone. Adding selonsertib to prednisone did not provide any benefit for survival at 24 weeks (70.3% vs 81.7%, respectively; $P = .18$) or liver function in terms of Lille response, bilirubin, and MELD score. Selonsertib also did not show any effect on infection when it was combined with prednisone.[68]

5. DUR-928

DUR-928 is a newly discovered endogenous molecule of 5-cholesten-3b, 23-diol 3 sulfate (25HC3S) that regulates multiple pathways in hepatic injury. It downregulates lipid metabolism via nuclear liver oxysterol receptor and sterol regulatory element binding proteins. It ameliorates inflammatory responses by reducing expression of proinflammatory cytokines and stabilizes mitochondria.[69] The safety and efficacy of DUR-928 were studied in an open-label, multicenter, phase 2a trial of 19 patients with AH. Of those, 78% of patients had sAH (MDF score ≥32). The drug was infused intravenously at day 1 and day 4 with different doses of 30 mg, 90 mg, or 150 mg. The study revealed an 89% overall response rate as measured by a Lille score less than 0.45. Among the patients with sAH, the overall response rate was 87% and the optimal dose was found to be 30 mg or 90 mg. Reduction of serum bilirubin and improvement in MELD score also were noticed at day 28. Contrasting historical data of Lille score in 145 AH patients in a study by Louvet and colleagues,[10,70] the DUR-928 provided better Lille score at day 7 after treatment.[71]

6. Extracorporeal liver assist device

The extracorporeal liver assist device (ELAD) is a liver-supportive therapy using human cells from the hepatoblastoma cell line (VTL C3A), which has numerous anti-inflammatory proteins and especially an expression of IL-1 receptor antagonist activity.[72,73] It also has some antioxidant activity and natural regeneration activity of hepatocytes. In a phase 3, randomized, placebo-controlled trial of 203 patients with sAH (MDF score $\geq$32), overall survival of patients receiving ELAD and standard-of-care was compared with that of those receiving standard-of-care alone. The overall survival rate was comparable between the 2 groups after a minimum of 91 days (51.1% vs 49.5%, respectively; $P = .9$). Subgroup analysis indicated lower mortality in patients with MELD score less than 28 and age less than 46.9 years. Coagulopathy and renal failure were found associated with worse outcomes, especially in patients with the MELD score greater than or equal to 28.[74] Based on the findings, a similar phase 3, randomized controlled trial (NTC02612428) was conducted in 151 sAH patients (MDF score $\geq$32) of younger age (18–49 years old), lower MELD score less than 30, and better renal and coagulation profiles (creatinine <1.3 and INR <2.5), comparing ELAD plus standard-of-care to standard-of-care alone. The study was terminated due to failure to achieve the primary endpoint, which was a comparison of survival rates between patients receiving ELAD and control, with additional survival data of pivotal trial VTL 308, including 203 patients from previous trial[74] up to 24 months until the time of database lock (ELAD, 70.5%, vs standard-of-care, 69.9%; $P = .76$).[75]

7. Other potential therapies

CCL2 (also known as monocyte chemoattractant protein-1 [MCP-1]) and CCL type 5 are involved in liver inflammation via the up-regulation of inflammatory mediators from the recruitment of macrophage and T cells.[76,77] The expression of both chemokines was increased in AH.[78] Moreover, MCP-1 (CCL2) deficiency was found to inhibit expression of inflammatory cytokines and oxidative stress and inhibit induction of genes linked to fatty acid metabolism in mice.[77] Cenicriviroc is an oral dual CCR2/5 antagonist, which is a potential therapy for AH. It was studied in the liver of alcohol-fed mice, which showed reduction of macrophage and T cell activation, reduction inflammatory cytokine production, and alleviation of cell death and steatosis.[76]

Alirocumab is a monoclonal antibody against proprotein convertase subtilisin/kexin type 9 (PCSK9) and is approved in familial hypercholesterolemia.[79] The liver expresses PCSK9, which is involved in the regulation of low-density lipoprotein cholesterol.[80] Alirocumab was found to mitigate hepatic inflammation via the regulation of mRNA expression of proinflammatory cytokines or chemokines and the infiltration of polymononuclear cells. It also was found to function in modulating the lipid metabolism via regulation of mRNA expression for fatty acid synthesis in rats.[81]

AGENTS WITH ANTIOXIDANT ACTIVITY

Alcohol induces liver injury through oxidative stress and hepatic mitochondrial production of reactive oxygen species, in particular superoxide anions, through high levels of TNF-α.[82] Alcohol also depletes the glutathione, which is the main antioxidant, causing hepatocytes to be more sensitive to TNF-α.[50,83] Silymarin is an antioxidant that inhibits lipid peroxidation and scavenges free radicals.[84] The randomized, double-blind, placebo-controlled trials of alcoholic cirrhosis patients treated with silymarin did not show any survival benefit or improvement in liver enzymes.[85,86] Vitamin E, an antioxidant, was compared with placebo for 3 months in patients with mild to moderate AH. There was no significant improvement in serum aminotransferase and bilirubin.[87] Phillips and colleagues investigated the efficacy of an antioxidant cocktail compared with prednisolone, 30 mg daily, in 101 patients with sAH. The antioxidant cocktail included β-carotene, vitamin C, vitamin E, selenium, methionine, allopurinol, desferrioxamine, and *N*-acetylcysteine (NAC). The patients receiving prednisolone, 30 mg daily, had a better 30-day mortality rate than those receiving the antioxidant cocktail, with an odds ratio of 2.4 in the antioxidant group.[88] Similarly, another small trial of an antioxidant cocktail (vitamins A–E, biotin, selenium, zinc, manganese, copper, magnesium, folic acid and coenzyme Q, for 6 months, and NAC, for 1 wk) was investigated in 36 patients with sAH. No survival benefit was observed in patients receiving either antioxidant therapy alone or in combination with corticosteroids.[89]

1. *N*-acetylcysteine

   NAC repletes the glutathione, the major antioxidant for hepatocytes.[90] A well-designed randomized controlled trial of 174 patients with sAH (MDF score ≥32) compared prednisolone plus NAC to prednisolone alone. The group receiving the combination therapy had lower short-term mortality compared with those receiving prednisolone alone (8% vs 24%, respectively; $P = .006$) but the effect was not seen in 3-month and 6-month mortality analysis (22% vs 34%, respectively; $P = .06$, and 27% vs 38%, respectively; $P = .07$). There were fewer incidences of hepatorenal syndrome and infection in the combination therapy group compared with the prednisolone alone group.[91] In another study of 57 sAH patients admitted to intensive care unit (ICU), an additional 90-day survival benefit of NAC to granulocyte colony-stimulating factor (G-CSF) was not found when the effect was compared with G-CSF alone. The details are described later.[92] Similarly, a recent retrospective analysis of 68 sAH patients demonstrated that an addition of intravenous NAC to prednisone did not provide any significant 90-day survival benefit compared with prednisone alone. The 90-day mortality was highest in patients with high MDF score and renal insufficiency.[93] Given a potential benefit of a lower infection rate in the NAC receiving group, an open-label, randomized controlled trial (NCT 03069300) has been recruiting patients with sAH to receive NAC plus prednisolone compared with prednisone alone to identify the mechanism of NAC in ameliorating infection.

2. Metadoxine

   Another antioxidant, metadoxine, is involved in glutathione synthesis.[94] A randomized, open-label trial of 70 sAH patients (MDF score >32) receiving metadoxine adjunct to prednisone was found to have 30-day and 90-day survival benefits compared with prednisone alone (74.3% vs 45.7%, respectively, and 68.6% vs 20.0%, respectively).[95] In an open-label, randomized controlled trial, the effect of metadoxine adjunct to either prednisone or pentoxyfylline was compared with prednisone alone or pentoxyfylline alone in 135 sAH patients. The 3-month survival of the combination group of metadoxine with either prednisone or pentoxyfylline was significantly better (68.6% vs 20%, respectively; $P = .0001$, and 59.4% vs 33.3%, respectively; $P = .04$) compared with prednisone alone or pentoxyfylline alone. Similarly, the 6-month survival of the combination group significantly outperformed than that of the groups receiving prednisone or pentoxyfylline alone (48.6% vs 20%, respectively; $P = .003$, and 50% vs 18.2%, respectively; $P = .003$). It also helped in the sustained abstinence from alcohol.[96]

3. Vitamin C

   Vitamin C is an antioxidant that shows hepatoprotective effect in animal studies via iron metabolic pathway.[97] Alcohol reduces hepcidin gene expression, leading to increase in iron absorption and macrophage iron release.[98] Both alcohol and iron cause oxidative stress and lipid peroxidation, leading to liver tissue injury.[99] Vitamin C also is found to be deficient in patients with alcohol use disorder.[100] Vitamin C was shown to protect the liver in alcohol-fed mice by decreasing the liver enzymes and hepatic iron overload via promoting the expression of hepcidin and reducing the expression of ferroportin.[97] Moreover, vitamin C modulates sepsis-induced inflammation and coagulation.[101] It also is shown to improve organ failure score in severe septic patients in ICU.[100] A randomized, double-blind, placebo-controlled trial (NCT03829683) has been recruiting 20 patients with AH and sepsis to assess safety and efficacy of vitamin C infusion compared with placebo with the primary endpoint of change in MELD score at 96 hours after infusion.

4. Omega-5 fatty acid (punicic acid)

Omega-5 fatty acid is a polyunsaturated fatty acid classified as a conjugated linolenic acid and has a hepatoprotective effect, with anti-inflammatory and antioxidant properties via peroxisome proliferator-activated receptor (PPAR)-γ and PPAR-δ, reducing lipid peroxidation, restoration of glutathione peroxidase, superoxide dismutase and catalase, and inhibiting the expression of proinflammatory cytokines in animal studies.[102–104] Currently, a randomized, double-blind placebo-controlled trial (NCT03723586) has been recruiting 40 patients with sAH (MDF score >32) to compare the 30-day survival of patients receiving omega-5 fatty acid adjunct to prednisone to those receiving prednisone alone.

AGENTS THAT MODULATE REGENERATIVE PATHWAYS

Proper hepatic regeneration is essential to the repair of injured livers. In AH, the inflammasome produced by the inflammatory cascade and incomplete differentiation of liver progenitor cells impairs mature hepatocyte proliferation.[105] Chronic alcohol consumption also limits mature hepatocyte in DNA synthesis and interferes in miRNA signaling during the regeneration process.[105,106] Novel agents that modulate hepatic regeneration thus became an interesting target for the development of therapeutic management.

1. Interleukin 22 infusion (F-652)

IL-22 is one of the cytokines from the IL-10 family, derived from the CD4$^+$ helper T cells. It not only modulates tissue proliferation, de novo lipogenesis, and inflammation but also has antioxidant and antiapoptosis effects. F-652 is a recombinant fusion protein of human IL-22 and IgG2 fragment crystallizable (Fc) fragments, having a mechanism similar to the native IL-22. The addition of human Fc fragments to the C-terminal of F-652 enhances pharmacokinetic and pharmacodynamics properties. F-652 repairs tissue after damage from inflammation or infection.[107–109] A phase 2a dose-escalating study of F-652 infusion, at doses of 10 μg/kg, 30 μg/kg, or 45 and μg/kg, at day 1 and day 7, was completed in 18 patients with sAH (MELD score 21–28). F-652 was shown to improve the MELD score and liver enzymes significantly at day 28 and day 42, and 83% of patients achieved a day 7 Lille score less than or equal to 0.45. F-652 was found to be safe without any significant side effects.[110] Further randomized placebo-controlled trials are necessary to investigate the efficacy.

2. Granulocyte colony-stimulating factor (filgrastim)

G-CSF is a cytokine that enhances hepatocyte repair and survival by mobilizing CD34$^+$ hemopoietic stem cells for differentiation of mature hepatocytes and stimulating hepatic progenitor cell proliferation.[111,112] A randomized study demonstrated the safety of G-CSF and its function of hepatic regeneration in 24 patients with alcoholic cirrhosis–superimposed steatohepatitis (MDF score 21–60).[113] An open-label, randomized pilot study of 46 patients with sAH showed that the 90-day survival of patients treated with G-CSF was significantly superior to the standard medical therapy using pentoxyfylline (78.3% vs 30.4%, respectively; $P = .001$). Moreover, G-CSF significantly improved the Child-Pugh, MELD, and MDF scores at 1 month, 2 months, and 3 months. Corticosteroids were not administered as standard-of-care.[114] Another open-label, randomized controlled trial of G-CSF alone compared with G-CSF plus NAC or standard medical therapy with pentoxifylline studied 57 patients with sAH admitted to ICU. There were improvements in MDF score at 1 month, 2 months, and 3 months (reductions of 60.36%, 75.36%, and 88.73%, respectively; $P = .02$, $P = .05$, and $P = .00$, respectively) as well as MELD score (reduction of 55.77%; $P = .01$) but not Child- Pugh score at 3 months in the G-CSF group compared with standard medical therapy. The 3-month survival rates were significantly better in the groups receiving either G-CSF alone or G-CSF combined with NAC compared with that of the group receiving standard-of-care ($P<.05$). There was no statistically significant difference in 3-month survival rates between the patients receiving G-CSF alone and those receiving G-CSF in combination with NAC ($P = .112$).[92] The efficacy of G-CSF in 28 steroid-nonresponder patients with sAH was studied in a double-blind, randomized placebo-controlled trial. The 90-day mortality (35.7% vs 71.4%, respectively; $P = .04$) as well as MELD and MDF scores at 90 days were improved significantly in patients who received G-CSF compared with placebo, although the 28-day mortality was comparable between the 2 groups (21.4% vs 28.6%, respectively; $P = .69$). The hazard ratio of receiving G-CSF was 0.37 (SD 0.14–0.98). The infection rate also was lower in the G-CSF group than in placebo group (28% vs 71%, respectively; $P<.001$). MELD score also was significantly improved in G-CSF group compared with placebo group ($P = .002$).[115] Owing to its promising efficacy without safety concerns, 3 randomized control trials currently are recruiting sAH patients to identify the efficacy of G-CSF either alone or adjunct to corticosteroids, as summarized in **Table 2**.

SUMMARY

The AH therapeutic armamentarium is limited. The only available therapeutic agents are corticosteroids, which provides only a short-term (28-day) survival benefit. Novel therapies currently are being explored, targeting different pathways in the pathogenesis of AH. Combinations of therapies are being investigated, possibly providing synergistic effect of compounds with different mechanisms of action. Given the high mortality rate, new safe and effective therapies are being sought under the sponsorship of the National Institute on Alcohol Abuse and Alcoholism in multiple consortia in the United States in order to assist patients with sAH. Based on available data on those emerging novel therapies, FMT, DUR-928, metadoxine, IL-22 infusion, and G-CSF might exhibit potential positive benefits in sAH patients. It still is early to make final conclusions on those novel therapies, however, because most of the clinical trials are emerging and ongoing.

CLINICS CARE POINTS

- The only current available pharmacotherapy for sAH is corticosteroids.
- Potential positive efficacy was found in GCSF, metadoxine, DUR-928, IL-22 infusion, and FMT.
- Consider combination therapies for synergistic effect.
- Further larger RCT phase 3 studies are required.

DISCLOSURE

All authors have nothing to disclose.

REFERENCE

1. Barritt ASt, Jiang Y, Schmidt M, et al. Charges for alcoholic cirrhosis exceed all other etiologies of cirrhosis combined: a national and state inpatient survey analysis. Dig Dis Sci 2019;64(6):1460–9.
2. Singal AK, Bataller R, Ahn J, et al. ACG clinical guideline: alcoholic liver disease. Am J Gastroenterol 2018;113(2):175–94.
3. Crabb DW, Bataller R, Chalasani NP, et al. Standard definitions and common data elements for clinical trials in patients with alcoholic hepatitis: recommendation from the NIAAA Alcoholic Hepatitis Consortia. Gastroenterology 2016; 150(4):785–90.
4. Lucey MR, Mathurin P, Morgan TR. Alcoholic hepatitis. N Engl J Med 2009; 360(26):2758–69.
5. Singal AK, Shah VH. Alcoholic hepatitis: prognostic models and treatment. Gastroenterol Clin North Am 2011;40(3):611–39.
6. Singal AK, Kamath PS, Gores GJ, et al. Alcoholic hepatitis: current challenges and future directions. Clin Gastroenterol Hepatol 2014;12(4):555–64 [quiz: e531–52].
7. Singal AK, Kodali S, Vucovich LA, et al. Diagnosis and treatment of alcoholic hepatitis: a systematic review. Alcohol Clin Exp Res 2016;40(7):1390–402.
8. Dunn W, Jamil LH, Brown LS, et al. MELD accurately predicts mortality in patients with alcoholic hepatitis. Hepatology 2005;41(2):353–8.
9. Maddrey WC, Boitnott JK, Bedine MS, et al. Corticosteroid therapy of alcoholic hepatitis. Gastroenterology 1978;75(2):193–9.
10. Louvet A, Naveau S, Abdelnour M, et al. The Lille model: a new tool for therapeutic strategy in patients with severe alcoholic hepatitis treated with steroids. Hepatology 2007;45(6):1348–54.
11. Thursz MR, Richardson P, Allison M, et al. Prednisolone or pentoxifylline for alcoholic hepatitis. N Engl J Med 2015;372(17):1619–28.
12. Louvet A, Thursz MR, Kim DJ, et al. Corticosteroids reduce risk of death within 28 Days for patients with severe alcoholic hepatitis, compared with pentoxifylline or placebo-a meta-analysis of individual data from controlled trials. Gastroenterology 2018;155(2):458–468 e8.
13. Mathurin P, Moreno C, Samuel D, et al. Early liver transplantation for severe alcoholic hepatitis. N Engl J Med 2011;365(19):1790–800.
14. Hasanin M, Dubay DA, McGuire BM, et al. Liver transplantation for alcoholic hepatitis: a survey of liver transplant centers. Liver Transpl 2015;21(11): 1449–52.
15. Marot A, Dubois M, Trepo E, et al. Liver transplantation for alcoholic hepatitis: a systematic review with meta-analysis. PLoS One 2018;13(1). e0190823.
16. Singal AK, Bashar H, Anand BS, et al. Outcomes after liver transplantation for alcoholic hepatitis are similar to alcoholic cirrhosis: exploratory analysis from the UNOS database. Hepatology 2012;55(5):1398–405.
17. Singal AK, Shah VH. Current trials and novel therapeutic targets for alcoholic hepatitis. J Hepatol 2019;70(2):305–13.
18. Szabo G. Gut-liver axis in alcoholic liver disease. Gastroenterology 2015; 148(1):30–6.

19. Wiest R, Lawson M, Geuking M. Pathological bacterial translocation in liver cirrhosis. J Hepatol 2014;60(1):197–209.

20. Lowe PP, Gyongyosi B, Satishchandran A, et al. Alcohol-related changes in the intestinal microbiome influence neutrophil infiltration, inflammation and steatosis in early alcoholic hepatitis in mice. PLoS One 2017;12(3). e0174544.

21. Keshavarzian A, Farhadi A, Forsyth CB, et al. Evidence that chronic alcohol exposure promotes intestinal oxidative stress, intestinal hyperpermeability and endotoxemia prior to development of alcoholic steatohepatitis in rats. J Hepatol 2009;50(3):538–47.

22. Konturek PC, Harsch IA, Konturek K, et al. Gut-liver axis: how do gut bacteria influence the liver? Med Sci (Basel) 2018;6(3):79.

23. Cassard AM, Ciocan D. Microbiota, a key player in alcoholic liver disease. Clin Mol Hepatol 2018;24(2):100–7.

24. Sarin SK, Pande A, Schnabl B. Microbiome as a therapeutic target in alcohol-related liver disease. J Hepatol 2019;70(2):260–72.

25. Yiu JH, Dorweiler B, Woo CW. Interaction between gut microbiota and toll-like receptor: from immunity to metabolism. J Mol Med (Berl) 2017;95(1):13–20.

26. Rathe M, Müller K, Sangild PT, et al. Clinical applications of bovine colostrum therapy: a systematic review. Nutr Rev 2014;72(4):237–54.

27. Sidhu S, Goyal O, Gupta A, et al. Corticosteroids and bovine colostrum in treatment of alcoholic hepatitis 'in Extremis': a pilot study. J Clin Exp Hepatol 2015; 5(Supplement 2):S19–20.

28. Available at: https://clinicaltrials.gov/ct2/show/results/NCT01968382. Assessed January 27, 2020.

29. Mohammad MK, Zhou Z, Cave M, et al. Zinc and liver disease. Nutr Clin Pract 2012;27(1):8–20.

30. Zhong W, Zhao Y, Sun X, et al. Dietary zinc deficiency exaggerates ethanol-induced liver injury in mice: involvement of intrahepatic and extrahepatic factors. PLoS One 2013;8(10):e76522.

31. Sun Q, Zhong W, Zhang W, et al. Zinc deficiency mediates alcohol-induced apoptotic cell death in the liver of rats through activating ER and mitochondrial cell death pathways. Am J Physiol Gastrointest Liver Physiol 2015;308(9): G757–66.

32. Szabo G, Mitchell M, McClain C, et al. IL-1 receptor antagonist in combination with pentoxifylline and zinc for severe alcoholic hepatitis: a multicenter randomized double- bind placebo-controlled clinical trial. Hepatology 2018;68(6): 1444A.

33. Bull-Otterson L, Feng W, Kirpich I, et al. Metagenomic analyses of alcohol induced pathogenic alterations in the intestinal microbiome and the effect of Lactobacillus rhamnosus GG treatment. PLoS One 2013;8(1):e53028.

34. Vergis N, Atkinson SR, Knapp S, et al. In patients with severe alcoholic hepatitis, prednisolone increases susceptibility to infection and infection-related mortality, and is associated with high circulating levels of bacterial DNA. Gastroenterology 2017;152(5):1068–77.e4.

35. Singal AK, Shah VH, Kamath PS. Infection in severe alcoholic hepatitis: yet another piece in the puzzle. Gastroenterology 2017;152(5):938–40.

36. Vlachogiannakos J, Viazis N, Vasianopoulou P, et al. Long-term administration of rifaximin improves the prognosis of patients with decompensated alcoholic cirrhosis. J Gastroenterol Hepatol 2013;28(3):450–5.

37. Vlachogiannakos J, Saveriadis AS, Viazis N, et al. Intestinal decontamination improves liver haemodynamics in patients with alcohol-related decompensated cirrhosis. Aliment Pharmacol Ther 2009;29(9):992–9.

38. Jimenez C, Ventura-Cots M, Sala M, et al. Use of rifaximin in alcoholic hepatitis: pilot study. J Hepatol 2018;69:S816.

39. Forsyth CB, Farhadi A, Jakate SM, et al. Lactobacillus GG treatment ameliorates alcohol-induced intestinal oxidative stress, gut leakiness, and liver injury in a rat model of alcoholic steatohepatitis. Alcohol. 2009;43(2):163–72.

40. Gu Z, Liu Y, Hu S, et al. Probiotics for alleviating alcoholic liver injury. Gastroenterol Res Pract 2019;2019:9097276.

41. Han SH, Suk KT, Kim DJ, et al. Effects of probiotics (cultured Lactobacillus subtilis/Streptococcus faecium) in the treatment of alcoholic hepatitis: randomized-controlled multicenter study. Eur J Gastroenterol Hepatol 2015;27(11):1300–6.

42. Philips CA, Pande A, Shasthry SM, et al. Healthy donor fecal microbiota transplantation in steroid-ineligible severe alcoholic hepatitis: a pilot study. Clin Gastroenterol Hepatol 2017;15(4):600–2.

43. Philips CA, Phadke N, Ganesan K, et al. Corticosteroids, nutrition, pentoxifylline, or fecal microbiota transplantation for severe alcoholic hepatitis. Indian J Gastroenterol 2018;37(3):215–25.

44. Dhiman RSA, Roy A, Premjumar M, et al. Role of fecal microbiota transplantation in severe alcoholic hepatitis: assessment of impact on prognosis and short-term outcomes. J Hepatol 2020;73:S179.

45. Afford SC, Fisher NC, Neil DA, et al. Distinct patterns of chemokine expression are associated with leukocyte recruitment in alcoholic hepatitis and alcoholic cirrhosis. J Pathol 1998;186(1):82–9.

46. Taïeb J, Mathurin P, Elbim C, et al. Blood neutrophil functions and cytokine release in severe alcoholic hepatitis: effect of corticosteroids. J Hepatol 2000;32(4):579–86.

47. Barnes MA, McMullen MR, Roychowdhury S, et al. Macrophage migration inhibitory factor contributes to ethanol-induced liver injury by mediating cell injury, steatohepatitis, and steatosis. Hepatology 2013;57(5):1980–91.

48. Minagawa M, Deng Q, Liu ZX, et al. Activated natural killer T cells induce liver injury by Fas and tumor necrosis factor-alpha during alcohol consumption. Gastroenterology 2004;126(5):1387–99.

49. Szabo G, Mandrekar P. A recent perspective on alcohol, immunity, and host defense. Alcohol Clin Exp Res 2009;33(2):220–32.

50. Louvet AMP. Alcoholic liver disease: mechanisms of injury and targeted treatment. Nat Rev Gastroenterol Hepatol 2015;12:231–42.

51. Iracheta-Vellve A, Petrasek J, Gyogyosi B, et al. Interleukin-1 inhibition facilitates recovery from liver injury and promotes regeneration of hepatocytes in alcoholic hepatitis in mice. Liver Int 2017;37(7):968–73.

52. Petrasek J, Bala S, Csak T, et al. IL-1 receptor antagonist ameliorates inflammasome-dependent alcoholic steatohepatitis in mice. J Clin Invest 2012;122(10):3476–89.

53. Orrock JE, Ilowite NT. Canakinumab for the treatment of active systemic juvenile idiopathic arthritis. Expert Rev Clin Pharmacol 2016;9(8):1015–24.

54. Sfriso P, Bindoli S, Doria A, et al. Canakinumab for the treatment of adult-onset Still's disease. Expert Rev Clin Immunol 2020;16(2):129–38.

55. Peeraphatdit TB, Simonetto DA, Shah VH. Exploring new treatment paradigms for alcoholic hepatitis by extrapolating from NASH and cholestasis. J Hepatol 2018;69(2):275–7.

56. Hartmann P, Hochrath K, Horvath A, et al. Modulation of the intestinal bile acid/ farnesoid X receptor/fibroblast growth factor 15 axis improves alcoholic liver disease in mice. Hepatology 2018;67(6):2150–66.

57. Verbeke L, Farre R, Trebicka J, et al. Obeticholic acid, a farnesoid X receptor agonist, improves portal hypertension by two distinct pathways in cirrhotic rats. Hepatology 2014;59(6):2286–98.

58. Nevens F, Andreone P, Mazzella G, et al. A placebo-controlled trial of obeticholic acid in primary biliary cholangitis. N Engl J Med 2016;375(7):631–43.

59. Neuschwander-Tetri BA, Loomba R, Sanyal AJ, et al. Farnesoid X nuclear receptor ligand obeticholic acid for non-cirrhotic, non-alcoholic steatohepatitis (FLINT): a multicentre, randomised, placebo-controlled trial. Lancet. 2015; 385(9972):956–65.

60. Barreyro FJ, Holod S, Finocchietto PV, et al. The pan-caspase inhibitor Emricasan (IDN-6556) decreases liver injury and fibrosis in a murine model of non-alcoholic steatohepatitis. Liver Int 2015;35(3):953–66.

61. Gracia-Sancho J, Manicardi N, Ortega-Ribera M, et al. Emricasan ameliorates portal hypertension and liver fibrosis in cirrhotic rats through a hepatocyte-mediated paracrine mechanism. Hepatol Commun 2019;3(7):987–1000.

62. Pockros PJ, Jeffers L, Afdhal N, et al. Final results of a double-blind, placebo-controlled trial of the antifibrotic efficacy of interferon-gamma1b in chronic hepatitis C patients with advanced fibrosis or cirrhosis. Hepatology 2007;45(3): 569–78.

63. Shiffman M, Freilich B, Vuppalanchi R, et al. Randomised clinical trial: emricasan versus placebo significantly decreases ALT and caspase 3/7 activation in subjects with non-alcoholic fatty liver disease. Aliment Pharmacol Ther 2019; 49(1):64–73.

64. Frenette CT, Morelli G, Shiffman ML, et al. Emricasan improves liver function in patients with cirrhosis and high model for end-stage liver disease scores compared with placebo. Clin Gastroenterol Hepatol 2019;17(4):774–83.e4.

65. Schuster-Gaul S, Geisler LJ, McGeough MD, et al. ASK1 inhibition reduces cell death and hepatic fibrosis in an Nlrp3 mutant liver injury model. JCI Insight 2020;5(2):e123294.

66. Wree A, McGeough MD, Pena CA, et al. NLRP3 inflammasome activation is required for fibrosis development in NAFLD. J Mol Med (Berl) 2014;92(10): 1069–82.

67. Wree A, Eguchi A, McGeough MD, et al. NLRP3 inflammasome activation results in hepatocyte pyroptosis, liver inflammation, and fibrosis in mice. Hepatology 2014;59(3):898–910.

68. Mathurin P, Dufour J, Bzowe NH, et al. Selonsertib in combination with prednisolone for the treatment of severe alcoholic hepatitis: a phase 2 randomized controlled trial. Hepatology 2018;68(S1):8A.

69. Ren S, Ning Y. Sulfation of 25-hydroxycholesterol regulates lipid metabolism, inflammatory responses, and cell proliferation. Am J Physiol Endocrinol Metab 2014;306(2):E123–30.

70. Louvet A, Labreuche J, Artru F, et al. Combining data from liver disease scoring systems better predicts outcomes of patients with alcoholic hepatitis. Gastroenterology 2015;149(2):398–406.e8 [quiz: e316–7].

71. Hassanein T, Stein L, Flamm S, et al. Safety AND Efficacy of DUR-928: a potential new therapy for acute alcoholic hepatitis. Hepatology 2019;70(6):1483A–4A.

72. Landeen LK, Van Allen J, Heredia N, et al. Expression of acute-phase proteins by ELAD C3A Cells. Transplantation 2015;99:208.

73. Bedard PW, Lapetoda J, Van Allen J, et al. ELAD VTL C3A cells may impact liver regeneration through secreted factors. Hepatology 2015;(suppl 1):1071A.

74. Thompson J, Jones N, Al-Khafaji A, et al. Extracorporeal cellular therapy (ELAD) in severe alcoholic hepatitis: a multinational, prospective, controlled, randomized trial. Liver Transpl 2018;24(3):380–93.

75. Pyrsopoulos N, Hassanein T, Subramanian R, et al. A study investigating the effect of extracorporeal cellular therapy with C3A cells on the survival of alcoholic hepatitis designed along the guidelines of the NIAAA. J Hepatol 2019;70:e282.

76. Ambade A, Lowe P, Kodys K, et al. Pharmacological inhibition of CCR2/5 signaling prevents and reverses alcohol-induced liver damage, steatosis, and inflammation in mice. Hepatology 2019;69(3):1105–21.

77. Mandrekar P, Ambade A, Lim A, et al. An essential role for monocyte chemoattractant protein-1 in alcoholic liver injury: regulation of proinflammatory cytokines and hepatic steatosis in mice. Hepatology 2011;54(6):2185–97.

78. Marra F, Tacke F. Roles for chemokines in liver disease. Gastroenterology 2014; 147(3):577–94.e1.

79. Blom DJ, Harada-Shiba M, Rubba P, et al. Efficacy and safety of Alirocumab in adults with homozygous familial hypercholesterolemia: the ODYSSEY HoFH trial. J Am Coll Cardiol 2020;76(2):131–42.

80. Lambert G, Sjouke B, Choque B, et al. The PCSK9 decade. J Lipid Res 2012; 53(12):2515–24.

81. Lee JS, Mukhopadhyay P, Matyas C, et al. PCSK9 inhibition as a novel therapeutic target for alcoholic liver disease. Sci Rep 2019;9(1):17167.

82. Hill DB, Devalaraja R, Joshi-Barve S, et al. Antioxidants attenuate nuclear factor-kappa B activation and tumor necrosis factor-alpha production in alcoholic hepatitis patient monocytes and rat Kupffer cells, in vitro. Clin Biochem 1999;32(7): 563–70.

83. Singal AKJS, Weinman SA. Antioxidants as therapeutic agents for liver disease. Liver Int 2011;31(10):1432–48.

84. Flora K, Hahn M, Rosen H, et al. Milk thistle (Silybum marianum) for the therapy of liver disease. Am J Gastroenterol 1998;93(2):139–43.

85. Parés A, Planas R, Torres M, et al. Effects of silymarin in alcoholic patients with cirrhosis of the liver: results of a controlled, double-blind, randomized and multicenter trial. J Hepatol 1998;28(4):615–21.

86. Lucena MI, Andrade RJ, de la Cruz JP, et al. Sánchez de la Cuesta F. Effects of silymarin MZ-80 on oxidative stress in patients with alcoholic cirrhosis. Results of a randomized, double-blind, placebo-controlled clinical study. Int J Clin Pharmacol Ther 2002;40(1):2–8.

87. Mezey E, Potter J, Rennie-Tankersley L, et al. A randomized placebo controlled trial of vitamin E for alcoholic hepatitis. J Hepatol 2004;40(1):40–6.

88. Phillips M, Curtis H, Portmann B, et al. Antioxidants versus corticosteroids in the treatment of severe alcoholic hepatitis—a randomised clinical trial 2006;2006(44):784–90.

89. Stewart S, Prince M, Bassendine M, et al. A randomized trial of antioxidaA randomized trial of antioxidant therapy alone or with corticosteroids in acute alcoholic hepatitis. J Hepatol 2007;47(2):277–83.

90. Rushworth GF, Megson IL. Existing and potential therapeutic uses for N-acetylcysteine: the need for conversion to intracellular glutathione for antioxidant benefits. Pharmacol Ther 2014;141(2):150–9.

91. Nguyen-Khac E, Thierry T, Piquet M, et al. Glucocorticoids plus N-acetylcysteine in severe alcoholic hepatitis. N Engl J Med 2011;365:1781–9.

92. Singh V, Keisham A, Bhalla A, et al. Efficacy of granulocyte colony-stimulating factor and N-acetylcysteine therapies in patients with severe alcoholic hepatitis. Clin Gastroenterol Hepatol 2018;16:1650–6.

93. Amjad W, Joseph A, Doycheva I, et al. A combination of n-acetylcysteine and prednisone has no bene t over prednisone alone in severe alcoholic hepatitis: a retrospective analysis. Dig Dis Sci 2020;65(12):3726–33.

94. Addolorato G, Ancona C, Capristo E, et al. Metadoxine in the treatment of acute and chronic alcoholism: a review. Int J Immunopathol Pharmacol 2003;16(3): 207–14.

95. Higuera-de la Tijera F, Servín-Caamaño AI, Cruz-Herrera J, et al. Treatment with Metadoxine and its impact on early mortality in patients with severe alcoholic hepatitis. Ann Hepatol 2014;13(3):343–52.

96. Higuera-de la Tijera F, Servín-Caamaño AI, Serralde-Zúñiga AE, et al. Metadoxine improves the three- and six-month survival rates in patients with severe alcoholic hepatitis. World J Gastroenterol 2015;21(16):4975–85.

97. Guo X, Li W, Xin Q, et al. Vitamin C protective role for alcoholic liver disease in mice through regulating iron metabolism. Toxicol Ind Health 2011;27(4):341–8.

98. Heritage ML, Murphy TL, Bridle KR, et al. Hepcidin regulation in wild-type and Hfe knockout mice in response to alcohol consumption: evidence for an alcohol-induced hypoxic response. Alcohol Clin Exp Res 2009;33(8):1391–400.

99. Flanagan JM, Peng H, Beutler E. Effects of alcohol consumption on iron metabolism in mice with hemochromatosis mutations. Alcohol Clin Exp Res 2007; 31(1):138–43.

100. Marik PE, Liggett A. Adding an orange to the banana bag: vitamin C deficiency is common in alcohol use disorders. Crit Care 2019;23(1):165.

101. Fujii T, Fowler R, Vincent JL. Vitamin C and thiamine for sepsis: time to go back to fundamental principles. Intensive Care Med 2020;46(11):2061–3.

102. Aruna P, Venkataramanamma D, Singh AK, et al. Health benefits of punicic acid: a review. Compr Rev Food Sci Food Saf 2016;15(1):16–27.

103. Celik I, Temur A, Isik I. Hepatoprotective role and antioxidant capacity of pomegranate (Punica granatum) flowers infusion against trichloroacetic acid-exposed in rats. Food Chem Toxicol 2009;47(1):145–9.

104. Shaban NZ, El-Kersh MA, El-Rashidy FH, et al. Protective role of Punica granatum (pomegranate) peel and seed oil extracts on diethylnitrosamine and phenobarbital-induced hepatic injury in male rats. Food Chem 2013;141(3): 1587–96.

105. Koteish A, Yang S, Lin H, et al. Chronic ethanol exposure potentiates lipopolysaccharide liver injury despite inhibiting Jun N-terminal kinase and caspase 3 activation. J Biol Chem 2002;277(15):13037–44.

106. Dippold RP, Vadigepalli R, Gonye GE, et al. Chronic ethanol feeding alters miRNA expression dynamics during liver regeneration. Alcohol Clin Exp Res 2013;37(Suppl 1):E59–69.

107. Kong X, Feng D, Mathews S, et al. Hepatoprotectiveandanti- fibrotic functions of interleukin-22: therapeutic potential for the treatment of alcoholic liver disease. J Gastroenterol Hepatol 2013;28(1):56–60.

108. Gao B, Xiang X. Interleukin-22 from bench to bedside: a promising drug for epithelial repair. Cell Mol Immunol 2019;16(7):666–7.

109. Yang L, Zhang Y, Wang L, et al. Amelioration of high fat diet induced liver lipogenesis and hepatic steatosis by interleukin-22. J Hepatol 2010;53(2):339–47.

110. Arab JP, Sehrawat TS, Simonetto DA, et al. An open-label, dose-Escalation study to assess the safety and efficacy of IL-22 agonist F-652 in patients with alcohol-associated hepatitis. Hepatology 2020;72(2):441–53.

111. Yannaki E, Athanasiou E, Xagorari A, et al. G-CSF-primed hematopoietic stem cells or G-CSF per se accelerate recovery and improve survival after liver injury, predominantly by promoting endogenous repair programs. Exp Hematol 2005; 33(1):108–19.

112. Theocharis SE, Papadimitriou LJ, Retsou ZP, et al. Granulocyte-colony stimulating factor administration ameliorates liver regeneration in animal model of fulminant hepatic failure and encephalopathy. Dig Dis Sci 2003;48(9):1797–803.

113. Spahr L, Lambert JF, Rubbia-Brandt L, et al. Granulocyte-colony stimulating factor induces proliferation of hepatic progenitors in alcoholic steatohepatitis: a randomized trial. Hepatology 2008;48(1):221–9.

114. Singh V, Sharma AK, Narasimhan RL, et al. Granulocyte colony-stimulating factor in severe alcoholic hepatitis: a randomized pilot study. Am J Gastroenterol 2014;109(9):1417–23.

115. Shasthry SM, Sharma MK, Shasthry V, et al. Efficacy of granulocyte colony-stimulating factor in the management of steroid-nonresponsive severe alcoholic hepatitis: a double-blind randomized controlled trial. Hepatology 2019;70(3): 802–11.

Current Trends in Liver Transplantation for Alcoholic Hepatitis

Sundus Bhatti, MD[a,b], Donghee Kim, MD, PhD[c], Aijaz Ahmed, MD[c], George Cholankeril, MD, MS[a,b,*]

KEYWORDS

- Alcoholic Hepatitis • Alcohol-related liver disease • Liver transplantation
- Alcohol relapse

KEY POINTS

- Patients with severe alcoholic hepatitis have limited treatment options and a high risk of mortality.
- Liver transplantation (LT) as a treatment in patients with corticosteroid refractory alcoholic hepatitis (AH) has demonstrated favorable outcomes.
- Risk of alcohol recidivism is a major concern when it comes to LT in patients with AH.
- This article outlines a pragmatic clinical algorithm that can be used to minimize the risk of recidivism and allow a pathway for LT as a treatment option in a subcohort of patients with AH who present with favorable variables.

INTRODUCTION

Alcohol use disorder (AUD) is responsible for nearly 3 million deaths each year, accounting for over 5% of all deaths worldwide.[1] Alcohol-related liver disease (ARLD) encompasses a broad spectrum of liver injury, including steatosis, steatohepatitis, fibrosis, and cirrhosis complicated by portal hypertension and risk of hepatic decompensation necessitating the need for liver transplantation (LT).[2] Alcohol-related or alcoholic hepatitis (AH), a severe acute syndrome superimposed on ARLD, can be associated with high morbidity and mortality. Because of the lack of effective medical

[a] Baylor College of Medicine, Section of Gastroenterology and Hepatology, 6620 Main Street, Suite 1450, Houston, TX 77030, USA; [b] Baylor College of Medicine, Division of Abdominal Transplantation, Houston, TX, USA; [c] Stanford University School of Medicine, Division of Gastroenterology and Hepatology, 750 Welch Road, #210, Stanford, CA 94304, USA
* Corresponding author. Baylor College of Medicine, Section of Gastroenterology and Hepatology, Liver Center, Division of Abdominal Transplantation, 6620 Main Street, Suite 1450, Houston, Texas 77030.
E-mail address: George.cholankeril@bcm.edu

Clin Liver Dis 25 (2021) 625–634
https://doi.org/10.1016/j.cld.2021.04.002
1089-3261/21/© 2021 Elsevier Inc. All rights reserved.
liver.theclinics.com

treatment options, patients with severe AH have early 28-day mortality surpassing 50%.[3] In a small minority of these patients, those who fail to respond to medical therapy, LT may be the only live-saving treatment option.

HISTORICAL JUSTIFICATION TO PERFORM LIVER TRANSPLANTATION IN ALCOHOL-RELATED LIVER DISEASE

In 1983, ARLD was listed as an indication for LT for the first time by the National Institutes of Health (NIH) in the United States. This indication was contingent on selecting patients who were judged as suitable candidates to abstain from alcohol and clinically expected to have a fatal outcome without LT. However, upon its approval as an indication for LT, ARLD constituted fewer than 10% of all LTs in the United States.[4] The role of LT for ARLD was promulgated by a landmark study by Thomas Starlz and colleagues in 1988, which reported a striking 1-year survival rate of 73% in 41 patients and low risk of alcohol recidivism during the short-term follow-up.[5] Subsequently, LT became a viable treatment option for patients with ARLD as long as each individual case was reviewed and approved by the liver transplant selection committee.

EVOLUTION OF ALCOHOL-RELATED LIVER DISEASE AS THE LEADING INDICATION FOR LIVER TRANSPLANTATION

Over the last 3 decades, LT for ARLD has gradually risen. By 2017, ARLD became the leading indication for LT in the United States, comprising of 29% of all LTs, with 1- and 5-year patient and graft survival rates comparable to those of other indications.[6,7] This trend was a reflection of rising prevalence of AUD in the population leading to a 45% increase in patients with ARLD on the waiting list for LT between 2004 and 2013.[8] At the same time, parallel trends were reported from Europe that led to ARLD catapulting to a leading indication for LT in 2019.[9]

DIAGNOSTIC CRITERIA FOR ALCOHOLIC HEPATITIS

Several diagnostic criteria for AH have been proposed. The NIH has classified AH as the onset of jaundice within 60 days in the setting of heavy alcohol consumption over 6 months with laboratory data demonstrating elevated serum total bilirubin more than 3 mg/dL, an aspartate aminotransferase (AST) level ranging from 50 U/L to 400 U/L (ie, more than 1.5 times higher than alanine aminotransferase level), and in which all other known etiologies of liver disease have been excluded.[10] AH patients with Maddrey discriminant function (MDF) greater than 32 or Model for End-Stage Liver Disease (MELD) greater than 20 are classified as severe AH. If medical therapy such as corticosteroid administration is not effective and/or there is progressive liver disease, LT remains the only life-saving intervention. However, LT as an indication for severe AH in the absence of 6 months of sobriety presents as a management challenge because of the historically conventional practice of documenting 6 months of sobriety with attendance at Alcoholic Anonymous meetings and random toxicology screening. Although some patients with AH may improve and not need a liver transplant surgery, others may not survive 6 months following hepatic decompensation.

EVIDENCE-BASED RATIONALE FOR LIVER TRANSPLANTATION IN ALCOHOLIC HEPATITIS

In a European pilot study, Mathurin and colleagues[11] observed that a subgroup of patients with severe AH who were able to demonstrate a strong psychosocial support

(PSS) and other favorable variables that were predictive of a low risk for relapse had a survival benefit. In the United States, however, LT for severe AH is contested without 6 months of abstinence.[12] Other barriers to LT for AH include variable transplant center practices, sociocultural barriers, scarcity of organs, and insurance policies.[12] It is important to respect opposing opinions regarding LT for patients who develop ARLD with or without AH without sobriety. However, this article will focus its discussion on identifying the evidence-based predictors that may provide comparable outcomes in the absence of 6 months of sobriety.[11,12] These studies support early evaluation for LT in patients with hepatic decompensation from AH that is refractory to medical therapy in the absence of: poorly controlled co-existing psychiatric comorbidities; fixed period of abstinence prior to LT; and psychosocial evaluation by a multidisciplinary team, including a social worker, an addiction specialist, and mental health professional with addiction and transplantation expertise. In addition, predictors of successful outcome include lack of history of previous attempts at addiction rehabilitation, absence of other substance dependency, adequate comprehension, psychosocial support, and willingness to commit to formal rehabilitation prior to and following LT. A comprehensive evaluation for LT even without 6 months of sobriety may provide comparable short-term and long-term survival outcome by assessing the predictors noted previously in a stepwise approach. Standardization of the approach at transplant centers must be made to maintain consistency during the liver transplant evaluation and to avoid disparity.

CONTROVERSIES IN DURATION OF SOBRIETY PRIOR TO LIVER TRANSPLANTATION FOR ALCOHOLIC HEPATITIS

A 6-month abstinence rule was proposed by the American Society of Transplant Physicians and the American Association for the Study of Liver Diseases prior to listing patients with ARLD for LT. This time can be used to observe clinical improvement, which may circumvent the need for LT and demonstrate clinical compliance via abstinence.[13] The 6-month abstinence rule is contentious, because curative treatment, LT, is withheld in patients with medication-refractory severe AH who have a 6-month mortality rate as high as 80%.[14] Furthermore, the 6-month abstinence period rule can be challenged because of a relapse rate of 20% at 5 years. The acceptance of AH as an indication for LT for AH may impact and shrink the already limited organ pool. Public opinion has been neutral, and LT for AH constitutes a mere 1% to 3% of all utilized donor livers.[11,12] AH is viewed as a self-induced disease from personal behavior choices with complicated psychosocial elements, but the attitude toward LT for this indication is quite the opposite to that of patients with viral hepatitis and nonalcoholic steatohepatitis (NASH) who exhibit noncompliance to diet and exercise regimens over years or patients who indulge in risky behaviors leading to hepatitis B and C viral infections.[13]

STEPWISE EVALUATION FOR LIVER TRANSPLANTATION IN ALCOHOLIC HEPATITIS

Beresford's introduction of a psychosocial assessment to gauge the risk of alcohol relapse in this group of patients introduced an integral aspect of favorable patient selection.[15] He prioritized 4 aspects a patient's psychosocial profile: social isolation, admittance and prior treatment of AUD, and presence of other psychiatric disorders.[16] Growing on this idea, several protocols and prognostic tools have been developed to assess the risk of alcohol relapse (**Table 1**). A recent multicenter study involving 9 centers performing LT in patients with AH contingent on 6-month abstinence criteria, proposed individualized patient selection derived from other more significant predictors of relapse. In this study, negative PSS emerged as the single criterion unanimously agreed upon by all the participating LT centers.[12] Important variables to consider are detailed in **Table 2**. Utilizing Maddrey discriminant function (MDF) greater than 32 aids in predicting patients with AH at risk for high short-term mortality who will benefit from treatment with corticosteroids. The Lille score ($\geq$0.45) can further be used as a prognostication tool to identify AH patients at high risk for mortality despite 7-day course of corticosteroids, who should be considered for other treatment options such as LT.[21] In summary, stepwise liver transplant evaluation is initiated by psychosocial assessment by a multidisciplinary team, including a social worker, an addiction specialist, and mental health professional with addiction and transplantation expertise, combined with medical assessment to document contraindication to steroids or failure of steroids after 7 days of treatment.

OUTCOMES FOR LIVER TRANSPLANTATION IN ALCOHOLIC HEPATITIS FROM EUROPE

Mathurin and colleagues[11] published the first French-Belgian landmark study at 7 participating centers, from 2005 to 2010. Twenty-six patients with medication-refractory severe AH received LT after undergoing stringent selection, with a median wait time of 2 weeks. Patients who received LT had favorable survival rates at 6 months and 2 years compared with the matched medication-refractory patients who did not undergo LT (77% vs 23% at 6 months and 71% vs 23% at 5 years). Three (<15%) patients relapsed, 2 patients at 24 months, and 1 patient at 37 months following LT; these rates are similar to relapse rates seen with alcohol-related cirrhosis. Of these 3 patients, only 1 patient adopted detrimental drinking habits, and the other 2 patients were social alcohol users. None of the 3 patients suffered from alcohol-related graft loss during the follow-up period.[11,22] On the basis of these findings, early LT as a definitive therapy is garnering favorable popularity at transplant centers and in public opinion.[12,23] In another study by Immordino and colleagues, 246 patients were assessed for ARLD from 1997 to 2007 at a liver transplant center in France. One hundred and thirty-three patients (54%) were listed, and 110 patients (45%) received LT. Post-transplant survival rates were 79%, 68%, and 64% at 1, 5, and 10 years, respectively. Explant pathology documented AH in 8 (7.2%) patients following LT. This study reported comparable survival outcomes and post-LT relapse in patients transplanted for AH when compared with the overall group of liver transplant recipients.[24] In a smaller study, Tomé and colleagues reported comparable survival outcomes for patients transplanted for alcohol use (n = 68) and patients with other causes of liver disease (n = 101). Interestingly, patients transplanted for alcohol-related cirrhosis and superimposed AH (n = 36) versus only cirrhosis (n = 32), and patients with mild (n = 26) versus severe (n = 10) AH, had comparable outcomes in their respective groups. Seven patients (10%) relapsed but did not suffer from graft loss or AH.[25]

OUTCOMES FOR LIVER TRANSPLANTATION IN ALCOHOLIC HEPATITIS FROM UNITED STATES

A retrospective study using the data from United Network of Organ Sharing (UNOS) between 2004 and 2010 compared 165 matched patients who received LT for alcoholic cirrhosis with 55 patients who underwent LT for AH.[26] Both groups had comparable 5-year graft survival (75% vs 73%, P=.97) and 5-year overall survival (80% vs

Table 1
Scoring tools to predict alcohol relapse

Tool	Factors Assessed	Relapse Prediction Score
Sustained Alcohol Use Post-Liver Transplantation (SALT) score[17]	1. Number of drinks 2. Failed rehabilitation attempts 3. AUD-related legal issues 4. Illicit drug use	SALT of ≥5 has 25% positive predictive value (PPV) (95% confidence interval [CI], 10%–47%) and 95% negative predictive value (NPV) (95% CI, 89%–98%) and specificity of 84% (95% CI, 76%–90%) for sustained alcohol use after LT Setting the cutoff at the maximum SALT score of 11 has a 50% PPV (95% CI, 1%–99%), 92% NPV (95% CI, 86%–96%), and specificity of 99% (95% CI, 95% –100%)
Stanford Integrated Psychosocial Assessment for Transplantation (SIPAT)[18]	1. Patient willingness (5 items) 2. Social support (3 items) 3. Psychological stability (5 items) 4. Lifestyle and effect of substance use (5 items)	Total SIPAT≥21 with a Pearson's coefficient of 0.853, $P<.001$
Alcohol Relapse Risk Assessment (ARRA)[19]	1. Absence of hepatocellular carcinoma 2. Tobacco dependence 3. Alcohol use after liver disease diagnosis 4. Low motivation for alcohol treatment 5. Poor stress management skills 6. No rehabilitation relationship 7. Limited social support 8. Lack of nonmedical behavioral consequences 9. Engagement in activities with alcohol present	The ARRA score was predictive of relapse to any alcohol use after liver transplant (log rank $\chi2 = 57.9$, $P<.001$) and relapse intensity for those who relapsed ($\chi2 = 15.7$, $P=.003$) ARRA I (score 0, relapse rate 0%) ARRA II (score 1–3, relapse rate 8%) ARRA III (score 4–6, relapse rate 57%) ARRA IV (score 7–9, relapse rate 75%) Supporting the clinical utility of the ARRA score is an area under the curve of 0.892, indicating that the probability that a patient who relapsed to alcohol use would have a higher ARRA score is 89.2%
High-Risk Alcoholism Relapse (HRAR)[20]	1. Duration of heavy drinking 2. Usual number of daily drinks 3. Number of prior inpatient alcohol treatments	Low HRAR score 0–3 High HRAR score 4–6 A high HRAR score was associated with a significantly higher risk of harmful alcohol use (odds ratio [OR], 10.7; 95% CI, 3.8–30.0) ($P<.005$)

Table 2
Inclusion and exclusion variables for liver transplantation in alcoholic hepatitis

Inclusion	Exclusion
Maddrey Discriminant Function >32 Model for End-stage Liver Disease (MELD) >20	Sepsis
Steroid non-responder (Lille $\geq$0.45) or ineligible for medical treatment	Severe comorbidities
Initial presentation of alcohol-related liver decompensation	Prior alcohol-related liver decompensating events
Favorable psychosocial profile	Poor psychosocial profile
Strong social support	Poor social support
Consensus of transplant selection committee	Severe psychiatric illness

From Im GY, Cameron AM, Lucey MR. Liver transplantation for alcoholic hepatitis. J Hepatol 2019;70(2):328-334. https://doi.org/10.1016/j.jhep.2018.11.007

78%, P=.90). There was no alcohol-related graft loss or liver transplant recipient mortality in either group.[26] A subsequent US study that utilized the UNOS database from 2011 to 2016, showed a fourfold rise in listing for patients with severe AH for LT.[27] In this study, early LT for severe AH showed comparable survival outcomes to those with medication-induced acute liver failure.[27] Although these data demonstrate favorable outcomes, alcohol use prior to and after LT is not captured in UNOS database and remains a limiting factor when analyzing these national data. In addition, other limiting factors include variability in diagnostic criteria for AH, avoidance of liver biopsy in the setting of severe AH leading to under-reporting, lack of national policy regarding LT as an indication for AH, and need for consensus among health care providers/insurance companies.

A study by Hasanin and colleagues investigated the LT trends for severe AH at 45 centers in the United States representing 45% of total US volume for LT from 2010 to 2015. A mere 12 of 45 centers (27%) were noted to list patients with AH for LT. Of these 12 centers, only 8 centers favored waitlisting for LT if it involved a patient with an initial episode of AH resulting in hepatic decompensation. The main differences in centers that waitlisted patients with severe AH for LT compared with centers that did not pivoted on the 6-month abstinence criteria, time to assess response to steroids, and improved natural course of disease. The predominant impediments against LT for AH were inadequate consensus between the members of liver transplant selection committee, lack of center protocol/policy for LT in patients with AH, paucity of donor organs, recidivism protocols, insurance approval, and psychosocial barriers.[12] The 12 centers unanimously agreed and prioritized 4 criteria in selecting patients with AH for LT: excellent PSS, steroid-refractory AH, initial episode of AH, and a signed contract for alcohol abstinence. Of the 12 centers, 6 implemented all 4 criteria to determine listing and LT of severe AH. Consequently, only 45 (1.4%) of 3290 liver transplant surgeries were performed for severe AH. The median time from waitlisting to LT was 4 weeks for severe AH. Of 45 liver transplant recipients for AH, 42, 40, and 31 patients reached 6-month, 1-year, and 5-year follow-up, respectively. The survival rates at these follow-ups were 93% (39/42), 93% (37/40), and 87%, respectively. Eight (18%) patients experienced relapse, which is comparable to that of LT for alcohol-related cirrhosis (15%–20%).[28]

Contrary to the comparable relapse rates, AH faces higher resistance as a widely accepted indication for LT.[12]

In 2018, the American Consortium of Early Liver Transplantation for Alcoholic Hepatitis (ACCELERATE-AH) reported the largest multicenter post-transplant experience in patients with AH. In this large, 12-center study, 147 patients with severe AH underwent LT from 2006 to 2017. Three-year post-transplant survival was 84%, similar to other leading indications for LT. Alcohol use was reported in nearly one-third of patients and was associated with over a threefold increase in mortality, further highlighting the importance of optimizing patient selection and management after LT.[29] Young age was found to be the sole predictor associated with any alcohol use. The only factor to indicate detrimental relapse was drinking more than 10 drinks per day at first presentation.[30] It is important to recognize the importance of close post-transplant follow-up needed to provide an adequate support system and psychosocial management to optimize outcomes in this patient population. Therefore, liver transplant centers evaluating patients with AH for LT must seek programmatic development and establish resources for post-transplant care of this special subpopulation.

In another single-center series experience, post-transplant outcomes and recidivism were evaluated in patients with severe AH without 6 months abstinence and were compared to those with alcoholic cirrhosis. As seen in prior studies, liver transplant recipient and graft survival were favorable in those with severe AH compared with alcoholic cirrhosis. Recidivism rates in AH group were observed to be higher but not statistically significant (28% vs 24%, $P=.8$).[31] In a case-control study of 36 severe AH patients who underwent LT, risk of recidivism in patients with at least 1-month (high-risk) and 3-month (medium-risk) sobriety were similar to those with alcoholic cirrhosis with at least 6-month sobriety.[32] A recent meta-analysis evaluated LT outcomes in 11 studies and further corroborated these outcomes. Patients who received LT for clinically severe AH and those who were incidentally found to have AH on the explant were included in this study. The overall 6-month survival rate was 85%. Six-month survival was 80% in the subgroup analysis that included only patients who underwent LT for clinically severe AH. The survival rate for LT of AH was similar to those transplanted for alcoholic cirrhosis. Despite strict criteria for LT candidacy, 14% of severe AH patients experienced relapse.[33] Factors incorporated in decision making included severity of alcohol use, failed attempts to remain abstinent, insight into unhealthy alcohol use, and psychiatric and social support. A uniform consensus is warranted to standardize criteria and guide centers in clinical assessment of patients with AH necessitating LT.[34]

SUMMARY

With the emerging data and findings from the reviewed literature, LT for AH provides an effective treatment option in patients with adequate psychosocial support and without a 6-month abstinence period. The survival rates and alcohol relapse rates for LT in properly selected patients with AH are comparable to those with alcoholic cirrhosis. A consensus conference to standardize the evaluation of patients with AH for LT is needed to develop practice guidelines. The development of practice guidelines will facilitate prompt diagnosis, optimize management, and promote uniform policies by health care insurance carriers with the goal of eliminating disparity.

CLINICS CARE POINTS

- Severe alcoholic hepatitis is associated with high short-term mortality rates. Liver transplantation is a curative therapy in patients who are refractory to corticosteroid therapy.
- Select patients with severe alcoholic hepatitis who have not responded to conventional medical therapy with a Maddrey discriminant function score > 32 or Model for End-Stage Liver Disease (MELD) score > 20 may be considered for liver transplantation.
- Early and expedient referral for liver transplantation is crucial for centers to assess potential psychosocial barriers and risk for recidivism. Several predictive scoring tools are readily available and can be integrated into the liver transplant evaluation to risk stratify candidates based on their psychosocial profile including the SALT and SIPAT scores.

DISCLOSURE

The authors have nothing to disclose.

REFERENCES

1. GBD 2016 Alcohol Collaborators. Alcohol use and burden for 195 countries and territories, 1990-2016: a systematic analysis for the Global Burden of Disease Study 2016 [published correction appears in Lancet. 2018 Sep 29;392(10153):1116] [published correction appears in Lancet. 2019 Jun 22;393(10190):e44]. Lancet 2018;392(10152):1015–35.
2. Frazier TH, Stocker AM, Kershner NA, et al. Treatment of alcoholic liver disease. Therap Adv Gastroenterol 2011;4(1):63–81.
3. Thursz MR, Richardson P, Allison M, et al, STOPAH Trial. Prednisolone or pentoxifylline for alcoholic hepatitis. N Engl J Med 2015;372(17):1619–28.
4. National Institutes of health consensus development conference statement: liver transplantation–June 20-23, 1983. Hepatology 1984;4(1 Suppl):107S–10S.
5. Starzl TE, Van Thiel D, Tzakis AG, et al. Orthotopic liver transplantation for alcoholic cirrhosis. JAMA 1988;260(17):2542–4.
6. Kim WR, Lake JR, Smith JM, et al. OPTN/SRTR 2017 annual data report: liver. Am J Transplan 2019;19(S2):184–283.
7. Cholankeril G, Ahmed A. Alcoholic liver disease replaces hepatitis C virus infection as the leading indication for liver transplantation in the United States. Clin Gastroenterol Hepatol 2018;16:1356–8.
8. Wong RJ, Aguilar M, Cheung R, et al. Nonalcoholic steatohepatitis is the second leading etiology of liver disease among adults awaiting liver transplantation in the United States. Gastroenterology 2015;148:547–55.
9. Burra P, Senzolo M, Adam R, et al. Liver transplantation for alcoholic liver disease in Europe: a study from the ELTR (European liver transplant registry). Am J Transplant 2010;10(1):138–48.
10. Crabb DW, Bataller R, Chalasani NP, et al. Standard definitions and common data elements for clinical trials in patients with alcoholic hepatitis: recommendation from the NIAAA alcoholic hepatitis consortia. Gastroenterology 2016;150(4): 785–90.
11. Mathurin P, Moreno C, Samuel D, et al. Early liver transplantation for severe alcoholic hepatitis. N Engl J Med 2011;365(19):1790–800.

12. Hasanin M, Dubay DA, McGuire BM, et al. Liver transplantation for alcoholic hepatitis: a survey of liver transplant centers. Liver Transpl 2015;21(11):1449–52.

13. Im GY, Cameron AM, Lucey MR. Liver transplantation for alcoholic hepatitis. J Hepatol 2019;70(2):328–34.

14. Singal AK, Kamath PS, Gores GJ, et al. Alcoholic hepatitis: current challenges and future directions. Clin Gastroenterol Hepatol 2014;12(4):555–64 [quiz e31-2].

15. Beresford T. Liver transplantation and alcoholism rehabilitation. Alcohol Health Res World 1994;18(4):310–2.

16. Beresford T. Psychological assessment of alcoholic candidates for liver transplantation. Cambridge: Cambridge University Press; 1994. p. 29–49.

17. Lee BP, Vittinghoff E, Hsu C, et al. Predicting low risk for sustained alcohol use after early liver transplant for acute alcoholic hepatitis: the sustained alcohol use post-liver transplant score. Hepatology 2019;69(4):1477–87.

18. Maldonado JR, Dubois HC, David EE, et al. The Stanford Integrated Psychosocial Assessment for Transplantation (SIPAT): a new tool for the psycho-social evaluation of pre-transplant candidates. Psychosomatics 2012;53(2):123–32.

19. Rodrigue JR, Hanto DW, Curry MP. The alcohol relapse risk assessment: a scoring system to predict the risk of relapse to any alcohol use after liver transplant. Prog Transplant 2013;23(4):310–8.

20. De Gottardi A, Spahr L, Gelez P, et al. A simple score for predicting alcohol relapse after liver transplantation: results from 387 patients over 15 years. Arch Intern Med 2007;167(11):1183–8.

21. Louvet A, Naveau S, Abdelnour M, et al. The Lille model: a new tool for therapeutic strategy in patients with severe alcoholic hepatitis treated with steroids. Hepatology 2007;45(6):1348–54.

22. Dew MA, DiMartini AF, Steel J, et al. Meta-analysis of risk for relapse to substance use after transplantation of the liver or other solid organs. Liver Transpl 2008;14(2):159–72.

23. Stroh G, Rosell T, Dong F, et al. Early liver transplantation for patients with acute alcoholic hepatitis: public views and the effects on organ donation. Am J Transpl 2015;15(6):1598–604.

24. Immordino G, Gelli M, Ferrante R, et al. Alcohol abstinence and orthotopic liver transplantation in alcoholic liver cirrhosis. Transpl Proc 2009;41(4):1253–5.

25. Tomé S, Martinez-Rey C, González-Quintela A, et al. Influence of superimposed alcoholic hepatitis on the outcome of liver transplantation for end-stage alcoholic liver disease. J Hepatol 2002;36(6):793–8.

26. Singal AK, Bashar H, Anand BS, et al. Outcomes after liver transplantation for alcoholic hepatitis are similar to alcoholic cirrhosis: exploratory analysis from the UNOS database. Hepatology 2012;55(5):1398–405.

27. Puri P, Cholankeril G, Myint TY, et al. Early liver transplantation is a viable treatment option in severe acute alcoholic hepatitis. Alcohol Alcohol 2018;53(6):716–8.

28. Singal AK, Chaha KS, Rasheed K, et al. Liver transplantation in alcoholic liver disease current status and controversies. World J Gastroenterol 2013;19(36):5953–63.

29. Lee BP, Mehta N, Platt L, et al. Outcomes of early liver transplantation for patients with severe alcoholic hepatitis. Gastroenterology 2018;155(2):422–30.e1.

30. Marot A, Moreno C, Deltenre P. Liver transplant for alcoholic hepatitis: a current clinical overview. Expert Rev Gastroenterol Hepatol 2020;14(7):591–600.

31. Weeks SR, Sun Z, McCaul ME, et al. Liver transplantation for severe alcoholic hepatitis, updated lessons from the World's largest series. J Am Coll Surg 2018;226(4):549–57.

32. Hajifathalian K, Humberson A, Hanouneh MA, et al. Ohio solid organ transplantation consortium criteria for liver transplantation in patients with alcoholic liver disease. World J Hepatol 2016;8(27):1149–54.

33. Marot A, Dubois M, Trépo E, et al. Liver transplantation for alcoholic hepatitis: a systematic review with meta-analysis. PLoS One 2018;13(1):e0190823.

34. Asrani SK, Trotter J, Lake J, et al. Meeting report: the dallas consensus conference on liver transplantation for alcohol associated hepatitis. Liver Transpl 2020;26:127–40.

Selection Criteria for Liver Transplantation for Acute Alcohol-Associated Hepatitis

Aparna Goel, MD*, Tami Daugherty, MD

KEYWORDS

- Transplant • Alcoholic hepatitis • Selection • Alcohol-associated liver disease
- Chronic liver disease • Alcohol use disorder

KEY POINTS

- Liver transplant selection criteria for severe acute alcohol-associated hepatitis vary across centers but there are important commonalities, such as nonresponse to medical therapy, a first liver-decompensating event, and the presence of strong caregiver support.
- Experienced psychiatrists or addiction medicine providers need to be involved in the assessment of potential candidates early in the liver transplant evaluation process.
- Selection criteria should identify candidates with good insight and conviction to pursue treatment for alcohol use disorder.

BACKGROUND

Alcohol-related liver disease (ALD) has become the leading indication for liver transplantation (LT) in the United States.[1] A distinct subset of ALD, alcohol-associated hepatitis (AH), is associated with a mortality rate upwards of 70% in the most severe cases that are refractory to medical treatment.[2,3] LT in this select population has markedly improved survival rates.[3]

The selection of patients with severe AH for LT can be extremely challenging. It is important to identify candidates that have a poor prognosis without transplantation and a high likelihood of long-term abstinence. The ability to predict both of these outcomes is imperfect with our current understanding of ALD and alcohol use disorder (AUD). As a result, selection practices and protocols for LT in severe patients with AH vary across transplant centers globally. Although varied demographic factors such as societal norms and payer systems drive some of these differences, an incomplete understanding of the disease and limited management options drive others. There is no resounding consensus on the single best selection protocol.[4] However,

Department of Medicine, Stanford University, 750 Welch Road, Suite 110, Palo Alto, CA 94304, USA
* Corresponding author. 430 Broadway Street, Pavillion C, Redwood City, CA 94063.
E-mail address: goela21@stanford.edu
Twitter: @AparnaGoelMD (A.G.)

Clin Liver Dis 25 (2021) 635–644
https://doi.org/10.1016/j.cld.2021.03.007
1089-3261/21/© 2021 Elsevier Inc. All rights reserved.

liver.theclinics.com

the increase in transplantation for severe AH at many liver transplant centers across the world has shed significant insight into the selection of such candidates.[3–7]

ETHICAL CONSIDERATIONS

Historically, a majority of LT centers in the United States mandated at least 6 months of abstinence before considering LT as a treatment option for ALD. This period of abstinence—coined the 6-month rule—intended to provide sufficient time for potential improvement in hepatic function and hence, prevent premature transplantation.[8,9] However, since its inception, the 6-month rule has been used as a surrogate marker for the predictability of alcohol relapse. In general, although the length of sobriety before LT is predictive of sobriety after LT, a defined period of 6 months does not correlate with survival, sobriety, or compliance after LT.[10–12]

When considering these patients for LT, the disproportionate weight placed on relapse risk in patients with ALD raises significant questions and should be reevaluated. AUD is no longer viewed a result of moral weakness and self-destructive behavior, but a chemical dependence with neurobiological roots influenced by social and psychological factors. AUD is a lifelong condition that can be characterized as a chronic relapsing disorder.[13,14] Similar to the risk of other chronic liver diseases such as nonalcoholic steatohepatitis, autoimmune hepatitis, and viral hepatitis which can recur after LT, there is a risk of recurrent ALD, albeit at a much lower rate than other liver diseases.[15,16] Although the rates of alcohol use in LT recipients with a history of ALD ranges from 20% to 50%, the risk of actual recurrent ALD is lower and the long-term post-transplant survival is comparable with, or even higher than, LT for other etiologies.[17–19] The low likelihood of graft loss and poor survival related to recurrent ALD should be balanced with the benefit of LT for an individual patient. Just as post-transplant care focuses on mitigating risks for recurrent nonalcoholic steatohepatitis, viral hepatitis, or autoimmune liver diseases, comparable treatment of the addiction in AUD should also be emphasized.[20,21]

Recognizing the absence of convincing data that mandated periods of abstinence can reliably predict which individuals will have harmful alcohol relapse after LT, policies restricting access to LT in patients with ALD based on abstinence periods alone raise important ethical concerns. The expectedly high mortality observed in patients with severe AH who do not improve with supportive care during a defined abstinence period heightens the ethical debate. Understandably, the central point of this controversy is the fairness of the allocation of scarce transplantation resources. The scarcity of organs imposes the need to incorporate equity, justice, usefulness, and benefit in the definition of priorities for organ allocation, concepts that may be in conflict and difficult to reconcile.[4] This conflict only highlights the need for uniform selection practices throughout the transplant community. Variance in selection practices will only exacerbate disparities in access to transplantation based on social or financial status.[22]

INTERNATIONAL EXPERIENCE WITH LIVER TRANSPLANTATION FOR ALCOHOL-ASSOCIATED HEPATITIS

The seminal article by Mathurin and colleagues[3] in 2011 demonstrated a significant survival benefit (77% vs 23%) with LT in those with severe AH nonresponsive to medical therapy. Influenced by these findings, several programs in the United States created center-specific protocols to identify appropriate candidates for LT. The limited published experience and data from these centers are detailed in **Table 1**.

Table 1
Post-transplant alcohol relapse and survival outcomes in studies evaluating LT for severe AH

Author, Year	No. of Patients	Follow-up	Relapse Rate (%)	Harmful Alcohol Relapse Rate (%)	Survival Rate (%)	Design
Mathurin et al,[3] 2011	26	2 y	10	4	72	Prospective
Im et al,[5] 2016	9	2 y	11	-	89	Retrospective single-center case series
Lee et al,[6] 2017	17	1.5 y	24	24	94	Retrospective single-center case series
Lee et al,[22] 2018	147	3 y	34	17	84	Retrospective multicenter

MEDICAL SELECTION CRITERIA

The selection of appropriate LT candidates is a lengthy process that seeks to optimize the allocation of a limited supply of donor grafts to a minority of patients who meet medical and psychosocial requirements to achieve a successful transplant outcome. Patients evaluated for LT for severe AH should follow the center's usual medical selection processes. This rigorous evaluation usually occurs stepwise (**Fig. 1**), although the urgency in evaluating candidates with severe AH will necessitate many steps occur concurrently. There should be a thorough assessment of contraindications to LT, such as frailty, debility, and multiorgan failure. Furthermore, given the importance of the psychosocial evaluation in assessing the severity of AUD and concomitant psychiatric illnesses, transplant social workers, and psychiatrists should be involved early in the evaluation process.[4] Even after there is consensus to waitlist a candidate for LT, it is critical to continue monitoring for signs of hepatic recovery, which would obviate the need for LT.

Selection protocols from individual centers for patients with ALD are variably described in the literature, although there are notable commonalities, including:

- Nonresponse to medical therapy[3,5,6]
- First liver-decompensating event[3,5,6]
- Presence of a strong support system[3,5,6]
- Absence of severe coexisting psychiatric disorders[3,5]
- Commitment to lifelong abstinence[3,5,6]
- Consensus agreement by transplant committee[3,6]

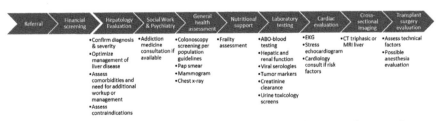

Fig. 1. Evaluation of candidacy for LT. CT, computed tomography; EKG, electrocardiogram.

Severity of Liver Disease

In terms of determining medical criteria for pursuing LT for severe AH, it is crucial to prevent the premature use of LT in those who will recover with supportive medical care. However, accurately predicting which patients will not recover with supportive care remains a challenge. Several models, including Lille and the Model for End-stage Liver Disease score, can predict those with a high likelihood of recovery, but not vice versa.[23]

The hepatologist's evaluation should provide a definitive diagnosis of AH and, if necessary, a liver biopsy should be performed. The practice of performing liver biopsies varies across centers globally. In the European study, a strict prospective protocol was followed where only those with liver biopsy-proven AH underwent evaluation for LT.[3] In the United States, a liver biopsy is used to establish a definitive diagnosis of AH when the clinical diagnosis remains uncertain.[22] The role of liver biopsy in the prognosis of patients with severe AH is not validated and requires further study.[24] To prevent bias in selecting candidates, centers should have consistency in determining the requirement for liver biopsy in their evaluation process.

Nonresponse to Medical Therapy

The definition and use of medical therapy in those with severe AH remains controversial. Thus, creating selection criteria based on nonresponse to medial therapy results in a heterogeneous pool of candidates. Glucocorticoid treatment may be offered to those with a Maddrey's discriminant function of 32 of higher and without contraindications including infection, renal failure, or gastrointestinal bleeding.[2] Nonresponse to such therapy is determined by a Lille score of greater than 0.45 or worsening liver function after 4 to 7 days of therapy.[25] A landmark trial evaluating the benefit of prednisolone or pentoxifylline in more than 1000 patients with severe AH revealed no improvement in survival with pentoxifylline and a nonsignificant reduction in 28-day mortality with prednisolone.[26] A subsequent meta-analysis of 4 controlled trials revealed a reduced risk of death within 28 days of glucocorticoid treatment but not in the following 6 months.[27] These data explain the variability in medical treatment across centers in the United States and globally. In the initial European study by Mathurin, 92% of patients received treatment with glucocorticoids, compared with 35% to 55% in studies from the United States.[3,5,6,22] To prevent bias in the selection of candidates, LT programs creating protocols for the evaluation of patients with severe AH should have standardized algorithms for medical treatment.

First Hepatic-Decompensating Event

A key criterion shared among all published experiences is the evaluation of only those presenting with their first hepatic decompensation. An LT evaluation should not proceed if a candidate with severe AH has had prior decompensated liver disease, such as jaundice, ascites, gastrointestinal bleeding, or hepatic encephalopathy.[4] This criterion serves as a reflection of a candidate's insight into their addiction, because ongoing or recurrent alcohol use despite prior hepatic decompensation portends a poor understanding of AUD.

Consensus Agreement by Transplant Committee

The need for consensus agreement for the successful selection of an LT candidate varies by center.[22] The initial European study required consensus agreement among all providers for a candidate to be waitlisted but not all US centers follow this protocol. Considerations to decrease bias include blinded voting in committee deliberations.

Comorbid Medical Conditions

Chronic alcohol use can result in multisystemic alcohol-related comorbidities and the presence of these conditions deserves careful evaluation in potential candidates with ALD. A thorough history and medical examination will elucidate many of these co-occurring diagnoses. Not all are a contraindication to pursue LT, but may require management both before and after LT. Notably, a nutrition assessment is crucial in all candidates because malnutrition is present in at least 50% of patients with AH and associated with high mortality.[28] These considerations include deficiencies in macronutrients and micronutrients along with marked loss of weight and muscle mass. The evaluating nutritionist should provide recommendations to optimize nutritional status, which may include enteral feeds. Potential comorbid conditions by system are noted in **Table 2**.[29]

PSYCHOSOCIAL SELECTION CRITERIA

The psychosocial assessment of candidates with severe AH should be performed by experienced social workers and psychiatrists, ideally with a background in transplantation and addiction medicine. This evaluation should occur early in the selection process. In addition to their evaluation and risk assessment, psychosocial assessors are critical in creating interventions and treatment plans for the management of AUD and coexistent psychiatric illnesses. It is usually not possible for patients with severe AH to undergo pre-LT rehabilitation owing to their severe, life-threatening illness; hence, stringent psychosocial selection criteria are prudent to ensure good outcomes after LT. Select candidates may be able to engage in online mutual support groups, which have significantly expanded access recently during the novel coronavirus disease 2019 pandemic.

To compliment criteria set forth by each transplant program, psychometric scales and instruments can be utilized to assist in the integration of data and recommendations. There have been various assessment tools utilized in this setting, including the Stanford Integrated Psychosocial Assessment for Transplantation (SIPAT), which is

Table 2 Multisystemic comorbidities related to alcohol use deserving careful evaluation during the transplant selection process	
Organ System	**Potential Comorbidities**
Neurologic	Brain atrophy Dementia Wernicke's encephalopathy Polyneuropathy
Cardiovascular	Cardiomyopathy Hypertension Supraventricular tachycardia
Gastrointestinal	Pancreatitis (acute and chronic) Gastropathy Bleeding (Mallory-Weiss tears or varices)
Hematopoietic	Anemia (iron deficiency, folate deficiency, sideroblastic) Thrombocytopenia
Malignancy	Head-neck cancer Esophageal squamous cell cancer

validated and widely used in multiple transplant centers.[30] Some have suggested a specific threshold SIPAT score (ie, <40) in patients with severe AH being considered for LT, although a specific cutoff has not been thoroughly studied or validated.[31]

Assessing Alcohol Use Disorder

The accurate assessment of AUD is challenging in an inpatient setting while a candidate is experiencing a life-threatening medical condition. There are limited time and evidence to assess a candidate's commitment to sobriety or compliance with recommended AUD treatment. Patients may be difficult to interview owing to feelings of guilt, fear, or pain. If a candidate is suffering from hepatic encephalopathy, a meaningful interview may become more difficult. Collateral information from family members and other clinical providers (such as a primary care provider, therapist, psychiatrist) can aid in providing a comprehensive picture of the patient's history, but cannot substitute for a direct interview with the patient. Some LT centers will not evaluate candidates who are intubated or have incapacitating encephalopathy.[4]

There is general agreement that an addiction specialist should assess the patient to ensure that patients with AH receive the full spectrum of AUD care. There are numerous treatment modalities for AUD and determining the appropriate fit for the individual patient with ALD requires expertise.[32] Treatment options include the following.

- Motivational enhancement therapy
- Cognitive behavior therapy
- Twelve-step facilitation
- Group therapies
- Intensive outpatient programs
- Inpatient and residential treatment
- Relapse prevention medications.

Recent surveys demonstrate a large gap in knowledge about approved and safe treatment options for AUD among hepatologists. Hence, incorporating an expert in AUD management is critical for the long-term care and outcomes of these patients.[21] When creating the appropriate AUD treatment plan, it is important to understand what resources are available based on payer coverage. The quality of the therapeutic alliance between the patient and the hepatologist is also likely to play a key role in the treatment of AUD.[32]

A maximum of 1 prior failed attempt at rehabilitation is suggested for primary listing criteria.[4] This criterion is to prevent penalizing the patient who has insight into their AUD and sought help previously. However, a candidate with repeated failed rehabilitation attempts should be excluded owing to the high risk of poor outcomes after LT. In subsequent follow-up, if a candidate demonstrates acceptable compliance with AUD treatment recommendations, they may be reevaluated and considered for LT under standard protocols.

Risk of Alcohol Relapse

Inherent in the psychosocial evaluation of patients with severe AH is calculating the risk of alcohol relapse. Predictive indices can be incorporated into the psychosocial evaluation, but they should not determine candidacy. Several studies have examined predictors of post-LT alcohol relapse. It is important to remember that the presence of a risk factor indicates that the likelihood of alcohol use is greater, not that it is certain.

There is no scoring system validated in LT candidates with severe AH.[4] The definition of relapse varies across the literature, with some studies including any alcohol use as a relapse and others only sustained alcohol use. The available predictive models were not created in cohorts that had optimal management of AUD, so perhaps the calculated risk would be modified with adequate treatment. A common theme is the increased risk of post-LT relapse with prior failed rehabilitation attempts. The predictive models for post-LT alcohol relapse are shown in **Table 3**. These models are not mutually exclusive and it is reasonable to incorporate more than 1 method in a psychosocial evaluation. Interestingly, the study used to create the psychosocial model also evaluated SIPAT and SALT scores in their cohort and found a SIPAT cutoff of greater than 21 and SALT score of greater than 7 was more predictive of alcohol relapse.[31]

Patients undergoing LT evaluation may be asked to sign an abstinence agreement or behavior contract. Although not legally binding, such contracts should further impress upon the patient and family that the management of the AUD is a priority, even after LT. A reluctance to sign such a contract raises a red flag on the commitment of the patient to participate in AUD treatment.

Comorbid Psychiatric Illness

Comorbid psychiatric illness occurs in nearly one-third of patients with ALD. Although selection policies at some centers exclude patients with severe AH with psychiatric illness from undergoing LT, most evaluate such candidates as long as a treating psychiatrist can manage the illness effectively.[35] Depression, anxiety disorders, and adjustment disorders tend to be particularly prevalent in this cohort, and alcohol is

Table 3 Models to predict alcohol use after LT		
Predictive Model	**Variables**	**Score**
High-Risk Alcoholism Relapse (HRAR)[33]	Duration heavy drinking, y ≤11 (0) 11–25 (1) ≥25 (2) Usual number of daily drinks ≤9 (0) 9–17 (1) ≥17 (2) Number of prior alcohol inpatient treatment attempts 0 (0) 1 (1) ≥1 (2)	Low (0–3) High (4–6)
Geneva Model[34]	HRAR score of 4–6 Presence of psychiatric comorbidity Sobriety <6 mo	No score
Sustained Alcohol use Post-LT (SALT)[35]	>10 drinks/d at presentation (+4) ≥ prior failed rehabilitation attempts (+4) Any history of prior alcohol-related legal issues (+2) History of non-THC illicit substance abuse (+1)	<5 predicts low risk
Psychosocial model[31]	Failure to engage in an intensive outpatient program despite recommendation Relapse after an initial attempt at sobriety Ongoing alcohol consumption after liver disease diagnosed	No score

commonly used as a method of treating symptoms of these diseases. Younger age, female sex, and Caucasians with ALD have the highest prevalence of psychiatric illness.[36] Often, these concurrent psychiatric illnesses are newly diagnosed during the LT evaluation process. If the psychiatric illness is not severe or incapacitating, a transplant evaluation can proceed. The management of an underlying psychiatric illness should be a priority of the transplant team, because inadequate management can significantly increase the risk of poor post-LT outcomes.

Additional Psychosocial Parameters

The psychosocial assessment for candidates with severe AH should also highlight the importance of insight into their AUD and the role of alcohol in their current presentation. Although some of this information can be gleaned from a patient's change in alcohol consumption after the diagnosis of liver disease, compliance with recommendations by the medical staff, forthcoming behavior related to AUD, and prior hepatic decompensation events, it can be difficult to truly ascertain insight when a patient is severely ill. The presence of close, supportive family members and caregivers is helpful when assessing a candidate's insight and is critical for a patient's recovery after LT.

PAYER COVERAGE

The financial authorization to evaluate a patient with severe AH for transplantation is one of the first steps in the selection process. Unfortunately, there is significant variability in payer coverage policies mandating a period of sobriety (usually 6 months). Although some payers have modified their policies based on recent medical data and institutional criteria, others have not. The result is increased health care disparities and unequal access to LT based on insurance coverage. Equally important is ensuring that the AUD treatment recommended by the transplant team is covered by a patient's insurance policy. Inability to access AUD treatment following LT poses a significant risk for poorer outcomes.

SUMMARY

Severe AH is associated with a very high mortality and LT in this select population has markedly improved survival rates. Although the selection criteria are not uniform across transplant centers, there is general guidance on which candidates are likely to have the best outcomes. Medical selection criteria should focus on other organ systems that are impacted by chronic alcohol use. Several instruments and predictive models are available to understand the severity of AUD and risk of relapse after LT. Equally important as the management of liver disease complications is the treatment of AUD with the input from experts in addiction medicine and psychiatry. As LT for this indication becomes increasingly common, it will be important for transplant centers to carefully assess outcomes and share this knowledge with the transplant community.

CLINICS CARE POINTS

- Severe AH that is non-responsive to medical therapy is associated with >70% mortality withing six months.

- Liver transplantation has been success and life-saving in highly select individuals.

- Treatment of alcohol use disorder (AUD) is critical in the overall management of patients with severe AH. Involvement of psychiatry and addiction medicine providers is paramount for successful outcomes.

DISCLOSURE

The authors have nothing to disclose.

REFERENCES

1. Cholankeril G, Ahmed A. Alcoholic liver disease replaces hepatitis C virus infection as the leading indication for liver transplantation in the United States. Clin Gastroenterol Hepatol 2018;16(8):1356–8.
2. Mathurin P. Corticosteroids for alcoholic hepatitis - what's next? J Hepatol 2005; 43(3):526–33.
3. Mathurin P, Moreno C, Samuel D, et al. Early liver transplantation for severe alcoholic hepatitis. N Engl J Med 2011;365(19):1790–800.
4. Asrani SK, Trotter J, Lake J, et al. Meeting report: the Dallas Consensus Conference on liver transplantation for alcohol associated hepatitis. Liver Transplant 2020;26(1):127–40.
5. Im GY, Kim-Schluger L, Shenoy A, et al. Early liver transplantation for severe alcoholic hepatitis in the United States–A single-center experience. Am J Transplant 2016;16(3):841–9.
6. Lee BP, Chen P-H, Haugen C, et al. Three-year results of a pilot program in early liver transplantation for severe alcoholic hepatitis. Ann Surg 2017;265(1):20–9.
7. Weeks SR, Sun Z, McCaul ME, et al. Liver transplantation for severe alcoholic hepatitis, updated lessons from the world's largest series. J Am Coll Surg 2018;226(4):549–57.
8. Dureja P, Lucey MR. The place of liver transplantation in the treatment of severe alcoholic hepatitis. J Hepatol 2010;52(5):759–64.
9. Ihori M. Acute alcoholic hepatitis. Nihon Rinsho 1976;34(11):3147–52.
10. DiMartini A, Day N, Dew MA, et al. Alcohol consumption patterns and predictors of use following liver transplantation for alcoholic liver disease. Liver Transplant 2006;12(5):813–20.
11. Lim JK, Keeffe EB. Liver transplantation for alcoholic liver disease: current concepts and length of sobriety. Liver Transplant 2004;10(10 Suppl. 2):S31–8.
12. Foster PF, Fabrega F, Karademir S, et al. Prediction of abstinence from ethanol in alcoholic recipients following liver transplantation. Hepatology 1997;25(6): 1469–77.
13. Cunningham JA, McCambridge J. Is alcohol dependence best viewed as a chronic relapsing disorder? Addiction 2012;107(1):6–12.
14. Moos RH, Moos BS. Rates and predictors of relapse after natural and treated remission from alcohol use disorders. Addiction 2006;101(2):212–22.
15. Cheung A, Levitsky J. Follow-up of the post-liver transplantation patient: a primer for the practicing gastroenterologist. Clin Liver Dis 2017;21(4):793–813.
16. Dew MA, DiMartini AF, Steel J, et al. Meta-analysis of risk for relapse to substance use after transplantation of the liver or other solid organs. Liver Transplant 2008; 14(2):159–72.
17. Bellamy COC, DiMartini AM, Ruppert K, et al. Liver transplantation for alcoholic cirrhosis: long term follow-up and impact of disease recurrence. Transplantation 2001;72(4):619–26.
18. Jain A, Reyes J, Kashyap R, et al. Long-term survival after liver transplantation in 4,000 consecutive patients at a single center. Ann Surg 2000;232(4):490–500.
19. Mackie J, Groves K, Hoyle A, et al. Orthotopic liver transplantation for alcoholic liver disease: a retrospective analysis of survival, recidivism, and risk factors predisposing to recidivism. Liver Transplant 2001;7(5):418–27.

20. Peeraphatdit T Bee, Kamath PS, Karpyak VM, et al. Alcohol rehabilitation within 30 days of hospital discharge is associated with reduced readmission, relapse, and death in patients with alcoholic hepatitis. Clin Gastroenterol Hepatol 2020; 18(2):477–85.e5.

21. Im GY, Mellinger JL, Winters A, et al. Provider attitudes and practices for alcohol screening, treatment and education in patients with liver disease: a survey from the AASLD ALD SIG. Clin Gastroenterol Hepatol 2020. https://doi.org/10.1016/j. cgh.2020.10.026.

22. Lee BP, Mehta N, Platt L, et al. Outcomes of early liver transplantation for patients with severe alcoholic hepatitis. Gastroenterology 2018;155(2):422–30.e1.

23. Forrest EH, Atkinson SR, Richardson P, et al. Application of prognostic scores in the STOPAH trial: discriminant function is no longer the optimal scoring system in alcoholic hepatitis. J Hepatol 2018;68(3):511–8.

24. Mookerjee RP, Lackner C, Stauber R, et al. The role of liver biopsy in the diagnosis and prognosis of patients with acute deterioration of alcoholic cirrhosis. J Hepatol 2011;55(5):1103–11.

25. Louvet A, Naveau S, Abdelnour M, et al. The Lille model: a new tool for therapeutic strategy in patients with severe alcoholic hepatitis treated with steroids. Hepatology 2007;45(6):1348–54.

26. Thursz MR, Richardson P, Allison M, et al. Prednisolone or pentoxifylline for alcoholic hepatitis. N Engl J Med 2015;372(17):1619–28.

27. Louvet A, Thursz MR, Kim DJ, et al. Corticosteroids reduce risk of death within 28 days for patients with severe alcoholic hepatitis, compared with pentoxifylline or placebo—a meta-analysis of individual data from controlled trials. Gastroenterology 2018;155(2):458–68.e8.

28. Higuera de la Tijera F, Servín Caamaño A, Servín Abad L, et al. Malnutrition is a key prognostic factor related to high mortality-rate in patients with severe alcoholic hepatitis. Nutr Hosp 2018;35(3):677–82.

29. Marroni CA, De Medeiros Fleck A, Fernandes SA, et al. Liver transplantation and alcoholic liver disease: history, controversies, and considerations. World J Gastroenterol 2018;24(26):2785–805.

30. Maldonado JR, Dubois HC, David EE, et al. The Stanford Integrated Psychosocial Assessment for Transplantation (SIPAT): a new tool for the psychosocial evaluation of pre-transplant candidates. Psychosomatics 2012;53(2):123–32.

31. Deutsch-Link S, Weinrieb RM, Jones LS, et al. Prior relapse, ongoing alcohol consumption, and failure to engage in treatment predict alcohol relapse after liver transplantation. Dig Dis Sci 2020;65(7):2089–103.

32. Mellinger JL, Winder GS. Alcohol use disorders in alcoholic liver disease. Clin Liver Dis 2019;23(1):55–69.

33. Yates WR, Booth BM, Reed DA, et al. Descriptive and predictive validity of a high-risk alcoholism relapse model. J Stud Alcohol 1993;54(6):645–51.

34. De Gottardi A, Spahr L, Gelez P, et al. A simple score for predicting alcohol relapse after liver transplantation: results from 387 patients over 15 years. Arch Intern Med 2007;167(11):1183–8.

35. Lee BP, Vittinghoff E, Hsu C, et al. Predicting low risk for sustained alcohol use after early liver transplant for acute alcoholic hepatitis: the sustained alcohol use post–liver transplant score. Hepatology 2019;69(4):1477–87.

36. Jinjuvadia R, Jinjuvadia C, Puangsricharoen P, et al. Concomitant psychiatric and nonalcohol-related substance use disorders among hospitalized patients with alcoholic liver disease in the United States. Alcohol Clin Exp Res 2018;42(2): 397–402.

Approaching Alcohol Use Disorder After Liver Transplantation for Acute Alcoholic Hepatitis

Peng-Sheng Ting, MD[a], Ahmet Gurakar, MD[b],*,
Jason Wheatley, MSW[c], Geetanjali Chander, MD, MPH[d],
Andrew M. Cameron, MD, PhD[e], Po-Hung Chen, MD[f]

KEYWORDS

- Alcohol use disorder • Hepatitis • Liver transplantation • Outcomes
- Pharmacologic therapy • Behavioral treatment • Motivational interviewing

KEY POINTS

- Severe alcoholic hepatitis carries a grim prognosis. It is increasingly considered an indication for liver transplantation in select candidates.
- A deliberate pretransplant assessment is the first step toward mitigating adverse posttransplant outcomes.
- The 3 pillars of post-liver transplant management specific to alcohol use disorder are destigmatized routine monitoring for alcohol relapse, pharmacologic therapy, and behavioral treatments.

INTRODUCTION

Severe alcoholic hepatitis (AH) is an acute manifestation of alcohol-related liver disease (ALD) with distinct histopathologic findings of steatohepatitis, pronounced cholestasis, and sclerosing hyaline necrosis; the latter 2 features help to distinguish severe AH from nonalcoholic steatohepatitis.[1] Severe AH carries a grim prognosis, even with

[a] Division of Gastroenterology and Hepatology, Johns Hopkins University School of Medicine, 1830 East Monument Street, Suite 431, Baltimore, MD 21287, USA; [b] Liver Transplant, Division of Gastroenterology and Hepatology, Johns Hopkins University School of Medicine, 720 Rutland Avenue, Ross Research Building, Suite 918, Baltimore, MD 21205, USA; [c] Department of Social Work, Johns Hopkins Hospital, 600 North Wolfe Street, Carnegie Suite 100, Baltimore, MD 21287, USA; [d] Division of General Internal Medicine, Johns Hopkins University School of Medicine, 1830 East Monument Street, Room 8047A, Baltimore, MD 21287, USA; [e] Division of Liver Transplant Surgery, Department of Surgery, Johns Hopkins University School of Medicine, 720 Rutland Avenue, Ross 765, Baltimore, MD 21205, USA; [f] Division of Gastroenterology and Hepatology, Johns Hopkins University School of Medicine, 1830 East Monument Street, Suite 429, Baltimore, MD 21287, USA
* Corresponding author.
E-mail address: aguraka1@jhmi.edu

Clin Liver Dis 25 (2021) 645–671
https://doi.org/10.1016/j.cld.2021.03.008
1089-3261/21/© 2021 Elsevier Inc. All rights reserved.

liver.theclinics.com

expert medical management.[2] Traditional risk factors for severe AH include female sex, younger age, obesity, and the presence of other liver disease such as hemochromatosis or hepatitis C.[3] On a genetic level, predisposition to severe AH involves a complex interplay between genes regulating inflammatory mediators via the commonly cited tumor necrosis factor pathway, genes regulating endotoxin response, genes involved in the balance of oxidative stress, genes involved in hepatic lipid metabolism such as PNPLA3, and epigenetic changes.[4] Major environmental risk factors include the quantity and pattern of alcohol consumption that may affect the CYP2E1 pathway that metabolizes alcohol to acetaldehyde, gut microbiota alterations leading to gut derived pathogen-associated molecular patterns and subsequent cytokine/chemokine release by Kupffer cells, and poor nutritional status.[4]

Traditionally, severe AH, defined as those with a Maddrey discriminant function of 32 or greater, is associated with a 28-day case fatality ratio of 50%.[5,6] Despite improvements in supportive care since the turn of the century, at least one-quarter of patients with severe AH still die within 90 days without liver transplantation (LT).[7] The 28-day case fatality ratio in corticosteroid nonresponders was 47% in a meta-analysis that defined nonresponders as patients who had a day 7 Lille score of 0.56 or higher.[8]

Early LT for AH is defined as LT performed without a 6-month period of pre-LT alcohol abstinence.[9] The combination of high mortality and lack of durably effective pharmaceuticals led major society guidelines to recommend LT evaluation for patients with severe AH who do not respond to medical therapy.[10,11] Notwithstanding its survival benefit for patients with severe AH, early LT remains controversial among health care providers.[12] Meanwhile, alcohol use disorder (AUD) has grown over 2 decades to a prevalence of 5.8% (14.4 million) in the US adult population in 2018, as reported by the National Survey on Drug Use and Health.[13] Early market data also showed more alcohol purchases nationwide after the coronavirus disease 2019 pandemic caused a plethora of socioeconomic disruptions.[14] This alcohol epidemic within a pandemic will likely lead to an increase in severe AH.

In this review, we provide a brief overview of the management of severe AH and outline methods to optimize transplant outcomes in early LT for severe acute AH.

DIAGNOSIS AND PRETRANSPLANT MEDICAL MANAGEMENT OF ALCOHOLIC HEPATITIS

To help standardize definitions in research, the American Association for the Study of Liver Diseases recommends categorizing the clinical syndrome of AH into 3 groups according to the consensus published in 2016: definite AH (biopsy proven), probable AH, and possible AH (should obtain a biopsy).[15] In practice, it is crucial early in the clinical course to distinguish between AH and decompensation of alcohol-related cirrhosis to guide medical treatment. The prompt administration of corticosteroids and complete abstinence may prevent LT in AH, but has less of an effect on the disease course of decompensated alcohol-related cirrhosis. At this time, there are no validated noninvasive tests that can differentiate between AH and decompensated alcohol-related cirrhosis. A liver biopsy can help in the event of diagnostic uncertainty.

There are no impressive pharmaceutical agents in the treatment of AH. Nonetheless, key aspects of pre-LT medical management must be emphasized both to limit the number of LT eventually needed for AH—thus preserving limited organ resources—and to optimize the LT candidate for major surgery. First, alcohol abstinence is the only proven treatment that leads to improved long-term outcomes and is also a necessary condition for LT candidacy in AH.[16] Second, corticosteroids are currently the only pharmaceuticals that decrease 28-day mortality, but the mortality benefit dissipates beyond 90 days.[7] Nonresponse to steroids is a common context within which providers may consider early LT for AH. It is worth noting that steroid therapy has been associated with a higher rate of serious infections, which can complicate LT. Biomarkers such as circulating bacterial DNA to predict infection may be helpful in guiding antibiotic therapy to improve outcomes.[17] Third, a comprehensive screening for infection including blood, urine, and peritoneal cultures at hospital admission is recommended.[18] Finally, a focus on nutrition and ensuring an enteral diet comprising 1 to 1.5 g protein/kg and 30 to 40 kcal/kg of body weight per day is a cornerstone of supportive care specifically in patients with encephalopathy.[18,19]

The appropriate management of potential LT candidates through the acute phase of severe AH as outlined in this article will not only optimize patients medically, but it will also maximize the use of nontransplant resources before resorting to LT as a life-saving measure.

THE ROLE FOR EARLY LIVER TRANSPLANTATION IN ALCOHOLIC HEPATITIS AND AVAILABLE CLINICAL EXPERIENCE

Transplant centers performing early LT in AH report excellent recipient and liver allo-graft survival, which we summarize in **Table 1**.[9,20-23] However, many transplant centers in the United States still use the 6-month rule for alcohol abstinence as a prerequisite to LT. The practice is problematic in the context of severe AH, where a significant proportion of patients die within 6 months of diagnosis.[24]

In Europe, Mathurin and colleagues[9] described 26 early LT recipients who had 6-month and 2-year post-LT survivals of 77% and 71%, respectively. Shortly thereafter, the United States began adopting this practice, and Lee and colleagues[22] described 147 early LT recipients across 12 US transplant centers who had 1-year and 3-year post-LT survivals of 94% and 84%, respectively. A mathematical simulation based in part on the aforementioned published US data estimated an average life expectancy of 6.55 years and 1.46 years for patients offered early and delayed LT for severe AH, respectively.[25] The increase in life expectancy was most pronounced in recipients with Model for End-Stage Liver Disease scores of 32 or more and Lille scores of 0.50 to 0.82 before LT.

Both the European and US cohorts had strict candidate selection criteria toward early LT, including nonresponse to medical management, social work evaluation for social support, and specialty assessment for substance use. In the European cohort and most US centers, there was an explicitly stated criterion for a consensus to transplant among all stakeholders on the liver transplant committee. One notable difference between the European and US experiences was the exclusion of patients with severe psychiatric comorbidities by European centers, whereas only 2 of 12 US centers explicitly excluded patients with psychiatric comorbidities.[22]

Not surprisingly, a measure emphasized on par with mortality in all of the aforementioned studies was post-LT alcohol relapse. The mathematical simulation discussed elsewhere in this article calculated a decrease of 7.23 life-years for LT recipients who relapse into sustained alcohol use.[25] Mathurin and colleagues[9] reported 3 transplant recipients (15%) who returned to any drinking after 2 years of follow-up, whereas Lee and colleagues[22] reported 10% and 17% of sustained alcohol use (defined as a minimum duration of 100 days of alcohol use) at 1 and 3 years, respectively. Despite differences in candidate selection criteria between the studies, the reported incidences of alcohol use were not notably different.

Although the past decade of experience with early LT for AH has been encouraging from the patients' perspective, intense controversy continues to surround the practice. This debate invariably distills down to balancing the prerogative of physicians

Table 1
Cohorts of early liver transplantation for AH

Author, Year Published	Location (No. of Participating Centers)	Sample Size	Proportion of Total Grafts Used for Severe AH Indication	Survival (Months after LT)	Graft Survival (Months after LT)	Alcohol Relapse	Definition of Alcohol Relapse per Study	Post-Transplant Alcohol Relapse Monitoring
Mathurin et al,[9] 2011	France and Belgium (7)	26	2.9%	77% (6), 71% (24)	N/A	12% at 24 mo after LT	Any alcohol use	Informal interviews with the patient (preferably with family present, although not required) with a median of 11 visits over 6 mo. Any alcohol was considered relapse and the frequency, type and amount of drinking would be recorded.
Im et al,[20] 2016[a]	United States (1)	9	3%	89% (6)	100% (6)	12.5%	4 or more drinks/d or 1 drink per day in 4 or more consecutive days	Assessment of relapse during outpatient follow-up visits in addition to random alcohol testing.
Weeks et al,[21] 2018[a]	United States (1)	46	8.8%	98% (6), 97% (12)	95% (6), 93% (12)	28% (any alcohol), 17% (harmful drinking)	Any alcohol use and presence of harmful drinking pattern	Assessed for both any alcohol relapse and presence of harmful drinking, defined as 4 or more days of drinking per week or 5 drinks/d for men or 4 drinks/d for women.

Lee et al,[22] 2018[a]	United States (12)	147	N/A	94% (12), 84% (36)	N/A	10% at 12 mo after LT, 17% at 36 mo after LT	Sustained alcohol use, defined as a minimum relapse duration of 100 d.	Assessment of alcohol use at every post-LT visit. Seven of 12 centers had routine urinary ethyl glucuronide or blood phosphatidylethanol testing.
Sundaram et al,[23] 2018	United States (1)	8	N/A	100% (10)	100% (10)	10% at 10 mo after LT	N/A	Median of 8 office visits at median follow-up time of 261 d.

All cohorts included only patients with nonresponse to medical management and stipulated pre-LT evaluation by social worker and addiction specialist.

Abbreviations: LT, liver transplantation.

[a] Redundancy present in these cohorts in the United States.

to save lives (ie, beneficence) against the other fundamental bioethical principles of justice, usefulness, and autonomy.[26,27] Ultimately, the patient selection process is paramount in both consolidating trust in the transplant selection process and optimizing post-transplant outcomes to maximize usefulness of precious graft resources.

OPTIMIZING TRANSPLANT OUTCOMES IN EARLY LIVER TRANSPLANTATION FOR SEVERE ALCOHOLIC HEPATITIS

Among centers offering early LT, there remain significant regional variations on the practice of early LT.[28] A consensus conference convened in Dallas, Texas, in April 2019 to establish recommendations for transplant centers.[29] The main goals were to (1) avoid LT in patients with AH who may recover with medical management (2) eliminate non–data-driven barriers to LT (ie, the 6-month sobriety requirement), in favor of a multidisciplinary evaluation, and (3) avoid creating or worsening health disparities through LT. These recommendations serve as a guide to standardize pre- and post-LT practices that ultimately could optimize outcomes for patients with AH.

Pretransplant Candidate Selection

An accurate diagnosis and medical management of severe AH, as summarized elsewhere in this article, is the first step in candidate selection. Patients with severe AH and nonresponse to medical management can then be evaluated for early LT. Response to medical management predicts survival and is best assessed by either changes in Model for End-Stage Liver Disease score alone or the combination of Model for End-Stage Liver Disease and the Lille Model (a dynamic measure).[29–31]

Once the physician identifies a medically appropriate candidate, selection shifts toward minimizing the risk of alcohol relapse after LT to optimize transplant outcomes. LT recipients who relapse to alcohol use not only develop significant hepatic steatosis and advanced fibrosis on histopathology, but they also have poorer graft and patient survival rates than those who remain abstinent.[25,32,33]

In severe AH, a frequent challenge is conducting an expeditious but accurate risk assessment for post-LT alcohol relapse within a limited window of opportunity for LT. To accomplish the task, the Dallas consensus conference recommended multidisciplinary psychosocial assessments by transplant social workers, addiction specialists, and other mental health professionals, as well as a consensus of medical and paramedical staff.[29] Existing LT literature supports identifying potential risk factors of adverse post-transplant outcomes. For example, Dew and colleagues[34] conducted a meta-analysis of 54 studies on solid organ transplantation (including 50 on LT) and found poor social support and family alcohol history associated with post-transplant relapse of alcohol use.

Numerous studies have proposed prediction models or guides that aim to predict poor psychosocial outcomes after LT, including alcohol relapse.[35,36] We summarize the most pertinent models in **Table 2**.[21,36–45] Of note, only the Sustained Alcohol Use post-LT score and the Hopkins Psychosocial Scale were developed specifically in patients who underwent early LT for severe AH; both instruments lack a consistent outcome measure and external validation.[21,37,38] The Harmful Alcohol Use post-LT score is a recently developed model that calculates the probability of alcohol relapse instead of providing a risk category.[36] The High-risk Alcoholism Relapse scale, originally developed in a Veterans Affairs population, was also studied in early LT for severe AH, but it was not predictive of alcohol relapse after LT.[21,38] The Alcohol Relapse Risk Assessment was developed in a cohort of 118 LT recipients who also had AUD, but only 38% had ALD as the primary cause of liver disease.[41] The Alcohol Relapse

Table 2
Selected prediction models for alcohol relapse after liver transplantation

Instrument	Scoring	Cohort Studied	Performance	Strengths	Limitations/Weaknesses
Sustained Alcohol use post-LT (SALT) score[37]	SALT score of <5 predicted abstinence >10 drinks/d at initial hospitalization (+4 points) Multiple prior rehabilitation attempts (+4 points) Prior alcohol-related legal issues (+2 points) Prior illicit substance abuse (+1 point)	Early liver transplantation for AH. Developed in 134 LT recipients.	NPV: 95% PPV: 25% c-statistic of 0.76. c-statistic of 0.73 on internal cross-validation.	Cohort is most relevant to early LT for AH Internally validated	Low PPV, which means high SALT score still may need full evaluation. Exclusion based on high SALT score may exclude suitable candidates. Arisen from retrospective data. Not externally validated.
Hopkins Psychosocial Scale (HPSS)[21,38]	HPSS score of <0 would predict sustained alcohol relapse.[a] Calculated according to protective characteristics and at risk characteristics. Protective characteristics: self-admission to hospital, drinks per day before abstinence, insight into diagnosis, marital status, abstinence period before transplant. At risk characteristics: psychiatric comorbidity, history of other substance abuse, history of failed rehab attempt, family history of alcoholism, employment immediately before presentation, legal issues related to alcohol.	Early LT for AH. Developed first in a cohort of 17 LT recipients.[38] Re-examined in an expanded cohort of 43 LT recipients, including the original 17 patients compared against LT recipients for ALD meeting 6 mo sobriety recruited during the same period.[21]	HPSS score of <0 had hazard ratio of 3.63 for any alcohol relapse.	Cohort is most relevant to early LT for AH Many variables considered thought to be more easily assessed objectively Combines unique characteristics of the AH population with established risk factors of relapse	Not internally or externally validated Single center Small sample size Complicated calculation

(continued on next page)

Table 2
(continued)

Instrument	Scoring	Cohort Studied	Performance	Strengths	Limitations/Weaknesses
Harmful Alcohol Use post-LT (HALT) score[36]	Multivariate regression model that calculates probability of harmful alcohol use after LT using the following variables: Age at LT Non–alcohol-related criminal history Pre-LT abstinence period Drinks per day	Developed in 241 LT recipients with ALD, including 59 patients with <6 mo of sobriety	Mean c-statistic of 0.74	Cohort includes early LT Internally validated Model output is a probability of relapse	Not externally validated Includes 74 (30.7%) patients with additional cause of liver disease or indication for LT
High-Risk Alcoholism Relapse (HRAR) scale[21,39,40]	HRAR of ≥4 predicted readmission within 6 mo for alcohol treatment 1. Duration of heavy drinking in years, <11 y = 0; 11–25 y = 1; >25 y = 2. 2. Usual daily number of standard drinks, <9 = 0; 9–17 = 1; >17 = 2. 3. Number of previous alcoholism inpatient treatments, 0 = 0; 1 = 1; >1 = 2.	Developed in 299 male patients in a VA population admitted to an alcohol treatment unit.[39] Reexamined in a prospective cohort of 387 LT recipients for ALD, which found association with harmful drinking.[40] Also reexamined in a single-center cohort of 46 LT recipients for AH, where HRAR was not predictive.[21]	HRAR of >3: OR = 4.0 (95% CI = 2.4–6.8) for readmission at 6 mo. HRAR of <4: OR = 2.5 (95% CI = 1.4–4.2) for abstinence at 6 mo.	Studied in many different cohorts specifically involving alcohol Easily calculated	Requires 25 y of heavy drinking to classify as highest risk assignment, which would limit usefulness in AH Has not been shown to be predictive in LT for AH when studied specifically in this population Skewed demographics including 100% male patients, which may not be generalizable

Alcohol Relapse Risk Assessment (ARRA) score[41]	ARRA score of ≥4 predicted any alcohol relapse. Each of these 9 parameters are given 1 point if present, and summed to a total ARRA score: absence of hepatocellular carcinoma (+1), tobacco dependence (+1), continued alcohol use after liver disease diagnosis (+1), low motivation for alcohol treatment (+1), poor stress management skills (+1), no rehabilitation relationship (+1), limited social support (+1), lack of nonmedical behavioral consequences (+1), and continued engagement in social activities with alcohol present (+1)	Developed in 118 LT recipients with history of AUD	NPV: 92% PPV: 87% c-statistic 0.892 $R^2 = 73\%$	Studied in LT recipients with AUD Classifies patients into 4 tiers of ARRA (I, II, III, and IV) based on score, which could be helpful in predicting intensity in alcohol relapse	Not internally or externally validated Single center Not specifically in the early LT for AH population and only 38% had ALD as the primary cause of liver disease leading to LT Skewed demographics, including 84% White and 86% male, which may not be generalizable Includes subjective parameters that may be difficult to reproduce or validate

(continued on next page)

Table 2
(continued)

Instrument	Scoring	Cohort Studied	Performance	Strengths	Limitations/Weaknesses
Stanford Integrated Psychosocial Assessment for Transplantation (SIPAT)[42,43]	SIPAT is used to predict positive or negative post-transplant outcome (rated by social worker and transplant coordinator) taking into account treatment adherence, psychosocial support system, recidivism, development of psychiatric problems, or graft failure. SIPAT score ranges from 0 to 110 and is calculated by assessing 4 domains: 1. Patient's readiness level and illness management. 2. Social support system level of readiness. 3. Psychosocial stability and psychopathology. 4. Lifestyle and effect of substance abuse.	Developed in 102 randomly selected cases of liver, heart, or lung transplant recipients.[42] Reexamined prospectively in same center that it was developed for 217 solid organ transplant recipients to find higher SIPAT scores predicted higher rates of rejection episodes, hospitalizations, psychiatric decompensation, and support system failure.[43]	c-statistic 0.70. High SIPAT scores correlated with negative outcomes.	Psychiatry-led development of model High interrater reliability, even between expert and novice raters	Not developed or validated in a pure LT population with AUD as the focus Single center Not validated to predict relapse of substance abuse

| Michigan Alcohol Prognostic Score (MAPS)[44,45] | MAPS ranges from 5 to 20. Scored by summating the following domains:
1. Acceptance of alcoholism: both patient and family (+4), patient only (+3), family only (+2), neither (+1)
2. Prognosis for sobriety: substitute activities (yes: +3, no: +1), behavioral consequences (yes: +3, no: +1), hope/self-esteem (yes: +3, no: +1), social relationship (yes: +3, no: +1)
3. Social stability: steady job (+1), stable residence (+1), does not live alone (+1), stable marriage (+1) | Developed in a cohort of 99 patients with AUD undergoing evaluation for LT, 45 of whom were deemed suitable for LT, but a fixed threshold or cutoff was not applied.[44] Reexamined in a validation study in a cohort of 50 LT recipients with AUD retrospectively and no differences found in MAPS between patients who relapsed and patients who abstained.[45] | Higher MAPS theoretically correlated with reduced rate of relapse. | Studied in LT recipients with AUD | Not found to be correlated with alcohol relapse in a later validation study
No threshold or estimation was published
Primarily used as a guide rather than a prediction model |

Abbreviations: NPV, negative predictive value; PPV, positive predictive value; VA, Veterans Affairs.

[a] Defined as alcohol use for a minimum duration of 100 d after LT.

Risk Assessment also has not undergone subsequent validation. The Stanford Integrated Psychosocial Assessment for Transplantation was developed in 102 randomly selected solid organ transplant recipients at a single transplant center to predict a range of post-transplant outcomes. In a later validation study, however, the Stanford Integrated Psychosocial Assessment for Transplantation was only moderately predictive of general psychosocial outcomes. It did not examine substance use outcomes owing to inadequate clinical documentation.[42,43] Finally, the Michigan Alcohol Prognostic Score originated from a cohort of 99 patients with AUD who were also undergoing LT evaluation.[44] However, a follow-up study by the same authors found no association between Michigan Alcohol Prognostic Score and post-LT alcohol relapse.[45]

Post-transplant Monitoring and Treatment: A Focus on Alcohol Use Disorder

Most aspects of post-LT medical management for the transplant indication of severe AH and other indications are the same.[46] However, early LT for severe AH often marks the beginning of the recipient's relationship with decompensated liver disease, whereas LT recipients for most other indications have struggled with liver disease for many years. The relatively brief disease awareness afforded to patients with severe AH leaves transplant practitioners justifiably concerned about the monitoring and treatment of alcohol relapse after LT.[27] We here review the 3 pillars of post-LT management specific to severe AH: monitoring for alcohol relapse, pharmacologic therapy, and behavioral treatment.

Monitoring for Alcohol Relapse

The importance of abstinence, or at least harm reduction, cannot be overstated. Although every patient with ALD will benefit from abstinence, early LT recipients stand to benefit the most with a new lease on life. Therefore, AUD treatment after LT is imperative. The optimal care for AUD begins with routine, destigmatized monitoring for relapse to alert clinicians to modify treatment as indicated.

In addition to regular screening for alcohol relapse by interview during scheduled post-LT visits (see **Table 1**), biomarkers of alcohol use can facilitate the early detection of relapse and initiation of treatment. Direct biomarkers are metabolites of alcohol; in contrast, indirect biomarkers reflect manifestations of the physiologic effects of alcohol.

Most indirect biomarkers of alcohol use such as the aspartate aminotransferase to alanine aminotransferase ratio and the mean corpuscular volume are good screening measures for heavy alcohol use that result in hepatitis or significant hepatic injury, but are insensitive to the occasional slip. Gamma-glutamyl transferase and carbohydrate deficient transferrin are indirect biomarkers that can detect alcohol use without hepatitis, but both can be elevated owing to other causes and confounders.

Select direct biomarkers such as blood alcohol level or alcohol breath tests are only useful for acute alcohol consumption. **Table 3** summarizes commonly used biomarkers in the post-LT setting.[10,47–51] Of note, phosphatidylethanol is a direct biomarker that was evaluated prospectively in 61 LT recipients and had 100% sensitivity for alcohol use in the preceding week.[48] The same study found ethyl glucuronide in hair to be useful in detecting alcohol use within the past 3 to 6 months.[48]

Given the differences in the window of detection and the level of drinking each test is designed to detect, a combination of biomarkers to maximize detection of both chronicity and low levels of alcohol consumption is ideal. For example, Staufer and colleagues[52] used the combination of urine ethyl glucuronide and carbohydrate

Table 3
Biomarkers for alcohol relapse in liver transplant recipients

Biomarker	Type of Biomarker	Specimens Tested	Detection Window	Drinking Pattern Designed to Detect	Potential Confounders
Ethanol[47]	Direct	Blood	Several hours, depending on the level of drinking	Any level	False elevations with blood ketones or non-ethanol alcohols (eg, isopropyl alcohol or methanol)
Phosphatidylethanol (PEth)[47,48]	Direct	Blood	2–4 wk	Moderate drinking (3–4 drinks/d)	No notable confounders[47]
Ethyl glucuronide (EtG)[47,48]	Direct	Hair (must be 3 cm or longer)	Up to 6 mo	Moderate drinking (2–3 drinks/d)	False positives in impaired renal function or EtG-containing hair treatments[47] False negatives in hair treatment involving dye, perm, or bleach[47]
		Urine	≤80 h	After a sitting of 1–2 drinks	False positives with nonbeverage alcohol use (eg, mouthwash) or impaired renal function[47] False negatives with diuretic use or urinary tract infection[47]
Carbohydrate deficient transferrin (CDT)[47,49]	Indirect	Blood	1–3 wk	Heavy drinking (3–5 drinks/d)	False positives with genetic variants, lower body mass index, or end-stage liver disease[49] False negatives with age <30, female sex, or obesity[49]
Gamma-glutamyl transferase (GGT)[50,51]	Indirect	Blood	2–4 wk	Moderate to heavy, chronic	Elevated in advanced hepatic fibrosis, regardless of cause False elevations by various medications (eg, phenytoin, furosemide, heparin)[51]

deficient transferrin in a cohort of 141 LT recipients to achieve a positive predictive value of 89.3% and negative predictive value of 98.9%.

There is no consensus on the intensity or duration of monitoring for alcohol relapse after LT. It may be reasonable to monitor more frequently for the first year after LT, during which 75% of all alcohol relapses occur.[22]

Pharmacologic Therapy

Pharmacologic treatments for AUD have seen slow application in patients with concurrent liver disease in part owing to a relative scarcity of empirical safety data; the studies on AUD pharmacotherapeutics often exclude patients with liver disease.[11] Unfortunately, data are even sparser in the post-LT scenario, although adverse effects are unlikely in theory because most transplant recipients have normal or near-normal liver function.

An ideal pharmacologic agent in the post-LT setting would have no hepatotoxicity, outstanding efficacy, and minimal interaction with antirejection medications. As mentioned elsewhere in this article, none of the presently available AUD pharmacotherapies possess safety or efficacy data in liver transplant recipients. Currently, there are 3 medications approved by the US Food and Drug Administration (FDA) for treating AUD: naltrexone, acamprosate, and disulfiram. Additionally, the American Psychiatric Association (APA) recommends gabapentin and topiramate for off-label use in AUD refractory to naltrexone and acamprosate.[53]

Naltrexone is a mu-opioid receptor antagonist that blocks euphoric effects of alcohol on the mesolimbic dopaminergic system. Initial naltrexone trials demonstrating reduced rates of relapse and fewer drinking days led to the medication's approval by the FDA in 1994. Subsequently, a Cochrane review of randomized controlled trials (RCTs) found a 17% reduction in heavy drinking and 4% reduction in drinking days with naltrexone treatment for AUD compared with placebo.[54] A potential concern in using naltrexone is the FDA boxed warning on naltrexone's capacity to cause hepatocellular injury "when given in excessive doses."[55]

Acamprosate is hypothesized to act on inhibitory N-methyl-D-aspartic acid receptors to attenuate the pleasurable effects of alcohol and prevent the uncomfortable effects of withdrawal and abstinence.[56] A Cochrane systematic review of 24 RCTs showed acamprosate to significantly increase cumulative abstinence duration compared with placebo.[57] The side effects of the medication include dose-dependent, typically transient diarrhea and suicidal ideation; however, rates of completed suicide were no higher in patients on acamprosate compared with placebo. Acamprosate is renally eliminated; it is contraindicated in patients with severe renal impairment.

Naltrexone and acamprosate may be good candidates for study in the post-LT setting given their relatively good safety profiles. In a meta-analysis by Jonas and colleagues,[58] the numbers needed to treat to prevent return to any drinking were 12 and 20 for acamprosate and oral naltrexone, respectively. The numbers needed to treat to prevent return to heavy drinking was 12 for oral naltrexone; the use of acamprosate did not result in statistically significant changes. In comparing naltrexone and acamprosate for AUD, another meta-analysis of 64 RCTs suggested naltrexone had a greater effect on the decreased of heavy drinking and acamprosate was more effective in maintaining abstinence.[59]

Disulfiram was the first medication approved by the FDA for treating AUD. Disulfiram inhibits aldehyde dehydrogenase, the enzyme responsible for metabolizing acetaldehyde downstream of the alcohol metabolic pathway. When one consumes alcohol while taking disulfiram, the accumulation of acetaldehyde results in aversive consequences, like severe nausea and vomiting. The negative reinforcement theoretically discourages subsequent alcohol use, but it requires patient insight on the risks with alcohol intake while on disulfiram.[53] Furthermore, disulfiram can lead to aminotransferase elevations in up to 25% of patients on chronic therapy. The acute liver injury is even occasionally fatal, which limits the use of disulfiram in the post-LT patient.[60] RCTs on disulfiram have differed greatly by primary outcomes. A meta-analysis on disulfiram efficacy suggested a higher chance of treatment success than different controls (Hedges' g = 0.58), but the authors detected possible publication bias in the literature.[61]

Anticonvulsant medications gabapentin and topiramate are not FDA approved for treating AUD, but the APA nonetheless recommends them as second-line treatments.[53] A Cochrane review found gabapentin and topiramate decrease heavy drinking and drinks per drinking day compared with placebo, but there was no improvement on continuous abstinence. The Cochrane authors acknowledged the difficulty in drawing conclusions from their meta-analysis given the heterogeneity of included studies.[62] A subsequent RCT illustrated a dose-dependent effect of gabapentin up to a daily dose of 1800 mg in maintaining abstinence and no heavy drinking.[63] One concern with gabapentin is its independent potential for abuse. Care providers should monitor its use by individuals with other substance use disorders in addition to AUD.[64]

Baclofen is the only anticraving medication that has been studied in advanced liver disease, although not in the post-LT setting. It is neither FDA approved nor recommended by the APA for treating AUD, although the American Association for the Study of Liver Diseases and the American College of Gastroenterology have endorsed using the medication in patients with ALD.[2,65] Existing data on baclofen's efficacy are conflicting; RCTs that examined the medication's effect on decreasing heavy drinking or increasing the duration of abstinence presented divergent conclusions.[66] The single RCT that enrolled patients with advanced liver disease—excluding those with hepatic encephalopathy or renal failure—suggested that baclofen has a relatively benign safety profile.[67] However, more recent national administrative data from France demonstrated a dose-dependent, positive association between the use of baclofen for AUD and increased risks of hospitalization and death.[68] Baclofen also can potentially cause encephalopathy.[2] Taken together, the risk–benefit ratio of using baclofen to treat AUD remains highly contested.

Table 4 summarizes the currently available AUD pharmacotherapeutics.[54,55,57–62,66–69] At this time, none can be recommended routinely for LT recipients given the absence of supporting literature. All of the AUD pharmacotherapies need further assessment in the post-LT setting.

In addition to the pharmacologic options discussed earlier, there are also some investigational medications for AUD. Nalmefene shares a similar chemical structure and pharmacologic mechanism with naltrexone and is potentially more efficacious at decreasing alcohol consumption. However, its oral formulations used in treating AUD is not available in the United States.[70,71] A recent meta-analysis of placebo-controlled RCTs involving participants with heavy drinking or AUD showed varenicline to attenuate alcohol craving but not reduce heavy drinking days, drinks per drinking day, or days abstinent.[72] Although its effect on AUD seems to be modest, varenicline may still have a role in patients with coexisting nicotine dependence. Aripiprazole decreased the number of drinks per drinking day, but did not improve abstinence in a large multicenter RCT for AUD.[73] Similar to varenicline, aripiprazole may still benefit select patients with AUD who have a concurrent psychiatric indication for the prescription. Finally, there are encouraging preliminary data on the use of ondansetron and

Table 4
Pharmacotherapeutics for AUD

Medication	Administration	Dosing	Efficacy Compared with Placebo	Level of Evidence for Efficacy	Common Side Effects	Safety in Liver Disease and Important Pharmacokinetics	FDA Approval for AUD
Naltrexone	PO, IM depot	PO: 50 mg once a day IM: 380 mg every 4 wk	Reduces risk of heavy drinking (RR, 0.83), drinks/drinking day (decrease by 3.89%), rate of relapse (decrease by 5%), and craving.[54,58,59]	RCTs and meta-analysis	Nausea, dyspepsia, loss of appetite	Not studied in patients with liver disease. Black box warning for hepatotoxicity.[55] Up to 25% on chronic therapy has mild aminotransferase elevation.[69]	Yes
Acamprosate	PO	666 mg 3 times a day, may decrease to twice a day for patients <60 kg (contraindicated in CrCl of <30)	Reduces risk of any drinking (RR, 0.86), rate of relapse (decrease by 5%), drinking days (decrease by 8.8%).[57,58]	RCTs and meta-analysis	Diarrhea, suicidality	Not studied in patients with liver disease. Not metabolized by liver. Renally excreted.	Yes
Disulfiram	PO	500 mg once daily for 1–2 wk, followed by 125–500 mg/d as maintenance	Maintenance of abstinence, but has mixed results.[58,61]	RCTs and meta-analysis	Gastrointestinal upset, headache, tremors, metallic taste, skin rash	Not studied in patients with liver disease. Hepatotoxicity. Up to 25% of patients on chronic disulfiram will have mild transaminase elevation.[60] Fatality rate is 10% when jaundice present.[60]	Yes
Gabapentin	PO	Daily dose of 600 mg to 1800 mg (dosage adjustment required for CrCl of <60)	Reduces heavy drinking (decrease by 0.45 SMD) and drinks/drinking days (2.14 less).[62]	RCTs and meta-analysis	Sedating, euphoria (potential for abuse)	Not studied in patients with liver disease. Rare reports of self-limited cholestatic liver enzyme elevations. Renally excreted.	No

Topiramate	PO	Reduces heavy drinking (decrease by 0.44 SMD) and drinks/drinking days (1.55 less).[62]	RCTs and meta-analysis	Dizziness, paresthesia, anorexia	Not studied in patients with liver disease. Rare reports of serum transaminase elevations. Approximately 70% renally excreted.	No
Baclofen	PO	Mixed results. Achieves and maintains abstinence (OR, 2.67).[66]	RCTs and meta-analysis	Sedation, dizziness, confusion	Single RCT in patients with ALD (excluding HE and renal failure) demonstrated safety.[67] However, French national claims data showed dose-dependent association with increased hospitalizations and deaths.[68] Limited hepatic metabolism. Up to 80% renally excreted.	No

Abbreviations: CrCl, creatinine clearance; FDA, US Food and Drug Administration; HE, hepatic encephalopathy; IM, intramuscular; PO, by mouth; RCT, randomized controlled trial; RR, relative risk; SMD, standardized mean differences.

zonisamide in treating AUD, but both medications require further studies to clarify their roles.[74,75]

Behavioral Treatment

Although total abstinence after LT may be the preferred goal, all relapses are not the same. Sustained alcohol use and harmful drinking patterns contribute most to deleterious outcomes.[22,76] Once alcohol relapse occurs, prompt intensive alcohol addiction treatment is paramount to mitigate harmful or sustained drinking and preserve allograft function. Behavioral treatment is the category of addiction treatment that identifies and modifies maladaptive behaviors. These strategies take root in traditional theories of psychology such as operant conditioning and cognitive theory.

The implementation of behavioral treatment in the post-LT setting can be conceptualized along 3 axes: the selected behavioral treatment strategies, the intensity of treatment, and the integration with the liver transplant clinic.[77] However, most of the data supporting behavioral treatment in LT recipients are extrapolations from observational studies of pre-LT patients with ALD.[78] **Fig. 1** illustrates our approach to behavioral treatment.

Behavioral treatment encompasses a spectrum of strategies from brief interventions conducted in the physician's office to recurring sessions of psychological interventions led by addiction therapists. Two of the best studied psychological interventions for AUD are cognitive behavioral therapy and motivational enhancement therapy. Cognitive behavioral therapy is the technique of first identifying a trigger that leads to drinking and then redirecting the response to said trigger toward nondrinking activities. The delivery of cognitive behavioral therapy often spans 10 or more sessions.[79] In a meta-analysis of 30 RCTs involving individuals with alcohol and other

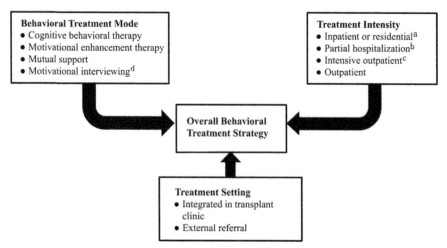

Fig. 1. Behavioral treatment for AUD. The 3 axes of overall behavioral treatment strategy is conceptualized in this diagram. The methods under each axis are listed in the order of preference in the posttransplant setting. [a]Trained counselors provide 24-hour care to stabilize imminent danger from addiction. [b]An organized outpatient treatment usually during the day, but does not provide 24-hour care. [c]Outpatient treatment typically occurring after work or school or on weekends. [d]Interviewing style aimed at fostering a constructive partnership between practitioner and patient. Can be part of a formal counseling program, or adapted to the transplant clinic setting.

substance use disorders (but not specifically ALD), cognitive behavioral therapy was more effective than minimal treatment controls across multiple outcome types and follow-up durations.[80] Motivational enhancement therapy is a focused, structured treatment using the principles of motivational interviewing (discussed elsewhere in this article) to evoke a patient's internal motivation for behavioral change. Instead of specialist-driven, unidirectional instructions, motivational enhancement therapy applies motivational feedback on a patient's personal circumstances to encourage concrete abstinence strategies.[56] In one of the few RCTs evaluating behavioral treatment in LT candidates, Weinrieb and colleagues[81] reported similar prevalence of self-reported relapse (approximately 25%) over 2 years of follow-up between 91 patients who received motivational enhancement therapy versus usual care (defined as referral to local addiction treatment services). However, among patients who relapsed, the motivational enhancement therapy group had fewer drinking days and fewer drinks per drinking day.

Relative to the more structured motivational enhancement therapy, motivational interviewing is a broader counseling philosophy that is nonjudgmental yet directive and focuses on the patient's internal recognition of the link between alcohol use and its consequences. The complete mastery of motivational interviewing challenges even addiction specialists, but nonspecialists (eg, transplant clinicians) can nonetheless learn to incorporate the essence of the motivational interviewing style in routine follow-up visits for patients with AUD.[77,82] As a harm reduction technique, motivational interviewing helps to establish a democratic, nonpunitive partnership between the clinician and the patient, where the clinician aspires to encourage and support behavioral change. The process facilitates constructive dialogue between the 2 parties should alcohol cravings arise, which hopefully promotes early recognition and treatment engagement. In a meta-analysis, Vasilaki and colleagues[83] examined RCTs on motivational interviewing interventions for excessive drinking and found motivational interviewing more efficacious than no treatment in reducing alcohol intake over the short term.

Although motivational interviewing is not a strictly structured behavioral treatment paradigm, it does take multiple encounters to show effect. The 5 guiding principles of motivational interviewing are to (1) express empathy to establish common ground with patients, (2) identify discrepancies between patients' stated goals and their current actions, (3) eschew direct confrontations, (4) roll with patient resistance, and (5) support self-efficacy.[84] Open-ended questions and reflective listening initially help the clinician to understand the patient's goals and then recognize discrepancies from actual behavior. Points of contention and resistance may arise as the clinician strives to guide the patient to perceive these discrepancies. It is vital to avoid arguments by shifting the focus away from confrontation. Affirming the patient's inner guide and encouraging self-motivational statements are 2 strategies to reinforce the patient's positive self-reflection.

Less structured behavioral treatment methods such as brief interventions or mutual support have a smaller—but not negligible—role in treating the severe AUD that may lead to severe AH or ALD.[56] Brief interventions are short sessions usually conducted by a clinician during a routine visit. Jointly, the provider and the patient set an achievable goal either to reduce or stop drinking and work on an action plan to that end. There is typically an agreement to reassess alcohol consumption on subsequent visits.[85] The US Preventive Services Task Force made a grade B recommendation in 2018 for conducting brief behavioral counseling in primary care settings to decrease unhealthy alcohol use, based on a mean decrease of 1.59 standard drinks per week in a meta-analysis of 37 trials involving 15,974 adults.[86] The summary of evidence notably excluded studies with pharmacologic treatment for severe AUD, which limited its extrapolation to patients with ALD.

Mutual support entails peer-led support groups that meet regularly and provide individuals with a beneficial social network and positive experiences in a sober environment.[87] Mutual support offers advantages like longitudinal therapy and low cost. Alcoholics Anonymous is perhaps the most visible among mutual support groups, but its spiritual foundations may not suit everyone. Self-Management And Recovery Training Recovery is a less spiritual alternative rooted in several of these behavioral treatment theories. The supportive social network adds a safety net not inherently available in cognitive behavioral therapy or motivational enhancement therapy, but mutual support alone may be insufficient for patients with severe AUD often seen in LT recipients for severe AH.[56] One reason may be the frequent lack of standardization between different sites, even among groups supposedly rooted in the same therapeutic tradition. Conversely, in 2 RCTs (1936 participants), standardized or manualized mutual support programs compared favorably with formal psychological interventions in achieving and maintaining sustained abstinence for 12 months.[88]

In addition to the behavioral treatment strategy selected either alone or in combination, treatment intensity should be personalized to each LT recipient. The American Society of Addiction Medicine (ASAM) offers a useful conceptual continuum that encompasses early intervention (ASAM level 0.5), outpatient services (ASAM level 1.0–2.5), and inpatient services (ASAM level 3.1–3.5).[89] Early intervention describes behavioral treatment before a confirmed AUD—or relapse of AUD for LT recipients—to gather information for assessment and prevent disease progression. Outpatient services comprise different time commitments ranging from less than 9 hours 1 week (ASAM level 1) to partial hospitalization without 24-hour staff availability (ASAM 2.5). Inpatient services offer varying levels of structured clinical time, but all patients live on-site with a 24-hour support staff. Although higher intensity arrangements may offer more resources in theory, they are typically costlier and still may be less optimal for a given individual. Factors such as time commitment, distance from home, privacy, and insurance coverage are all important considerations in light of multiple competing priorities in the first year after LT, including postsurgical complications and financial obligations.[90,91] Thus, the decision of optimal treatment intensity ideally involves a thoughtful discussion between the patient, transplant providers, social workers, and addiction specialists.

Integrated (defined as co-locating in the same physical space) care delivery models that combine behavioral treatment with the standard transplant practice may be the most effective in treating AUD and reducing post-LT relapse.[92] The close physical proximity enhances the communication between transplant and addiction care providers. Addolorato and colleagues[93] compared post-LT alcohol outcomes before versus after the 2002 establishment of an Alcohol Addiction Unit within their Liver Transplant Center in Rome, Italy. The LT recipients who received integrated treatment had significantly lower prevalence of alcohol relapse and death (16.4% and 14.5%) than the recipients who received nonintegrated care (35.1% and 37.8%). Similarly, the RCT by Weinrieb and colleagues[81] demonstrated the effectiveness of integrated motivational enhancement therapy on decreasing the quantity and frequency of post-LT drinking relative to a nonintegrated approach.

Extrapolating from the pre-LT literature, behavioral treatment interventions likely have the potential to maintain abstinence and mitigate harmful drinking in early LT recipients with AH. Unfortunately, the current literature lacks detailed descriptions of behavioral treatment strategies in the post-LT setting. A prospective therapeutic trial is under way.[94,95]

SUMMARY

LT is an exercise of public trust bestowed upon the transplant team by society. The present article proposed several strategies to manage AUD after early LT for AH. For the high-stakes scenario of LT where harmful alcohol relapse can lead to devastating post-LT outcomes, frequent follow-ups within an integrated/co-locating clinical practice combining transplant and addiction specialists may prove to be the most effectual approach. Prospective investigations are in progress to elucidate and elevate our care for these vulnerable patients.

CLINICS CARE POINTS

- Alcohol abstinence is the only proven treatment for alcoholic hepatitis that leads to improved long-term outcomes.
- The management of liver transplantation recipients for alcoholic hepatitis centers around monitoring and early detection of alcohol relapse, and pharmacologic and behavioral treatment of alcohol use disorder.
- An ideal pharmacologic agent for alcohol use disorder in the post-liver transplant setting would have no hepatotoxicity, outstanding efficacy, and minimal interaction with antirejection medications. None of the presently available alcohol use disorder pharmacotherapies possess all of these characteristics.
- Behavioral treatment for alcohol use disorder should be offered to all liver transplant recipients for alcoholic hepatitis. Substance abuse specialists ideally would be integrated with the transplant clinic and provide recurrent structured treatment sessions employing methods such as cognitive behavioral therapy or motivational enhancement therapy.

DISCLOSURE

This independent work was supported by the National Institute on Alcohol Abuse and Alcoholism of the National Institutes of Health under award numbers K24AA027483 (G. Chander), P50AA027054 (A.M. Cameron and G. Chander), and K23AA028297 (P.-H. Chen); Gilead Sciences Research Scholars Program in Liver Disease—The Americas (Chen); and Johns Hopkins University Clinician Scientist Award (P.-H. Chen). The content is solely the responsibility of the authors and does not necessarily represent the official views of the National Institutes of Health.

REFERENCES

1. Theise ND. Histopathology of alcoholic liver disease. Clin Liver Dis (Hoboken) 2013;2(2):64–7.
2. Crabb DW, Im GY, Szabo G, et al. Diagnosis and treatment of alcohol-associated liver diseases: 2019 practice guidance from the American Association for the Study of Liver Diseases. Hepatology 2020;71(1):306–33.
3. Yeluru A, Cuthbert JA, Casey L, et al. Alcoholic hepatitis: risk factors, pathogenesis, and approach to treatment. Alcohol Clin Exp Res 2016;40(2):246–55.
4. Seitz HK, Bataller R, Cortez-Pinto H, et al. Alcoholic liver disease. Nat Rev Dis Primers 2018;4(1):18.
5. Maddrey WC, Boitnott JK, Bedine MS, et al. Corticosteroid therapy of alcoholic hepatitis. Gastroenterology 1978;75(2):193–9.

6. Carithers RL Jr, Herlong HF, Diehl AM, et al. Methylprednisolone therapy in patients with severe alcoholic hepatitis. A randomized multicenter trial. Ann Intern Med 1989;110(9):685–90.

7. Thursz MR, Richardson P, Allison M, et al. Prednisolone or pentoxifylline for alcoholic hepatitis. N Engl J Med 2015;372(17):1619–28.

8. Mathurin P, O'Grady J, Carithers RL, et al. Corticosteroids improve short-term survival in patients with severe alcoholic hepatitis: meta-analysis of individual patient data. Gut 2011;60(2):255–60.

9. Mathurin P, Moreno C, Samuel D, et al. Early liver transplantation for severe alcoholic hepatitis. N Engl J Med 2011;365(19):1790–800.

10. EASL clinical practice guidelines: management of alcohol-related liver disease. J Hepatol 2018;69(1):154–81.

11. Lucey MR, Im GY, Mellinger JL, et al. Introducing the 2019 American Association for the Study of Liver Diseases Guidance on alcohol-associated liver disease. Liver Transpl 2020;26(1):14–6.

12. Alsahhar JS, Mehta A, Lepe R. Con: liver transplantation should not be performed in patients with acute alcoholic hepatitis. Clin Liver Dis (Hoboken) 2019;13(5): 144–7.

13. SAMHSA. National Survey on Drug Use and Health (NSDUH). Substance Abuse and Mental Health Services Administration. 2018. Available at: https://www.samhsa.gov/data/sites/default/files/cbhsq-reports/NSDUHDetailedTabs2018R2/NSDUHDetTabsSect5pe2018.htm#tab5-4b. Accessed May 20, 2020.

14. Rebalancing the 'COVID-19 effect' on alcohol sales. Chicago: Nielson Global Media; 2020. Available at: https://www.nielsen.com/us/en/insights/article/2020/rebalancing-the-covid-19-effect-on-alcohol-sales/. Accessed July 17, 2020.

15. Crabb DW, Bataller R, Chalasani NP, et al. Standard definitions and common data elements for clinical trials in patients with alcoholic hepatitis: recommendation from the NIAAA alcoholic hepatitis consortia. Gastroenterology 2016;150(4): 785–90.

16. Potts JR, Goubet S, Heneghan MA, et al. Determinants of long-term outcome in severe alcoholic hepatitis. Aliment Pharmacol Ther 2013;38(6):584–95.

17. Vergis N, Atkinson SR, Knapp S, et al. In patients with severe alcoholic hepatitis, prednisolone increases susceptibility to infection and infection-related mortality, and is associated with high circulating levels of bacterial DNA. Gastroenterology 2017;152(5):1068–77.e4.

18. Mitchell MC, Friedman LS, McClain CJ. Medical management of severe alcoholic hepatitis: expert review from the clinical practice updates committee of the AGA institute. Clin Gastroenterol Hepatol 2017;15(1):5–12.

19. Antar R, Wong P, Ghali P. A meta-analysis of nutritional supplementation for management of hospitalized alcoholic hepatitis. Can J Gastroenterol 2012;26(7): 463–7.

20. Im GY, Kim-Schluger L, Shenoy A, et al. Early liver transplantation for severe alcoholic hepatitis in the United States–A single-center experience. Am J Transplant 2016;16(3):841–9.

21. Weeks SR, Sun Z, McCaul ME, et al. Liver transplantation for severe alcoholic hepatitis, updated lessons from the world's largest series. J Am Coll Surg 2018;226(4):549–57.

22. Lee BP, Mehta N, Platt L, et al. Outcomes of early liver transplantation for patients with severe alcoholic hepatitis. Gastroenterology 2018;155(2):422–30.e1.

23. Sundaram V, Wu T, Klein AS, et al. Liver transplantation for severe alcoholic hepatitis: report of a single center pilot program. Transplant Proc 2018;50(10): 3527–32.

24. Kubiliun M, Patel SJ, Hur C, et al. Early liver transplantation for alcoholic hepatitis: ready for primetime? J Hepatol 2018;68(3):380–2.

25. Lee BP, Samur S, Dalgic OO, et al. Model to calculate harms and benefits of early vs delayed liver transplantation for patients with alcohol-associated hepatitis. Gastroenterology 2019;157(2):472–80.e5.

26. Solga SF, Goldberg DS, Spacek LA, et al. Early liver transplantation for alcoholic hepatitis. Gastroenterology 2019;156(1):284–5.

27. Wu T, Morgan TR, Klein AS, et al. Controversies in early liver transplantation for severe alcoholic hepatitis. Ann Hepatol 2018;17(5):759–68.

28. Cotter TG, Sandikci B, Paul S, et al. Liver transplantation for alcoholic hepatitis in the United States: excellent outcomes with profound temporal and geographic variation in frequency. Am J Transplant 2021;21(3):1039–55.

29. Asrani SK, Trotter J, Lake J, et al. Meeting report: the Dallas consensus conference on liver transplantation for alcohol associated hepatitis. Liver Transpl 2020;26(1):127–40.

30. Louvet A, Labreuche J, Artru F, et al. Combining data from liver disease scoring systems better predicts outcomes of patients with alcoholic hepatitis. Gastroenterology 2015;149(2):398–406.e8 [quiz: e16–7].

31. Merion RM, Wolfe RA, Dykstra DM, et al. Longitudinal assessment of mortality risk among candidates for liver transplantation. Liver Transpl 2003;9(1):12–8.

32. Rice JP, Eickhoff J, Agni R, et al. Abusive drinking after liver transplantation is associated with allograft loss and advanced allograft fibrosis. Liver Transpl 2013;19(12):1377–86.

33. Dumortier J, Dharancy S, Cannesson A, et al. Recurrent alcoholic cirrhosis in severe alcoholic relapse after liver transplantation: a frequent and serious complication. Am J Gastroenterol 2015;110(8):1160–6.

34. Dew MA, DiMartini AF, Steel J, et al. Meta-analysis of risk for relapse to substance use after transplantation of the liver or other solid organs. Liver Transpl 2008; 14(2):159–72.

35. Lim J, Sundaram V. Risk factors, scoring systems, and interventions for alcohol relapse after liver transplantation for alcoholic liver disease. Clin Liver Dis (Hoboken) 2018;11(5):105–10.

36. Satapathy SK, Thornburgh C, Heda R, et al. Predicting harmful alcohol relapse after liver transplant: the HALT score. Clin Transplant 2020;34(9):e14003.

37. Lee BP, Vittinghoff E, Hsu C, et al. Predicting low risk for sustained alcohol use after early liver transplant for acute alcoholic hepatitis: the sustained alcohol use post-liver transplant score. Hepatology 2019;69(4):1477–87.

38. Lee BP, Chen PH, Haugen C, et al. Three-year results of a pilot program in early liver transplantation for severe alcoholic hepatitis. Ann Surg 2017;265(1):20–9.

39. Yates WR, Booth BM, Reed DA, et al. Descriptive and predictive validity of a high-risk alcoholism relapse model. J Stud Alcohol 1993;54(6):645–51.

40. De Gottardi A, Spahr L, Gelez P, et al. A simple score for predicting alcohol relapse after liver transplantation: results from 387 patients over 15 years. Arch Intern Med 2007;167(11):1183–8.

41. Rodrigue JR, Hanto DW, Curry MP. The alcohol relapse risk assessment: a scoring system to predict the risk of relapse to any alcohol use after liver transplant. Prog Transplant 2013;23(4):310–8.

42. Maldonado JR, Dubois HC, David EE, et al. The Stanford Integrated Psychosocial Assessment for Transplantation (SIPAT): a new tool for the psychosocial evaluation of pre-transplant candidates. Psychosomatics 2012;53(2):123–32.

43. Maldonado JR, Sher Y, Lolak S, et al. The Stanford Integrated Psychosocial Assessment for Transplantation: a prospective study of medical and psychosocial outcomes. Psychosom Med 2015;77(9):1018–30.

44. Lucey MR, Merion RM, Henley KS, et al. Selection for and outcome of liver transplantation in alcoholic liver disease. Gastroenterology 1992;102(5):1736–41.

45. Lucey MR, Carr K, Beresford TP, et al. Alcohol use after liver transplantation in alcoholics: a clinical cohort follow-up study. Hepatology 1997;25(5):1223–7.

46. Lucey MR, Terrault N, Ojo L, et al. Long-term management of the successful adult liver transplant: 2012 practice guideline by the American Association for the Study of Liver Diseases and the American Society of Transplantation. Liver Transpl 2013;19(1):3–26.

47. Allen JP, Wurst FM, Thon N, et al. Assessing the drinking status of liver transplant patients with alcoholic liver disease. Liver Transpl 2013;19(4):369–76.

48. Andresen-Streichert H, Beres Y, Weinmann W, et al. Improved detection of alcohol consumption using the novel marker phosphatidylethanol in the transplant setting: results of a prospective study. Transpl Int 2017;30(6):611–20.

49. Fleming MF, Anton RF, Spies CD. A review of genetic, biological, pharmacological, and clinical factors that affect carbohydrate-deficient transferrin levels. Alcohol Clin Exp Res 2004;28(9):1347–55.

50. The role of biomarkers in the treatment of alcohol use disorders, 2012 revision. Substance Abuse and Mental Health Services Administration (SAMHSA). 2012. Available at: https://etg.weebly.com/uploads/7/4/7/5/74751/samsha_biomarker_advisory_may_2012.pdf. Accessed November 15, 2020.

51. Salaspuro M. Conventional and coming laboratory markers of alcoholism and heavy drinking. Alcohol Clin Exp Res 1986;10(6 Suppl):5S–12S.

52. Staufer K, Andresen H, Vettorazzi E, et al. Urinary ethyl glucuronide as a novel screening tool in patients pre- and post-liver transplantation improves detection of alcohol consumption. Hepatology 2011;54(5):1640–9.

53. Reus VI, Fochtmann LJ, Bukstein O, et al. The American Psychiatric Association practice guideline for the pharmacological treatment of patients with alcohol use disorder. Am J Psychiatry 2018;175(1):86–90.

54. Rosner S, Hackl-Herrwerth A, Leucht S, et al. Opioid antagonists for alcohol dependence. Cochrane Database Syst Rev 2010;(12):CD001867.

55. Alkermes. Vivitrol (naltrexone) [package insert]. U.S. Food and Drug Administration Website; 2010. Available at: https://www.accessdata.fda.gov/drugsatfda_docs/label/2010/021897s015lbl.pdf. Accessed November 7, 2020.

56. Ray LAPD, Bujarski SPD, Grodin EPD, et al. State-of-the-art behavioral and pharmacological treatments for alcohol use disorder. Am J Drug Alcohol Abuse 2019; 45(2):124–40.

57. Rosner S, Hackl-Herrwerth A, Leucht S, et al. Acamprosate for alcohol dependence. Cochrane Database Syst Rev 2010;(9):CD004332.

58. Jonas DE, Amick HR, Feltner C, et al. Pharmacotherapy for adults with alcohol use disorders in outpatient settings: a systematic review and meta-analysis. JAMA 2014;311(18):1889–900.

59. Maisel NC, Blodgett JC, Wilbourne PL, et al. Meta-analysis of naltrexone and acamprosate for treating alcohol use disorders: when are these medications most helpful? Addiction 2013;108(2):275–93.

60. LiverTox. Clinical and research information on drug-induced liver injury. Bethesda (MD): National Institute of Diabetes and Digestive and Kidney Diseases; Disulfiram; 2018. Available at: https://www.ncbi.nlm.nih.gov/books/NBK548103/.

61. Skinner MD, Lahmek P, Pham H, et al. Disulfiram efficacy in the treatment of alcohol dependence: a meta-analysis. PLoS One 2014;9(2):e87366.

62. Pani PP, Trogu E, Pacini M, et al. Anticonvulsants for alcohol dependence. Cochrane Database Syst Rev 2014;(2):CD008544.

63. Mason BJ, Quello S, Goodell V, et al. Gabapentin treatment for alcohol dependence: a randomized clinical trial. JAMA Intern Med 2014;174(1):70-7.

64. Smith RV, Havens JR, Walsh SL. Gabapentin misuse, abuse and diversion: a systematic review. Addiction 2016;111(7):1160-74.

65. Singal AK, Bataller R, Ahn J, et al. ACG clinical guideline: alcoholic liver disease. Am J Gastroenterol 2018;113(2):175-94.

66. Rose AK, Jones A. Baclofen: its effectiveness in reducing harmful drinking, craving, and negative mood. A meta-analysis. Addiction 2018;113(8):1396-406.

67. Addolorato G, Leggio L, Ferrulli A, et al. Effectiveness and safety of baclofen for maintenance of alcohol abstinence in alcohol-dependent patients with liver cirrhosis: randomised, double-blind controlled study. Lancet 2007;370(9603): 1915-22.

68. Chaignot C, Zureik M, Rey G, et al. Risk of hospitalisation and death related to baclofen for alcohol use disorders: comparison with Nalmefene, acamprosate, and naltrexone in a cohort study of 165 334 patients between 2009 and 2015 in France. Pharmacoepidemiol Drug Saf 2018;27(11):1239-48.

69. LiverTox. Clinical and research information on drug-induced liver injury. Bethesda (MD): National Institute of Diabetes and Digestive and Kidney Diseases; 2020. Naltrexone. 2012. Available at: https://www.ncbi.nlm.nih.gov/books/NBK548583/.

70. Soyka M, Friede M, Schnitker J. Comparing Nalmefene and Naltrexone in alcohol dependence: are there any differences? Results from an indirect meta-analysis. Pharmacopsychiatry 2016;49(2):66-75.

71. Soyka M, Rosner S. Nalmefene for treatment of alcohol dependence. Expert Opin Investig Drugs 2010;19(11):1451-9.

72. Gandhi KD, Mansukhani MP, Karpyak VM, et al. The impact of varenicline on alcohol consumption in subjects with alcohol use disorders: systematic review and meta-analyses. J Clin Psychiatry 2020;81(2):19r12924.

73. Anton RF, Kranzler H, Breder C, et al. A randomized, multicenter, double-blind, placebo-controlled study of the efficacy and safety of aripiprazole for the treatment of alcohol dependence. J Clin Psychopharmacol 2008;28(1):5-12.

74. Correa Filho JM, Baltieri DA. A pilot study of full-dose ondansetron to treat heavy-drinking men withdrawing from alcohol in Brazil. Addict Behav 2013;38(4): 2044-51.

75. Arias AJ, Feinn R, Oncken C, et al. Placebo-controlled trial of zonisamide for the treatment of alcohol dependence. J Clin Psychopharmacol 2010;30(3):318-22.

76. DiMartini A, Dew MA, Day N, et al. Trajectories of alcohol consumption following liver transplantation. Am J Transplant 2010;10(10):2305-12.

77. Ting PS, Wheatley J, Chen PH. Behavioral treatment for patients with alcohol-related liver disease: a primer for hepatologists. Clin Liver Dis (Hoboken) 2020; 15(1):31-5.

78. Schlagintweit HE, Lynch MJ, Hendershot CS. A review of behavioral alcohol interventions for transplant candidates and recipients with alcohol-related liver disease. Am J Transplant 2019;19(10):2678-85.

79. Magill M, Ray LA. Cognitive-behavioral treatment with adult alcohol and illicit drug users: a meta-analysis of randomized controlled trials. J Stud Alcohol Drugs 2009;70(4):516–27.

80. Magill M, Ray L, Kiluk B, et al. A meta-analysis of cognitive-behavioral therapy for alcohol or other drug use disorders: treatment efficacy by contrast condition. J Consult Clin Psychol 2019;87(12):1093–105.

81. Weinrieb RM, Van Horn DH, Lynch KG, et al. A randomized, controlled study of treatment for alcohol dependence in patients awaiting liver transplantation. Liver Transpl 2011;17(5):539–47.

82. Emmons KM, Rollnick S. Motivational interviewing in health care settings. Opportunities and limitations. Am J Prev Med 2001;20(1):68–74.

83. Vasilaki EI, Hosier SG, Cox WM. The efficacy of motivational interviewing as a brief intervention for excessive drinking: a meta-analytic review. Alcohol Alcohol 2006;41(3):328–35.

84. Center for Substance Abuse Treatment. Enhancing motivation for change in substance abuse treatment. Rockville (MD): Substance Abuse and Mental Health Services Administration (US); 1999 (Treatment Improvement Protocol (TIP) Series, No. 35.) Chapter 3—Motivational Interviewing as a Counseling Style. Available at: https://www.ncbi.nlm.nih.gov/books/NBK64964/.

85. Centers for Disease Control and Prevention. Planning and implementing screening and brief intervention for risky alcohol use: a step-by-step guide for primary care practices. Atlanta: Centers for Disease Control and Prevention, National Center on Birth Defects and Developmental Disabilities; 2014. Available at: https://www.cdc.gov/ncbddd/fasd/documents/AlcoholSBIImplementation Guide-P.pdf. Accessed November 7, 2020.

86. U.S.P.S.T.F., Curry SJ, Krist AH, et al. Screening and behavioral counseling interventions to reduce unhealthy alcohol use in adolescents and adults: US preventive services task force recommendation statement. JAMA 2018;320(18): 1899–909.

87. Kelly JF, Yeterian JD. The role of mutual-help groups in extending the framework of treatment. Alcohol Res Health 2011;33(4):350–5.

88. Kelly JF, Humphreys K, Ferri M. Alcoholics anonymous and other 12-step programs for alcohol use disorder. Cochrane Database Syst Rev 2020;(3):CD012880.

89. What are the ASAM levels of care? American Society of Addiction Medicine. 2019. Available at: https://www.asamcontinuum.org/knowledgebase/what-are-the-asam-levels-of-care/. Accessed November 7, 2020.

90. Jones JB. Liver transplant recipients' first year of posttransplant recovery: a longitudinal study. Prog Transplant 2005;15(4):345–52.

91. Rodrigue JR, Reed AI, Nelson DR, et al. The financial burden of transplantation: a single-center survey of liver and kidney transplant recipients. Transplantation 2007;84(3):295–300.

92. Khan A, Tansel A, White DL, et al. Efficacy of psychosocial interventions in inducing and maintaining alcohol abstinence in patients with chronic liver disease: a systematic review. Clin Gastroenterol Hepatol 2016;14(2):191–202.e1-4 [quiz: e120].

93. Addolorato G, Mirijello A, Leggio L, et al. Liver transplantation in alcoholic patients: impact of an alcohol addiction unit within a liver transplant center. Alcohol Clin Exp Res 2013;37(9):1601–8.

94. Multidisciplinary approach to study of patients with Severe Alcoholic Hepatitis Undergoing Liver Transplantation. Grantome. 2019. Available at: https://grantome.com/grant/NIH/P50-AA027054-01. Accessed November 7, 2020.
95. Project 2-optimization of post-transplant care via biomarkers and behavioral interventions. Grantome. 2019. Available at: https://grantome.com/grant/NIH/P50-AA027054-02-5362. Accessed November 7, 2020.

Moving?

Make sure your subscription moves with you!

To notify us of your new address, find your **Clinics Account Number** (located on your mailing label above your name), and contact customer service at:

Email: journalscustomerservice-usa@elsevier.com

800-654-2452 (subscribers in the U.S. & Canada)
314-447-8871 (subscribers outside of the U.S. & Canada)

Fax number: 314-447-8029

**Elsevier Health Sciences Division
Subscription Customer Service
3251 Riverport Lane
Maryland Heights, MO 63043**

*To ensure uninterrupted delivery of your subscription, please notify us at least 4 weeks in advance of move.

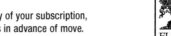

Printed and bound by CPI Group (UK) Ltd, Croydon, CR0 4YY

03/10/2024

01040470-0019